DATE DUE

			PRINTED IN U.S.A.

HEALTH TECHNOLOGY
SOURCEBOOK

SECOND EDITION

Health Reference Series

HEALTH TECHNOLOGY
SOURCEBOOK

SECOND EDITION

Provides Basic Consumer Health Information about Medicine and Technology, Telehealth, Telemedicine and E-health, Information Technology and Medicine, Preventive Medicine and Health Technology, Medical Devices, Screening and Detection Technologies, Diagnostic Technology, Nanotechnology, Neurologic, Health Information Technology, Artificial Intelligence (AI), Augmented Reality (AR), Virtual Reality (VR), Stem Cell Research, and Assistive Devices

Along with Information about Digital Innovations in Healthcare, Medical Technology Laws, Policy, Legislation, and Regulations, a Glossary of Related Terms, and a List of Resources for Additional Help and Information

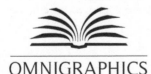

OMNIGRAPHICS

615 Griswold St., Ste. 520, Detroit, MI 48226

Bibliographic Note

Because this page cannot legibly accommodate all the copyright notices,
the Bibliographic Note portion of the Preface constitutes an extension
of the copyright notice.

* * *

OMNIGRAPHICS
Kevin Hayes, *Managing Editor*

* * *

Library of Congress Cataloging-in-Publication Data

Names: Hayes, Kevin (Editor of health information), editor.

Title: Health technology sourcebook: basic consumer health Information about medicine and technology, telehealth, telemedicine and E-health, information technology and medicine, preventive medicine and health technology, medical devices, screening and detection technologies, diagnostic technology, nanotechnology, neurologic, health information technology, artificial Intelligence (AI), augmented reality (AR), virtual reality (VR), stem cell research, and assistive devices ; along with Information about digital innovations in healthcare, medical technology laws, policy, legislation, and regulations, a glossary of related terms, and a list of resources for additional help and information / edited by Kevin Hayes.

Description: Second edition. | Detroit, MI : Omnigraphics, [2021] | Series: Health reference series | Includes bibliographical references and index. | Summary: "Provides consumer health information about the medicine and technology, telehealth, medical devices, screening and detection technologies, nanotechnology, health information technology, artificial intelligence (AI), stem cell research, and medical technology laws, policy, legislation, and regulations. Includes index, glossary of related terms, and a list of resources for additional help and information"-- Provided by publisher.

Identifiers: LCCN 2021021291 (print) | LCCN 2021021292 (ebook) | ISBN 9780780819115 (library binding) | ISBN 9780780819122 (ebook)

Subjects: LCSH: Medical technology. | Medical care--Data processing.

Classification: LCC R855.3.H437 2021 (print) | LCC R855.3 (ebook) | DDC 610.285--dc23

LC record available at https://lccn.loc.gov/2021021291
LC ebook record available at https://lccn.loc.gov/2021021292

∞

This book is printed on acid-free paper meeting the ANSI Z39.48 Standard. The infinity symbol that appears above indicates that the paper in this book meets that standard.

Printed in the United States

Table of Contents

Preface

ABOUT THIS BOOK

Technology has revolutionized the way healthcare is being delivered today, from preventive medicine to rehabilitation. Future technological innovations will transform healthcare, helping health-care professionals provide better services with enhanced precision. More than anything, technology drives healthcare, enabling good health and wellness to people all over the world. The emergence of health information technology (HIT) has made things easier, faster, and simpler for health-care professionals. It provides information they need with the click of a button. According to the Office of the National Coordinator for Health Information Technology (ONC), in 2018 a majority of individuals (84 percent) are confident that their medical records are safe from unauthorized viewing but (66 percent) have concerns when health information is electronically exchanged. More individuals are now confident that their records are safe from unauthorized viewing, compared to 2017.

Health Technology Sourcebook, Second Edition provides facts about health technology, telehealth, its expansion benefits, and uses during COVID-19, telemedicine technology, digital health, innovations in preventive medicine, screening and detection, imaging, and patient monitoring services. It further discusses medical and surgical treatment technologies, new cancer technologies, nutrigenomics, nanotechnology, robotics, rehabilitation, assistive devices, and health information technology. In addition, it details ethical and legal concerns of medical technology, cloning and cloning laws, and the future of health technology. The book concludes with a glossary of related terms and a directory of resources for additional information.

HOW TO USE THIS BOOK

This book is divided into parts and chapters. Parts focus on broad areas of interest. Chapters are devoted to single topics within a part.

Part 1: Introduction to Health Technology gives an overview of medical technology, telehealth, and its uses during COVID-19, telemedicine, and e-health concepts. It also provides information about health technology assessment, and technology and healthcare-related expenditures. The part also details on blockchain technology and the Internet of Things (IoT).

Part 2: Technology and Preventive Healthcare begins with information on the types of telemedicine technology and goes on to discuss the use of technology in preventive healthcare. It offers detailed information about digital-health concepts and innovations namely sensors, body area networks (BANs), wearables and safety, etc. It also gives insights on medical device data systems, medical device interoperability, and clinical decision support systems. Additionally, it discusses the use of big data in healthcare and screening and detection technologies such as advanced molecular detection (AMD), DNA microarray technology, genetic testing, AI-assisted medical devices, etc.

Part 3: Diagnostic Technology deals with various technologies used in the field of diagnoses such as imaging, diagnostic testing, precision medicine, cinematic rendering and digital twin technology, and wireless patient monitoring systems. It also discusses various advanced imaging concepts, the application of digital technology in the COVID-19 pandemic, and other innovations in diagnostic technology.

Part 4: Role of Technology in Treatment provides information about medical and surgical treatment technologies such as computer-assisted surgical systems, robotic angiography gantry, smart operating rooms of the future, and much more. Nanomedicine, genomic medicine, nutrigenomics, nanotechnology, and robotics are also discussed. In addition, it provides details on various advanced therapies such as tissue and cartilage engineering, regenerative medicine, and light therapy.

Part 5: Rehabilitation and Assistive Technologies discusses various rehabilitative and assistive technologies such as prosthetic engineering, cybernetics, robotic wheelchairs, and vision, hearing, and mobility aids. It further discusses the role of electrical signals and stimulations in rehabilitation and research and scientific advances in the field.

Part 6: Health Information Technology and Its Future deals with the basics and benefits of health information technology and trends in its use. Facts about information and communication technologies, digital-health records, and other aspects are also discussed. It also gives insight into the various health technologies of the future such as artificial brain, artificial intelligence, augmented reality, virtual reality, computational modeling, stem cell research, genome sequencing, and photonic dosimetry. Additionally, it provides information on medical applications of 3D printing and microneedle patches for flu vaccination.

Part 7: Medical Technology – Legal and Ethical Concerns discusses medical records privacy, confidentiality, and health information privacy law and policy. It also provides details about health IT legislation and regulations, and cloning and law.

Part 8: Additional Help and Information provides a glossary of important terms related to health technology and a directory of agencies that offers information related to health technology.

BIBLIOGRAPHIC NOTE

This volume contains documents and excerpts from publications issued by the following U.S. government agencies: ADA.gov; Agency for Healthcare Research and Quality (AHRQ); Argonne National Laboratory (ANL); Center for Limb Loss and Mobility (CLiMB); Centers for Disease Control and Prevention (CDC); Centers for Medicare & Medicaid Services (CMS); Congressional Research Service (CRS); Education Resources Information Center (ERIC); *Eunice Kennedy Shriver* National Institute of Child Health and Human Development (NICHD); Federal Trade Commission (FTC); Fogarty International Center (FIC); HealthIT.gov; MedlinePlus; National Aeronautics and Space Administration (NASA); National Cancer Institute (NCI); National Center for Biotechnology Information (NCBI); National Cybersecurity Center of Excellence (NCCoE); National Eye Institute (NEI); National Human Genome Research Institute (NHGRI); National Institute for Occupational Safety and Health (NIOSH); National Institute of Allergy and Infectious Diseases (NIAID); National Institute of Biomedical Imaging and Bioengineering (NIBIB); National Institute of Dental and Craniofacial Research (NIDCR); National Institute of Diabetes and Digestive and Kidney Diseases (NIDDK); National Institute of Mental Health (NIMH); National Institute of Standards and Technology (NIST); National Institute on Aging (NIA); National Institute on Deafness and Other Communication Disorders (NIDCD); National Institutes of Health (NIH); Networking and Information Technology Research and Development (NITRD); *NIH News in Health*; Office of Disease Prevention and Health Promotion

(ODPHP); Office on Women's Health (OWH); U.S. Consumer Product Safety Commission (CPSC); U.S. Department of Energy (DOE) Office of Science; U.S. Department of Health and Human Services (HHS); U.S. Department of Homeland Security (DHS); U.S. Department of Veterans Affairs (VA); U.S. Food and Drug Administration (FDA); U.S. National Library of Medicine (NLM); and U.S. Senate Special Committee on Aging.

It also contains original material produced by Omnigraphics and reviewed by medical consultants.

ABOUT THE *HEALTH REFERENCE SERIES*

The *Health Reference Series* is designed to provide basic medical information for patients, families, caregivers, and the general public. Each volume provides comprehensive coverage on a particular topic. This is especially important for people who may be dealing with a newly diagnosed disease or a chronic disorder in themselves or in a family member. People looking for preventive guidance, information about disease warning signs, medical statistics, and risk factors for health problems will also find answers to their questions in the *Health Reference Series*. The *Series*, however, is not intended to serve as a tool for diagnosing illness, in prescribing treatments, or as a substitute for the physician–patient relationship. All people concerned about medical symptoms or the possibility of disease are encouraged to seek professional care from an appropriate healthcare provider.

A NOTE ABOUT SPELLING AND STYLE

Health Reference Series editors use *Stedman's Medical Dictionary* as an authority for questions related to the spelling of medical terms and *The Chicago Manual of Style* for questions related to grammatical structures, punctuation, and other editorial concerns. Consistent adherence is not always possible, however, because the individual volumes within the *Series* include many documents from a wide variety of different producers, and the editor's primary goal is to present material from each source as accurately as is possible. This sometimes means that information in different chapters or sections may follow other guidelines and alternate spelling authorities. For example, occasionally a copyright holder may require that eponymous terms be shown in possessive forms (Crohn's disease vs. Crohn disease) or that British spelling norms be retained (leukaemia vs. leukemia).

MEDICAL REVIEW

Omnigraphics contracts with a team of qualified, senior medical professionals who serve as medical consultants for the *Health Reference Series*. As necessary, medical consultants review reprinted and originally written material for currency and accuracy. Citations including the phrase "Reviewed (month, year)" indicate material reviewed by this team. Medical consultation services are provided to the *Health Reference Series* editors by:

Dr. Vijayalakshmi, MBBS, DGO, MD
Dr. Senthil Selvan, MBBS, DCH, MD
Dr. K. Sivanandham, MBBS, DCH, MS (Research), PhD

HEALTH REFERENCE SERIES UPDATE POLICY

The inaugural book in the *Health Reference Series* was the first edition of *Cancer Sourcebook* published in 1989. Since then, the *Series* has been enthusiastically received by librarians and in the medical community. In order to maintain the standard of providing high-quality health information for the layperson the editorial staff at Omnigraphics felt it was necessary to implement a policy of updating volumes when warranted.

Medical researchers have been making tremendous strides, and it is the purpose of the *Health Reference Series* to stay current with the most recent advances. Each decision to update a volume is made on an individual basis. Some of the considerations include how much new information is available and the feedback we receive from people who use the books. If there is a topic you would like to see added to the update list, or an area of medical concern you feel has not been adequately addressed, please write to:

Managing Editor
Health Reference Series
Omnigraphics
615 Griswold St., Ste. 520
Detroit, MI 48226

Part 1 | Introduction to Health Technology

Chapter 1 | **Understanding Medical Technology**

The advancement of basic science about human health and the onset of diseases have been so rapid in the second half of the twentieth century that we have been labeled as "living in a biological revolution." It is with the help of technology and strategy that the field of healthcare is flourishing.

Medical technology is the application of science, research, and organized knowledge to create solutions to health concerns. It involves the usage of devices, procedures, vaccines, and medicines to identify health problems, prevent diseases, monitor good health, and improve the quality of life (QOL).

Medical technology is the key to a hospital's positioning and understanding in the dynamic healthcare world. Every year, plenty of exciting new biomedical instruments and technologies are being unveiled. Since the advent of eyeglasses and the stethoscope, medical research has advanced significantly. The growth of a more wealthy middle class, as well as an aging world population, are both pushing transformations in the healthcare market, and the infrastructure that supports it is transforming faster than ever before.

The COVID-19 pandemic in 2020 pushed healthcare forward, and as a result, many promising medical innovations were put to the test on a large scale. The challenge in the forthcoming years is how such innovations will be combined in a postpandemic environment. The following are a few advancements of technology in the medical field.

ADVANCED TELEMEDICINE

During the COVID-19 pandemic, telemedicine made significant progress. In January 2020, it was reported that 24 percent of health-care institutions had a telehealth service in place. The nation was on track to complete over a billion virtual treatment visits by the end of the year. Many of telehealth's regulatory hurdles have been lifted as a result of its forced implementation, and healthcare providers now have almost a year's worth of research on how to assess and develop telehealth systems.

DEVELOPMENT OF DRUGS

One of the greatest scientific achievements in human history could be the discovery of several safe and reliable COVID-19 vaccines in less than a year. The procedure was accelerated not only by regulatory expediting but also by advancements in the way drug trials are performed.

NANOMEDICINE

Nanomedicine has applications in imaging, sensing, detection, and dissemination by medical devices, and the potential is enormous for anything so small.

CONNECTIVITY

A secure and lightning-fast internet access is the base for cutting-edge technologies such as artificial intelligence (AI), Internet of Things (IoT), and big data to achieve their maximum potential in healthcare. The most immediate benefits of a secure real-time link can be seen in telemedicine, which will increase access to treatment for millions of people. More embedded sensors with authentic data streams open the door to a healthcare revolution.

CLUSTERED REGULARLY INTERSPACED SHORT PALINDROMIC REPEATS

Clustered regularly interspaced short palindromic repeats (CRISPR) is the most sophisticated gene-editing technique available that functions by using the immune systems of invading virus-infected bacteria cells, which are then able to "cut out" infected deoxyribo-nucleic acid (DNA) strands. This cutting of DNA has the potential to revolutionize the way we approach disease. Any of the most serious risks, such as cancer and HIV, can be resolved in a couple of years by altering genes.

TELEHEALTH

Many healthcare providers will be concentrating their efforts on how to better align telehealth systems with traditional physical ones. Virtual visits can continue to be used to enhance collaboration with hospitals, long-term care facilities, dialysis centers, and mental-health providers, as well as to expand access to primary care and urgent care.

In today's technologically advanced world, instead of waiting for face-to-face visits with their doctor, telehealth helps people to access medical attention from their digital devices. For instance, highly personalized smartphone applications are being created that enable patients to communicate remotely with doctors and other medical professionals in order to obtain an immediate diagnosis and medical advice. Telehealth is particularly beneficial to people who are undergoing treatment for chronic illnesses because it provides them with regular, convenient, and cost-effective care.

WEARABLE DEVICES

Wearable devices have increased in popularity in recent years, especially after the release of Bluetooth in 2000. People nowadays use their phones to keep track of everything from their walking steps, exercise, calories burnt, and heartbeat to their sleeping habits. These wearable devices are advancing in tandem with the rise of chronic diseases such as diabetes and cardiovascular disease (CVD), and they seek to tackle them by assisting patients in monitoring and improving their health.

ROBOTIC SURGERY

In minimally invasive operations, robotic surgery is used to assist with accuracy, stability, and flexibility. Robotic surgery allows surgeons to perform very complicated operations that would either be impractical or very difficult. While some fear that the invention will ultimately replace human surgeons, it is more likely to be used to aid and improve surgeons' practice in the future.

SMART INHALERS

Inhalers are the most common medication for asthma, and if used properly, they will help 90 percent of patients. Bluetooth-enabled smart inhalers have been designed to assist asthma sufferers in properly managing their illnesses. The inhaler has a small tracker attached to it that tracks proper administration and date and duration of each dosage. This information is then sent to the patients' smartphones, allowing them to monitor and maintain their health. Clinical research revealed that those who used the smart inhaler system used a lesser amount of medication than the conventional inhaler.

VIRTUAL REALITY AND AUGMENTED REALITY

Virtual reality (VR) has uses in fields such as emotional trauma, where it can relieve phobias and posttraumatic stress disorder (PTSD) by personalized exposure and care. Cambridge Consultants created augmented reality (AR) glasses for operating rooms that enable surgeons to see within a patient's body by superimposing data from 3-D (three-dimensional) scans and computerized axial tomography (CAT) scans. This allows for unprecedented exposure during minimally invasive "keyhole surgeries" and needs almost no extra preparation.

References

1. David, Yadin; Zambuto Peter, Raymond. "Medical Technology," Science Direct, December 2, 2018.
2. "The Ten Hottest Medical Technologies in 2021," Medical Technology Schools, January 15, 2019.
3. "Top 10 New Medical Technologies of 2019," Proclinical, February 27, 2019.
4. "10 Ways Technology Is Changing Healthcare," The Medical Futurist, March 3, 2020.

Chapter 2 | Basics of Telehealth

Chapter Contents

Section 2.1 | **Understanding Telehealth**

This section includes text excerpted from documents published by three public domain sources. Text under the headings marked 1 are excerpted from "Telehealth," National Institute of Biomedical Imaging and Bioengineering (NIBIB), August 2020; Text under the headings marked 2 are excerpted from "What Is Telehealth?" Telehealth.HHS.gov, U.S. Department of Health and Human Services (HHS), May 19, 2021; Text under the heading marked 3 is excerpted from "Telehealth and Telemedicine: Frequently Asked Questions," Congressional Research Service (CRS), March 12, 2020.

WHAT IS TELEHEALTH?[1]

Telehealth is broadly defined as the use of communications technologies to provide healthcare at a distance. Telehealth has become a valuable tool thanks to combined advances in communications, computer science, informatics, and medical technologies.

Telehealth often involves remote monitoring of blood pressure, heart rate, and other measurements obtained by a device worn by the patient and electronically sent to medical personnel. Smartphones and other smart personal devices are increasingly utilized for the collection, dissemination, and even analysis of health status due to their increasing presence around the globe, even in remote, underserved communities.

In the last several years, virtual visits between doctors and patients have become very common, especially with the onset of the COVID-19 pandemic. The willingness of physicians, patients, and insurers to embrace virtual medicine is likely to cause it to remain a popular option in healthcare.

WHAT TYPES OF CARE CAN YOU GET USING TELEHEALTH?[2]

You might be surprised by the variety of care you can get through telehealth. Services such as medication management and online counseling are particularly suited to telehealth as consistent and regular visits improve outcomes. Your doctor will decide whether telehealth is right for your health needs.

If you need care – especially during COVID-19 – it is worth checking to see what your telehealth options are.

For example, you may meet with a doctor in real time to discuss:
- Lab test or x-ray results
- Therapy and online counseling

- Recurring conditions such as migraines or urinary tract infections
- Skin conditions
- Prescription management
- Urgent care issues such as colds, coughs, and stomach complaints
- Postsurgical follow-up

Doctors may ask you to:
- Send blood pressure, blood sugar, or other condition monitoring information
- Send images of how a wound, eye, or skin condition is healing
- Document symptoms
- Request medical records sent to another doctor (e.g., x-rays to a physical therapist)

Doctors can send information to you such as:
- Notifications to remind you to do rehabilitation exercises or take a critical medication
- Encouragement to stick with your treatment plan
- New suggestions for improving diet, mobility, or stress management
- Detailed instructions on how to continue your care at home

HOW CAN TELEHEALTH TECHNOLOGIES IMPROVE MEDICAL CARE?[1]
Teleconsultations

This allows a physician in a remote area to receive advice from a specialist at a distant location about special or complex patient conditions. Such consultations can be as simple as a phone call. Increasingly, they involve sophisticated sharing of medical information such as computed tomography (CT), magnetic resonance imaging (MRI), or ultrasound scans. These images can be taken by the local physician, incorporated into an electronic medical record, and sent to the specialist for diagnosis and treatment recommendations.

Remote Patient Monitoring

It enables patient monitoring outside of clinical settings, such as at home. Patients use or wear sensors that wirelessly collect and transmit physiological data to health professionals. Remote patient monitoring (RPM) can significantly improve an individual's quality of life. For example, in diabetes management, the real-time transmission of blood glucose readings enables health-care providers to intervene when needed and avoid acute events and hospitalizations.

Telehomecare

It provides the remote care needed to allow people with chronic conditions, dementia, or those at high risk of falling, to remain living in their own homes. The approach focuses on reacting to emergency events and raising a help response quickly. Sensors monitor changes in chronic conditions as well as other risks including floods, fires, and gas leaks. Sensors can also alert caregivers if a person with dementia leaves the house. When a sensor is activated, a monitoring center is alerted to take appropriate action such as contacting a caregiver or sending emergency services.

Point of Care

Medicine relies on diagnostic devices that can perform at the time and place of patient care, which includes at home, in doctor's offices and clinics, and in remote areas without electricity or laboratory equipment. Point-of-care (POC) devices can detect micronutrient deficiencies, anemia, infectious agents, and even some cancers. Combined with telehealth, POC technologies allow health-care workers to test patients and rapidly obtain results without the need for a complex laboratory setting which can result in significant cost-reduction.

BENEFITS OF TELEHEALTH[2]

Although virtual visits may not be as common as traditional in-person doctor's appointments, there are many benefits that explain why this type of care is growing in popularity.

- Limiting physical contact reduces everyone's exposure to COVID-19
- Visiting virtually can address health issues wherever patients are, even from the comfort of home
- Staying put cuts down on commuting, travel in bad weather, time off from work, need for child care
- Using virtual health-care tools can shorten wait times to see a provider and expand the range of access to specialists who live further away

Telehealth is not a perfect fit for everyone or every medical condition. Make sure you discuss any disadvantages or risks with your doctor.

FREQUENTLY ASKED QUESTIONS ABOUT TELEHEALTH[3]
Telehealth Modalities
WHAT IS A TELEHEALTH MODALITY?

A telehealth modality refers to the mode in which a telehealth service transpires. There are four common telehealth modalities: (1) clinical video telehealth or live video, (2) mobile health, (3) remote patient monitoring, and (4) store-and-forward technology. Other telehealth modalities include the use of the telephone and facsimile (fax) machine.

HOW DOES THE CLINICAL VIDEO TELEHEALTH MODALITY FUNCTION?

The clinical video telehealth (CVT) modality allows a health-care provider who is not located in the same location as a patient to view, diagnose, monitor, and treat medical conditions of the patient in real time. The CVT modality functions by allowing a health-care provider and the patient to see each other via interactive live video technology.

HOW DOES THE MOBILE HEALTH MODALITY FUNCTION?

The mobile health (mHealth) modality allows a provider to deliver educational materials and other health-care resources to patients through a mobile application. Patients who use mHealth can access health-care information such as disease-specific resources and mental-health resources on their mobile devices.

HOW DOES THE REMOTE PATIENT MONITORING MODALITY FUNCTION?

The remote patient monitoring (RPM) modality allows a health-care provider who is not located in the same location as a patient to provide the patient with daily case management services for the patient's chronic medical conditions, such as chronic heart disease (CHD) or diabetes.

HOW DOES THE STORE-AND-FORWARD TECHNOLOGY MODALITY FUNCTION?

The store-and-forward technology (SFT) modality facilitates the interpretation of clinical information. SFT enables a health-care provider who is not in the same location as a patient to assist a health-care provider who is in the same location and who has provided in-person care to the patient. The SFT modality is similar to the exchange of videos, pictures, and files through an e-mail or personal mobile device. However, the exchange within a telehealth encounter is sent from a health information technology (HIT) system; for example, when a patient's electronic health record (EHR) is sent to the consulting provider's HIT system.

Telehealth Services
WHAT TYPES OF HEALTH-CARE SERVICES CAN HEALTH-CARE PROVIDERS PROVIDE THROUGH TELEHEALTH?

Health-care providers generally can provide any health-care service via telehealth that the provider can provide in person. Such health-care services include dietician services, disease management, genetic counseling, palliative care, psychological assessment, and speech therapy. However, federal and state laws prohibit health-care providers from delivering certain services via telehealth. For example, Medicare providers can provide only telehealth services authorized by the Centers for Medicare and Medicaid Services (CMS), of the U.S. Department of Health and Human Services (HHS), such as diabetes management and counseling for tobacco use. Medical abortions are another heath-care service regulated by law; some states have or are considering measures to either allow or prohibit medical abortions via telehealth.

WHAT IS A DIRECT-TO-CONSUMER TELEHEALTH SERVICE?

A direct-to-consumer (DTC) telehealth service refers to a health-care service provided on-demand via a clinical video telehealth modality to a patient, upon the patient's request. Patients generally can access DTC telehealth services 24 hours a day on any day of the week. DTC telehealth services typically consist of urgent care services for illnesses such as headaches, sore throats, and urinary tract infections (UTIs). Some DTC telehealth organizations offer the same behavioral health-care services as DTC telehealth services.

Two aspects of a DTC telehealth service make it convenient. First, a patient does not have to be enrolled in a health-care facility to receive services. The patient generally receives telehealth service from a health-care provider who has contracted with a DTC telehealth organization such as American Well or Teladoc. A patient can access DTC telehealth services from a local health-care facility, her or his workplace, or a school that has chosen to integrate DTC telehealth services into the respective facility.

Second, a patient can access a DTC telehealth service immediately at the time of her or his request. The patient can also schedule a future DTC telehealth service with her or his health-care provider. The provider does not have to be located in the same location as the patient when the telehealth service transpires, withstanding state licensing laws for the delivery of telehealth services across state lines. The health-care provider can prescribe medications, withstanding federal and state licensing laws for the prescribing of medications across state lines.

Section 2.2 | **Telemedicine and E-health**

Telemedicine uses telecommunication technology to help healthcare professionals remotely diagnose and treat patients in a virtual setting and deliver medical services. Technology in telemedicine is used to provide services such as managing medications, and chronic conditions, along with consultations from specialists. Telemedicine has made healthcare accessible, affordable, and engaging. Telemedicine is beneficial to the rural and senior citizen faction of the population. A health insurance portability and accountability act (HIPAA, 1996) compliant video conferencing software is the most basic requirement for telemedicine services. There are three types of telemedicine services such as:

- Interactive medicine – live video or synchronous virtual visits between a person and their caregiver, using telecommunications technology
- Remote patient monitoring
- Store and forward or asynchronous virtual visits
- Mobile health, often called "mHealth" or "eHealth"

Present-day applications of telemedicine include remote post-hospitalization care, assisted living support, school-based telehealth, and preventive care, sharing medical information, reducing the load on hospital emergency rooms, access to multiple medical opinions, access to specialist consultations for fragile medical cases such as premature babies, providing disaster relief, and mobile health. Fields that utilize telemedicine are radiology, pediatric, mental health, and dermatology. Medical care devices that are easy to use and install at home help practitioners monitor vitals and other parameters such as blood glucose levels. Some devices that can stream their data over long distances are digital stethoscopes, EKGs, pulse oximeters, dermatoscope, otoscopes, and ultrasounds. Telemedicine is a continuously improving industry and was estimated at a value of $35 billion in 2020.

BENEFITS OF TELEMEDICINE

Telemedicine provides a wide range of benefits for patients and providers, such as:

- **Convenience.** Telemedicine allows patients to access medical care from the comfort of their homes. Accessing healthcare services through telemedicine does not interfere with work schedules which is beneficial for patients.
- Preventive care through telemedicine leads to better health outcomes since people with low incomes or rural areas who cannot afford to make in-person doctor appointments can access preventative care options.
- **Lower costs.** Healthcare services obtained through telemedicine lead to reduced overall costs such as fuel costs, child care costs, and lower consultation fees as video consultations only incur data usage charges.
- Better access to quality healthcare for those with a disability, at a disadvantage such as under-house arrest or in prison, or solitary senior citizens
- **Safety.** During a pandemic, or to protect individuals with low immunity caused by conditions such as HIV/AIDS or cancer, or for people who are highly susceptible to infections, it can be the safest option to harness the services of telemedicine technology and enlist medical services remotely.
- For health-care providers, telemedicine offers a more significant revenue or return on investment (ROI) since they can reach many more patients than what a physical clinic could accommodate.
- Telemedicine providers can ensure customer satisfaction as going mobile helps them offer various services to the customers on a single platform rather than outsourcing services. Customers look for convenience and a one-stop solution to all their healthcare needs which can quickly be delivered through telemedicine.
- Health-care providers can save costs by avoiding overhead expenses such as customer support expenses or extra office space.

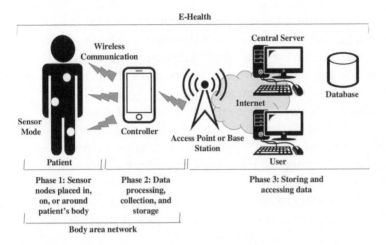

Figure 2.1. Architecture of the WBAN and E-healthcare System

E-health is the use of the Internet along with information and communication technology (ICT) in the delivery of healthcare services. E-health specifically combines intuitive data aggregating technology and coordination of clinical referrals. E-health is beneficial in managing disease care for the patient. Telehealth and telemedicine are services under e-health along with electronic medical records, health IT systems, consumer health IT data, virtual healthcare, electronic health records (EHRs), and big data systems. E-health is involved in improving the overall efficiency of healthcare. It allows medical practitioners to access and manage patient health records through electronic channels for better patient care. E-health permits patients to be actively involved in their treatment, understand their condition better and manage it efficiently.

BENEFITS OF E-HEALTH

The key benefits of e-health include:

- Improves self-care. Services provided under e-health encourage patients to take better care of their health conditions, and it helps them recognize if they need medical attention. This also helps in reducing the load on the healthcare system.

- Helps save time. Telemedicine and other similar services help cut waiting times drastically, which patients can use for other daily activities. The direct approach employed by health IT removes the need and time spent on mediatory services.
- Administrative processes are more secure and more manageable with the induction of e-health services such as electronic health records. Such approaches can avoid cumbersome paperwork and are a more sustainable method.
- Enables patients to stay informed about their diagnoses and prescriptions and any other services or diagnostic services that may be required
- Encourages transparency in services from providers to transactions for payments from patients. Patients require precise information on their medical history, and EHRs help provide the same.
- Services under e-health can sometimes prevent unnecessary deaths by providing remote medical interventions in the form of paramedic help through telemedicine.
- E-health allows for earlier detection, diagnosis, and subsequent treatment, which can improve overall health outcomes.
- Removes geographical barriers to quality healthcare and helps bridge the gap between medical services and access to the same, especially among minorities, low-income groups, and rural populations

Telemedicine and e-health come with some disadvantages, such as not being considered by insurance and health coverage providers, susceptibility to cybercrime, or delays in immediate care. It must be noted that these types of healthcare services are digitally relevant and highly beneficial. Both services aid in improving healthcare delivery, increasing the quality of services, and help to reinforce patient–physician interactions. For patients, these services help instill a sense of confidence in the physician and a stronger sense of healthcare responsibility in both.

References

1. "What Is Telemedicine?" Chiron Health, March 4, 2016.
2. "What Is Telemedicine?" VSee, October 13, 2012.
3. "eHealth," Innovate Med Tec, May 29, 2016.
4. "What Is eHealth?" USF Health, April 19, 2021.
5. "Dividing E-health, Telehealth and Telemedicine," Electronic Health Reporter, March 20, 2018.
6. Villines, Zawn. "Telemedicine Benefits: For Patients and Professionals," *Medical News Today,* April 20, 2020.

Section 2.3 | Uses of Telehealth during COVID-19

This section contains text excerpted from the following sources: Text in this section begins with excerpts from "Uses of Telehealth during COVID-19 in Low Resource Non-U.S. Settings," Centers for Disease Control and Prevention (CDC), July 21, 2020; Text beginning with the heading "The Role of Telehealth in the COVID-19 Crisis" is excerpted from "Telehealth and Patient Safety during the COVID-19 Response," Agency for Healthcare Research and Quality (AHRQ), U.S. Department of Health and Human Services (HHS), May 14, 2020.

Changes in the way that healthcare is delivered during the COVID-19 pandemic have occurred to reduce staff and patient exposure to sick people, preserve personal protective equipment (PPE), and minimize the impact of patient surges on facilities. Health-care systems may need to adjust the way they triage, evaluate, and care for patients using methods that do not rely on in-person encounters. Telehealth services help provide necessary care to patients while minimizing the transmission risk of SARS-CoV-2, the virus that causes COVID-19, to health-care workers and patients.

Telehealth modalities include:
- **Synchronous.** Real-time telephone or live audio-video interaction, typically with a patient, using a smartphone, tablet, or computer.
  - In some cases, peripheral medical equipment (e.g., digital stethoscopes, otoscopes, ultrasounds) can be used by another health-care provider (e.g., nurse, medical assistant) physically with the patient, while

the consulting medical provider conducts a remote evaluation.

- **Asynchronous.** The provider and patient communication does not happen in real time. For example, "store and forward" technology allows messages, images, or data to be collected at one point in time and interpreted or responded to later. Patient portals can facilitate this type of communication between provider and patient through secure messaging.
- **Remote patient monitoring.** This allows direct transmission of a patient's clinical measurements from a distance (may or may not be in real time) to their health-care provider.

WHAT ARE POTENTIAL USES OF TELEHEALTH DURING COVID-19?
Triaging and Screening for COVID-19 Symptoms

Telehealth can be used to screen for COVID-19 symptoms and assess patients for potential exposure. Phone screening, online screening tools, mobile applications, or virtual telemedicine visits can be used to evaluate patients for COVID-19 symptoms, assess the severity of their symptoms, and decide whether the patient needs to be seen for evaluation, admitted to the hospital, or can be managed at home. Screening algorithms can be used in telehealth communication. For patients who may need to be hospitalized, mobile phones and tablets or other telehealth technology can be used by mobile home health-care units, community health volunteers/workers, or emergency services to communicate with health-care providers at a health facility.

Health-care providers can use telehealth to conduct a remote evaluation of the patient's medical condition and determine if the patient needs to be in a regular hospital bed or in an intensive care unit. Making this decision remotely can avoid rushing the patient through the emergency room upon arrival at the hospital, limiting the exposure of emergency department personnel and other health-care workers, and preserving PPE. Telehealth can also be used to screen patients before they visit the health-care facility for non-COVID-19 care. If COVID-19 symptoms are reported during the telehealth interview, patients could be advised to delay nonemergent care and first seek testing for COVID-19.

Contact Tracing

Telehealth, especially via phone, can be used to interview patients with COVID-19 to determine who they were in contact with during the time they were potentially infectious, and to follow up with their contacts to inform them of the need to quarantine, assess whether they have any symptoms, and tell them what to do if symptoms develop.

Monitoring COVID-19 Symptoms

Patients with mild or moderate COVID-19 symptoms can often isolate and be monitored at home to avoid overcrowding in health-care facilities and save hospital beds for more severe cases. Using telehealth technology such as phones or apps, health-care providers can check in with patients frequently to monitor their condition, provide advice, and determine if the patient's condition is deteriorating and they need to be evaluated for in-person care, such as hospitalization.

Providing Specialized Care for Hospitalized Patients with COVID-19

Patients who are hospitalized with COVID-19 may require care from a diverse team (e.g., nurses, respiratory therapists, physicians). One member of the team can enter the patient's room and consult with the rest of the team using telehealth technology (tablets, phones) to assess the condition of the patient, adjust respiratory and other therapy, adjust the treatment plan, and manage complications.

In addition, health facilities can use telehealth to consult with physicians who have specialized training or expertise in respiratory infections such as COVID-19. Teleintensive care unit platforms, which consist of real-time audio, visual, and electronic connections between remote critical care teams (intensivists and critical care nurses) and patients in distant ICUs, can also be used to monitor critically ill patients and provide expert guidance for care. Tele-radiology can also be used to consult with radiologists at remote locations. Telehealth can also be used to provide online training on COVID-19 for medical professionals and health-care workers.

Providing Access to Essential Healthcare for Non-COVID-19 Patients

Telehealth can be used as a strategy to maintain continuity of care, to the extent possible, to avoid negative consequences from preventive, chronic, or routine care that might otherwise be delayed due to COVID-19 concerns. Telehealth visits can help determine when it is reasonable to defer an in-person visit or service. Follow-up visits can be conducted by phone or Internet to reduce the number of in-person visits and overcrowding in outpatient settings.

Providers can use Internet-based drug prescriptions and provide multimonth dispensing of medications to further reduce the need for in-person encounters. Remote access can also help assure health-care access when an in-person visit is not practical or feasible due to COVID-19 concerns. To mitigate stress during COVID-19, mental- and behavioral-health services can be provided to the population through hotlines or virtual provider-patient visits.

Monitoring Recovering COVID-19 Patients

After COVID-19 patients are discharged from the hospital, health-care providers can use telehealth technology to follow up with those who might need to continue isolation at home or be monitored for any sudden deterioration or long-term health effects due to COVID-19.

THE ROLE OF TELEHEALTH IN THE COVID-19 CRISIS

In March 2020, the U.S. Department of Health and Human Services (HHS) issued a series of new rules and temporary waivers designed to assist the medical community in addressing the COVID-19 pandemic. This has included several provisions related to the use of telehealth, including the expansion of what services may be provided virtually. Private insurers are also taking steps to support the use of telehealth, such as expanding lists of eligible services, waiving cost-sharing, and providing monitoring devices to patients. Through necessity and as a result of these emergency provisions, the use of telehealth technologies, and broader application of telehealth concepts outside of the CMS technical standards, has rapidly increased. Its expanded use has served as a means of ensuring the safety of both patients and frontline providers, as well as conserving the use of critical PPE supplied.

Ensuring Patient Safety

Telehealth can be an effective way of limiting patient exposure to individuals who have – or may have – contracted the virus that causes COVID-19. One approach is to use telehealth in place of traditional in-person visits for care unrelated to COVID-19 that cannot be postponed, such as required monitoring of medications for chronic disease. This allows patients to receive care from the safety of their homes and avoid exposure to the virus during transit or at in-person appointments.

Another approach is to use telehealth as a means of performing an initial evaluation and triage of patients with COVID-19 symptoms. Such virtual triage processes can protect other patients by directing potentially infected individuals to the most appropriate location to seek care or testing and keep them out of primary care waiting rooms.

Ensuring Provider Safety

In addition to the more "traditional" uses of telehealth, the COVID-19 crisis has necessitated creative thinking about how telehealth technology can help protect providers. For example, approaches such as video conferencing and remote diagnostic tools can allow hospital and ambulatory care providers to employ telehealth best practices and patient evaluation techniques that avoid direct patient contact, while still treating the patient on-site. Telemedicine using remote monitoring technologies can facilitate treatment and even decrease the frequency of virtual and in-person patient encounters.

Using these remote and virtual capabilities can reduce the number of providers that need to come into direct contact with a patient in the hospital and can conserve single-use PPE.

While telehealth is providing powerful approaches for protecting patients and providers during the COVID-19 outbreak, its increased and evolving use raises other potential patient safety concerns. First, providers need to understand the limitations of delivering care remotely and the implications on their diagnostic capabilities, particularly among providers who have limited prior telehealth experience.

Secondly, strategies need to be in place for connecting with patients and caregivers who are less technologically enabled, have multiple comorbid conditions, do not have access to broadband, and/or have low health or digital-health literacy.

In addition, providers will need to ensure reasonable accommodations are in place for patients who are deaf, hard of hearing, are blind, or have low vision. They will also need to be responsive to linguistic minorities who may have limited English proficiency.

Finally, in the effort to maximize the use of telehealth services and minimize the risk of patient exposure to the virus, remote evaluations allow providers to recommend more judicious use of ancillary services, recognizing that there is a continued need to ensure patients are able to receive all necessary services when appropriate (e.g., labs, x-rays, procedures).

ALLEVIATING PATIENT SAFETY CONCERNS
Rapidly accelerating telehealth capabilities may be necessary for many institutions as the health-care community tackles the COVID-19 epidemic. However, there are critical precautions that can be taken to minimize the risk to patient safety.

Establishing Escalation Protocols
Institutions should establish escalation protocols that dictate when a patient receiving telehealth services should be transitioned to urgent in-person follow-up care, or even to receiving emergency services. Follow-up care can continue to occur remotely, but

consideration should be made for conditions in which the patient may require in-person services, particularly in more vulnerable populations. Escalation protocols should be identified, developed, and applied in the context of a given practice and should cover the range of scenarios that practice may encounter, including the need for a higher level of care, such as an emergency visit, or the need for diagnostic studies. The protocols should align with existing clinical workflows and take into consideration the level of comfort and familiarity physicians have with practicing telehealth.

These types of guidance documents help to ensure that patients are receiving telehealth and in-person care in a consistent way, that the capabilities and limitations of telehealth are communicated effectively, and can ease the adjustment for providers with minimal prior experience performing telehealth. All clinical staff within a given institution should be aware of these guidance documents and of when to use them.

Encourage Precharting of Upcoming Patient Visits

Providers should be encouraged to conduct a detailed review of their upcoming patient appointments and determine if any can be appropriately converted to telehealth appointments. This may require additional communication and outreach to the patient by nurses or medical assistants to review and update information regarding the patient's medical history, validate that the reason for their visit is complete, accurate, and identifies the need for any necessary ancillary services (i.e., lab work, imaging), and ensure that the patient understands what to expect if they will be participating in a telehealth visit.

It may be necessary, in some cases, to arrange for patients to obtain remote monitoring devices in advance of more complex virtual assessments. Where ever possible, maintain in-person pediatric visits for vaccinations so children remain on schedule.

Quality Assurance Plan

As with in-person visits, a quality assurance plan should be in place for telehealth visits. Medical staff should hold patient safety huddles to discuss cases with both positive and negative patient safety outcomes. It is important for institutions to maintain good patient safety culture and ensure that providers have the opportunity to learn from what went right and what went wrong in telehealth cases.

Provider Tutorials of Telehealth Basics

Telehealth tutorials can provide awareness of basic telehealth communication best practices. Understanding such fundamentals, such as regulating speech patterns or positioning the video camera, lighting, and location can make the experience more user-friendly for the patient and facilitate a smooth and effective visit.

If implemented appropriately, telehealth can be an incredibly effective approach to ensuring patient and provider safety during this unprecedented outbreak. This unique opportunity to implement innovative and creative approaches to patient care will have long-lasting impacts on the future of telehealth. As providers and patients become more familiar with the technical aspects of telehealth, and as patients' understanding of both the benefits and limitations of telehealth increases, telehealth will become a part of standard practice for delivering safe, high-quality healthcare.

Chapter 3 | **Health Technology Assessment**

Technological innovation has yielded truly remarkable advances in healthcare during the last five decades. In recent years, breakthroughs in a variety of areas have helped to improve health-care delivery and patient outcomes, including antivirals, anticlotting drugs, antidiabetic drugs, antihypertensive drugs, antirheumatic drugs, vaccines, pharmacogenomics, and targeted cancer therapies, cardiac rhythm management (CRM), diagnostic imaging, minimally invasive surgery, joint replacement, pain management, infection control, and health information technology (HIT).

The proliferation of health-care technology and its expanding uses have contributed to burgeoning health-care costs, and the former has been cited as "culprit" for the latter. However, this relationship is variable, complex, and evolving. In the U.S., the Congressional Budget Office (CBO) concluded that "roughly half of the increase in health-care spending during the past several decades was associated with the expanded capabilities of medicine brought about by technological advances."

Few patients or clinicians are willing to forego access to state-of-the-art health-care technology. In the wealthier countries and those with growing economies, adoption and use of technology have been stimulated by patient and physician incentives to seek any potential health benefit with limited regard to cost, and by third-party payment, provider competition, effective marketing of technologies, and consumer awareness.

This chapter includes text excerpted from "HTA 101: Introduction to Health Technology Assessment," U.S. National Library of Medicine (NLM), July 22, 2019.

In this era of increasing cost pressures, restructuring of health-care delivery and payment, and heightened consumer demand – yet continued inadequate access to care for many millions of people – technology remains the substance of healthcare. Culprit or not, technology can be managed in ways that improve patient access and health outcomes while continuing to encourage useful innovation. The development, adoption, and diffusion of technology are increasingly influenced by a widening group of policymakers in the health-care sector. Health product makers, regulators, clinicians, patients, hospital managers, payers, government leaders, and others increasingly demand well-founded information to support decisions about whether or how to develop technology, to allow it on the market, to acquire it, to use it, to pay for its use, to ensure its appropriate use, and more. The growth and development of health technology assessment (HTA) in government and the private sector reflect this demand.

Health technology assessment methods are evolving and their applications are increasingly diverse. This chapter introduces fundamental aspects and issues of a dynamic field of inquiry. Broader participation of people with multiple disciplines and different roles in healthcare is enriching the field. The heightened demand for HTA, in particular from the for-profit and not-for-profit private sectors as well as from government agencies, is pushing the field to evolve more systematic and transparent assessment processes and reporting to diverse users. The body of knowledge about HTA cannot be found in one place and is not static. Practitioners and users of HTA should not only monitor changes in the field but have considerable opportunities to contribute to its development.

ORIGINS OF TECHNOLOGY ASSESSMENT

Technology assessment (TA) arose in the mid-1960s from an appreciation of the critical role of technology in modern society and its potential for unintended, and sometimes harmful, consequences. Experience with the side effects of a multitude of chemical, industrial and agricultural processes, and such services as transportation, health, and resource management contributed to this understanding. Early assessments concerned such topics as offshore oil drilling, pesticides, automobile pollution, nuclear power plants, supersonic airplanes, weather modification, and the artificial heart. TA was conceived as a way to identify the desirable first-order, intended effects of technologies as well as the higher-order, unintended social, economic, and environmental effects.

The term "technology assessment" was introduced in 1965 during deliberations of the Committee on Science and Astronautics of the U.S. House of Representatives. Congressman Emilio Daddario emphasized that the purpose of TA was to serve policymaking, "technical information needed by policymakers is frequently not available, or not in the right form. A policymaker cannot judge the merits or consequences of a technological program within a strictly technical context. He has to consider social, economic, and legal implications of any course of action."

Congress commissioned independent studies by the National Academy of Sciences, the National Academy of Engineering (NAE), and the Legislative Reference Service of the Library of Congress that significantly influenced the development and application of TA. These studies and further congressional hearings led the National Science Foundation to establish a TA program and, in 1972, Congress to authorize the congressional Office of Technology Assessment (OTA), which was founded in 1973, became operational in 1974 and established its health program in 1975.

Many observers were concerned that TA would be a means by which government would impede the development and use of technology. However, this was not the intent of Congress or of the agencies that conducted the original TAs. In 1969, an NAE report to Congress emphasized that technology assessment would aid Congress to become more effective in assuring that broad public, as well as private interests, are fully considered while enabling technology to make the maximum contribution to our society's welfare.

With somewhat different aims, private industry used TA to aid in competing in the marketplace, for understanding the future business environment, and for producing options for decision-makers.

Technology assessment methodology drew upon a variety of analytical, evaluative, and planning techniques. Among these were systems analysis, cost-benefit analysis, consensus development methods (e.g., Delphi method), engineering feasibility studies, clinical trials, market research, technological forecasting, and others. TA practitioners and policymakers recognized that TA is evolving, flexible, and should be tailored to the task.

EARLY HEALTH TECHNOLOGY ASSESSMENT

Health technologies had been studied for safety, effectiveness, cost, and other concerns long before the advent of HTA. The development of TA as a systematic inquiry in the 1960s and 1970s coincided with the introduction of some health technologies that prompted widespread public interest in matters that transcended their immediate health effects. Health-care technologies were among the topics of early TAs. Multiphasic health screening was one of three topics of "experimental" TAs conducted by the NAE at the request of Congress. In response to a request by the National Science Foundation (NSF) to further develop the TA concept in the area of biomedical technologies, the National Research Council (NRC) conducted TAs on in vitro fertilization, predetermination of the sex of children, retardation of aging, and modifying human behavior by neurosurgical, electrical or pharmaceutical means. The OTA issued a report on drug bioequivalence in 1974, and the OTA Health Program issued its first formal report in 1976.

Since its early years, HTA has been fueled in part by the emergence and diffusion of technologies that have evoked social, ethical, legal, and political concerns. Among these technologies are contraceptives, organ transplantation, artificial organs, life-sustaining technologies for critically or terminally ill patients, and, more recently, genetic testing, genetic therapy, ultrasonography for fetal sex selection, and stem cell research. These technologies have challenged certain societal institutions, codes, and other norms regarding fundamental aspects of human life such as parenthood, heredity, birth, bodily sovereignty, freedom and control of human behavior, and death.

Despite the comprehensive approach originally intended for TA, its practitioners recognized early on that "partial TAs" may be preferable in circumstances where selected impacts are of particular interest or where necessitated by resource constraints. In practice, relatively few TAs have encompassed the full range of possible technological impacts; most focus on certain sets of impacts or concerns.

FACTORS THAT REINFORCE THE MARKET FOR HEALTH TECHNOLOGY

- Advances in science and engineering
- Intellectual property, especially patent protection
- Aging populations
- Increasing prevalence of chronic diseases
- Emerging pathogens and other disease threats
- Third-party payment, especially fee-for-service payment
- Financial incentives of technology companies, clinicians, hospitals, and others
- Public demand driven by direct-to-consumer advertising, mass media reports, social media, and consumer awareness and advocacy
- Off-label use of drugs, biologics, and devices
- "Cascade" effects of unnecessary tests, unexpected results, or patient or physician anxiety
- Clinician specialty training at academic medical centers
- Provider competition to offer state-of-the-art technology
- Malpractice avoidance
- Strong or growing economies

Chapter 4 | **Technology and Healthcare Expenditure**

Healthcare expenditure measurements provide an estimate of the final consumption of medical goods and services in a country. This is also known as the "current health expenditure." Healthcare expenditure estimates include various spending policies for medical services such as government-run programs, insurance, or personal expenditures. Estimating healthcare expenditure must include unintended spending such as for training, support, and power outages. Expenses associated with population health, prevention programs, and health system administration are also included while estimating total healthcare expenditures. The total healthcare expenditure for the United States in 2019 was estimated to be around $3.8 trillion.

Technological innovations in medical technology have improved survival rates in the United States and increased healthcare expenditure concerning the gross domestic product (GDP) compared to other countries, according to a study published by the Journal of Economic Literature in 2012. In 2015, healthcare expenditure contributed to 17.8 percent of the GDP in the United States as studied by the Centers for Medicare and Medicaid Services (CMS). In 2015, the cost of healthcare per person in the United States was estimated to be around $9,990. The common trend observed in the United States is that the country spends a large amount of dollars on healthcare, and the strain is observed in the U.S. economy.

Technology in medicine has been highly beneficial, especially in the last decade, but it has also increased the price of healthcare. The cost of these technological advances contributes to the high price of healthcare. New medical technology is responsible for a 40–50 percent increase in the annual cost of healthcare. High prices of medical services and increased use of technology are the drivers of increased spending on healthcare. Over the years, as technology has improved, services have improved in efficiency and patient care. On another note, it has also fueled rising health costs. Since the United States has increased cases of obesity, the need for associated medical services is also higher, which contributes to high spending potential for healthcare. A report published in 2018 by AdvaMed estimated that in 2016, medical devices constituted a small but consistent share in the national health expenditure. The study concluded that in-house diagnostic services and medical device spending cost $173.1 billion and contributed 5.2 percent of the national health expenditure. In 2019, the United States spent 17.7 percent of the GDP on health-care services.

Though healthcare technology can be expensive for medical technologies, the benefits exceed the costs of productivity, efficiency, and reduced disabilities. In 2018, overall healthcare expenditure in the United States per resident amounted to $10,000. This was estimated to be higher than other OECD (Organization for Economic Co-operation and Development) countries. The general notion that technology can help reduce costs in healthcare is challenged by years of surveys and studies that show that innovation is not helping to reduce healthcare costs. Increased costs in healthcare in the United States can lead to deferred care. Though the U.S. healthcare system encourages innovation, this does not help combat price rise. This effect can be due to reduced net productivity

DEVICES AND TECHNOLOGIES UNDER HEALTHCARE EXPENDITURE

The healthcare technology market has various solutions to serve patients. Between 2016 and 2021, the health technology industry was estimated to reach a value of $280 billion with a compound annual growth rate (CAGR) of 15.9 percent. In 2018, the United States exported medical devices in critical categories amounting to $43 billion. The export potential for medical devices from the United States is estimated to reach $208 billion in 2023. The most significant healthcare technologies and their expenditure shares include:

- **Internet of Medical Things (IoMT).** The market share for Internet of Things for healthcare is likely to touch $158.1 billion in 2022, and $534.3 billion in 2025.
- **Telehealth.** The remote patient monitoring market stood at $15.871 billion in 2017.
- **Cloud computing.** In 2019, the cloud computing market reached $23.4 billion.
- **mHealth.** As of 2018, there were 47,911 mHealth apps available for use. Growth in the mHealth app market in the United States is at a rate of 35 percent.
- Data breaches in healthcare are expensive, causing expenses 2.5 times higher than the global average. In 2018, the U.S. Department of Health and Health Services (HHS) collected $28.7 million from healthcare agencies and insurance providers for inadequate handling of data breaches.
- **Augmented reality/virtual reality (AR/VR).** AR/VR market share was estimated to be $2.14 billion in 2018.
- **Big data analytics.** If big data analytics is implemented on a system-wide basis, it can reduce U.S. healthcare spending by $300–450 billion annually. In 2017, the North American big data market reached a value of $9.36 billion.

Other leading technologies that come under medical services costing higher are:
- Diagnostic testing such as genetic testing
- Advanced imaging equipment such as teleradiology, PET scans, CT scans, MRIs, and ultrasound imaging
- Single-use implant devices such as pacemakers, stents, and artificial joints
- Laparoscopic surgeries
- Electronic medical records (EMRs) and patient portals
- Supply management systems

The United States spends more than any other country on healthcare technology. Rising healthcare costs are attributed to an aging population, a split healthcare system, lack of care coordination, and medical innovation. With higher expenditures, health outcomes are lower, and life expectancy is considerably low. Approaches to reduce costs, improve affordable access, and addressing risk factors such as obesity and other chronic conditions can help the nation to reduce healthcare technology expenditure.

References

1. Chandra, Amitabh, et al. "Technology Growth and Expenditure Growth in Health Care," *Journal of Economic Literature (JEL)*, September 2012.
2. Cahan, Eli M., et al. "Why Is Not Innovation Helping Reduce Health Care Costs?" Health Affairs, June 4, 2020.
3. Clemens, Maria. "Technology and Rising Health Care Costs," *Forbes*, October 26, 2017.
4. Monegain, Bernie. "Technology Helps Drive High Cost of U.S. Healthcare," Healthcare I.T. News, May 3, 2012.
5. Donahoe, Gerald. "Estimates of Medical Device Spending in the United States," AdvaMed, November 2018.
6. "The Ultimate List of Healthcare I.T. Statistics for 2020," Arkenea, January 15, 2021.
7. "Health Expenditure Per Capita," OECD iLibrary, The Organization for Economic Co-operation and Development (OECD), November 7, 2019.
8. Kamal, Rabah, et al. "How Has U.S. Spending on Healthcare Changed Over Time?" Health System Tracker, December 23, 2020.
9. "The Impact of Medical Technology on Medicare Spending," Avalere Health, September 2015.
10. Tikkanen, Roosa, et al. "U.S. Health Care from a Global Perspective, 2019: Higher Spending, Worse Outcomes?" The Commonwealth Fund, January 30, 2020.

Chapter 5 | **Digital Health**

The broad scope of digital health includes categories such as mobile health (mHealth), health information technology (HIT), wearable devices, telehealth and telemedicine, and personalized medicine.

From mobile medical apps and software that support the clinical decisions doctors make every day to artificial intelligence (AI) and machine learning, digital technology has been driving a revolution in healthcare. Digital-health tools have the vast potential to improve our ability to accurately diagnose and treat disease and to enhance the delivery of healthcare for the individual.

Digital-health technologies use computing platforms, connectivity, software, and sensors for healthcare and related uses. These technologies span a wide range of uses, from applications in general wellness to applications as a medical device. They include technologies intended for use as a medical product, in a medical product, as companion diagnostics, or as an adjunct to other medical products (devices, drugs, and biologics). They may also be used to develop or study medical products.

WHAT ARE THE BENEFITS OF DIGITAL-HEALTH TECHNOLOGIES?

Digital tools are giving providers a more holistic view of patient health through access to data and giving patients more control over their health. Digital health offers real opportunities to improve medical outcomes and enhance efficiency.

These technologies can empower consumers to make better-informed decisions about their own health and provide new options for facilitating prevention, early diagnosis of life-threatening

This chapter contains text excerpted from the following sources: Text in this chapter begins with excerpts from "What Is Digital Health?" U.S. Food and Drug Administration (FDA), September 22, 2020; Text under the heading "Digital Health Center of Excellence" is excerpted from "Digital Health Center of Excellence," U.S. Food and Drug Administration (FDA), March 24, 2021.

diseases, and management of chronic conditions outside of traditional health-care settings. Providers and other stakeholders are using digital-health technologies in their efforts to:

- Reduce inefficiencies
- Improve access
- Reduce costs
- Increase quality
- Make medicine more personalized for patients

Patients and consumers can use digital-health technologies to better manage and track their health and wellness-related activities.

The use of technologies, such as smartphones, social networks, and Internet applications, is not only changing the way we communicate but also providing innovative ways for us to monitor our health and well-being and giving us greater access to information. Together, these advancements are leading to a convergence of people, information, technology, and connectivity to improve healthcare and health outcomes.

THE FDA's FOCUS IN DIGITAL HEALTH

Many medical devices now have the ability to connect to and communicate with other devices or systems. Devices that are already U.S. Food and Drug Administration (FDA) approved, authorized, or cleared are being updated to add digital features. New types of devices that already have these capabilities are being explored.

Many stakeholders are involved in digital-health activities, including patients, health-care practitioners, researchers, traditional medical device industry firms, and firms new to the FDA regulatory requirements, such as mobile application developers.

The FDA's Center for Devices and Radiological Health (CDRH) is excited about these advances and the convergence of medical devices with connectivity and consumer technology. The following are topics in the digital-health field on which the FDA has been working to provide clarity using practical approaches that balance benefits and risks:

- Software as a Medical Device (SaMD)

- Artificial Intelligence and Machine Learning (AI/ML) in Software as a Medical Device
- Cybersecurity
- Device Software Functions, including Mobile Medical Applications
- Health IT
- Medical Device Data Systems
- Medical Device Interoperability
- Telemedicine
- Wireless Medical Devices

As another important step in promoting the advancement of digital-health technology, CDRH has established the Digital Health Center of Excellence which seeks to empower digital-health stakeholders to advance healthcare.

DIGITAL HEALTH CENTER OF EXCELLENCE

The Digital Health Center of Excellence aims to empower stakeholders to advance healthcare by fostering responsible and high-quality digital-health innovation with an objective to:
- Connect and build partnerships to accelerate digital-health advancements.
- Share knowledge to increase awareness and understanding, drive synergy, and advance best practices.
- Innovate regulatory approaches to provide efficient and least burdensome oversight while meeting the FDA standards for safe and effective products.

Through fulfilling these objectives, the FDA anticipates the following advancements across digital health:
- Strategically advance science and evidence for digital-health technologies that meet the needs of stakeholders
- Efficient access to a highly specialized expertise, knowledge, and tools to accelerate access to digital-health technology

- Aligned regulatory approach to harmonize international regulatory expectations and industry standards
- Increased awareness and understanding of digital-health trends
- Consistent application of digital-health technology policy and oversight approaches
- Reimagined medical device regulatory paradigm tailored for digital-health technologies

Chapter 6 | **Blockchain Technology**

Due to improvements in genetic research and the advancement of precision medicine, healthcare is witnessing an innovative approach to disease prevention and treatment that incorporates an individual patient's genetic makeup, lifestyle, and environment. Simultaneously, IT advancement has produced large databases of health information, provided tools to track health data, and engaged individuals more in their own healthcare. Combining these advancements in healthcare and information technology would foster transformative change in the field of health IT.

The American Recovery and Reinvestment Act (ARRA) required all public and private health-care providers to adopt electronic medical records (EMRs) by January 1, 2014, in order to maintain their existing Medicaid and Medicare reimbursement levels. This EMR mandate spurred significant growth in the availability and utilization of EMRs. However, the vast majority of these systems do not have the capacity to share their health data.

Blockchain technology has the potential to address the interoperability challenges currently present in health IT systems and to be the technical standard that enables individuals, health-care providers, health-care entities, and medical researchers to securely share electronic health data.

Interoperability is also a critical component of any infrastructure supporting Patient-Centered Outcomes Research (PCOR)

This chapter includes text excerpted from "Blockchain for Health Data and Its Potential Use in Health IT and Health-Care Related Research," HealthIT.gov, Office of the National Coordinator for Health Information Technology (ONC), March 8, 2021.

and the Precision Medicine Initiative (PMI). A national health IT infrastructure based on blockchain has far-reaching potential to promote the development of precision medicine, advance medical research, and invite patients to be more accountable for their health.

UNDERLYING FUNDAMENTALS OF BLOCKCHAIN TECHNOLOGY

Blockchain is a peer-to-peer (P2P) distributed ledger technology for a new generation of transactional applications that establishes transparency and trust. Blockchain is the underlying fabric for Bitcoin and is a design pattern consisting of three main components: a distributed network, a shared ledger, and digital transactions.

Distributed Network Blockchain

A decentralized P2P architecture with nodes consisting of network participants. Each member in the network stores an identical copy of the blockchain and contributes to the collective process of validating and certifying digital transactions for the network.

Shared Ledger Members

A distributed network records digital transactions into a shared ledger. To add transactions, members in the network run algorithms to evaluate and verify the proposed transaction. If a majority of the members in the network agree that the transaction is valid, the new transaction is added to the shared ledger. Changes to the shared ledger are reflected in all copies of the blockchain in minutes or, in some cases, seconds. After a transaction is added it is immutable and cannot be changed or removed. Since all members in the network have a complete copy of the blockchain no single member has the power to tamper or alter data.

Digital Transactions

Any type of information or digital asset can be stored in a blockchain, and the network implementing the blockchain defines the type of information contained in the transaction. Information is encrypted and digitally signed to guarantee authenticity and accuracy. Transactions are structured into blocks and each block contains a cryptographic hash to the prior block in the blockchain. Blocks are added in a linear, chronological order.

A BLOCKCHAIN MODEL FOR HEALTHCARE

Any blockchain for healthcare would need to be public and would also need to include technological solutions for three key elements: scalability, access security, and data privacy.

Scalability

A distributed blockchain that contains health records, documents, or images would have data storage implications and data through-put limitations. If modeled after the Bitcoin blockchain, every member in the distributed network of the health-care blockchain would have a copy of every health record for every individual in the United States and this would not be practical from a data storage perspective. Because health data is dynamic and expansive, replicating all heath records to every member in the network would be bandwidth-intensive, wasteful on network resources, and pose data throughput concerns. For healthcare to realize benefits from blockchain, the blockchain would need to function as an access-control manager for health records and data.

The information contained in a health blockchain would be an index, a list of all the user's health records, and health data. The index is similar to a card catalog in a library. The card catalog contains metadata about the book and a location where the book can be found. The health blockchain would work the same way. Transactions in the blocks would contain a user's unique identifier, an encrypted link to the health record, and a timestamp for when the transaction was created. To improve data access efficiency, the transaction would contain the type of data contained in the health record and any other metadata that would facilitate frequently used queries (the metadata could be added as tags). The health blockchain would contain a complete indexed history of all medical data, including formal medical records as well as health data from mobile applications and wearable sensors, and would follow an individual user throughout their life.

All medical data would be stored off blockchain in a data repository called a "data lake." Data lakes are highly scalable and can store a wide variety of data, from images to documents to key value stores. Data lakes would be valuable tools for health research and would be used for a variety of analyses including mining for factors that impact outcomes, determining optimal treatment options based on genetic markers, and identifying elements that influence preventative medicine. Data lakes support interactive queries, text mining, text analytics, and machine learning. All information stored in the data lake would be encrypted and digitally signed to ensure the privacy and authenticity of the information.

When a health-care provider creates a medical record (prescription, lab test, pathology result, MRI) a digital signature would be created to verify the authenticity of the document or image. The health data would be encrypted and sent to the data lake for storage. Every time information is saved to the data lake a pointer to the health record is registered in the blockchain along with the user's unique identifier. The patient is notified that health data was added to their blockchain. In the same fashion, a patient would be able to add health data with digital signatures and encryption from mobile applications and wearable sensors.

Access Security and Data Privacy

The user would have full access to their data and control over how their data would be shared. The user would assign a set of access permissions and designate who can query and write data to their blockchain. A mobile dashboard application would allow the user to see who has permission to access their blockchain. The user would also be able to view an audit log of who accessed their blockchain, including when and what data was accessed. The same dashboard would allow the user to give and revoke access permissions to any individual who has a unique identifier.

Access control permissions would be flexible and would handle more than "all-or-nothing" permissions. The user would set up specific, detailed transactions about who has access, the allotted time frame for access, and the particular types of data that can be accessed. At any given time, the user may alter the set of permissions. Access control policies would also be securely stored on a blockchain and only the user would be allowed to change them. This provides an environment of transparency and allows the user to make all decisions about what data is collected and how the data can be shared. After a health-care provider is granted access to a user's health information, she or he queries the blockchain for the user's data and utilizes the digital signature to authenticate the data. The health-care provider could utilize a customized best-of-breed application to analyze the health data.

Identity authentication would follow the best practices established by financial institutions and regulators. Ideally, biometric identity systems would be utilized as they offer enhanced security over password and token (smartcard) based methods for identity authentication.

Given this model, the user has singular control over their data and the power to grant access to specific health-care providers and/or health-care entities for communication and collaboration in disease treatment and prevention. The decentralized nature of the blockchain combined with digitally signed transactions ensures that an adversary cannot pose as the user or corrupt the network as that would imply the adversary forged a digital signature or gained control over the majority of the network's resources. Similarly, an adversary would not be able to learn anything from the shared public ledger as only hashed pointers and encrypted information would be contained within the transactions.

TECHNICAL ADVANTAGES OF A HEALTHCARE BLOCKCHAIN
Blockchain technology offers many advantages for healthcare IT. Blockchain is based on open-source software, commodity hardware, and an open application programming interface (API). These components facilitate faster and easier interoperability between systems and can efficiently scale to handle larger volumes of data and more blockchain users. The architecture has built-in fault tolerance and disaster recovery, and the data encryption and cryptography technologies are widely used and accepted as industry standards.

The health blockchain would be developed as open-source software. Open-source software is peer-reviewed software developed by skillful experts. It is reliable and robust under fast- 7 changing conditions that cannot be matched by closed, proprietary software. Open-source solutions also drive innovations in the applications market. Health providers and individuals would benefit from the wide range of application choices and could select options that matched their specific requirements and needs.

Blockchain would run on widely used and reliable commodity hardware. Commodity hardware provides the greatest amount of useful computation at a low cost. The hardware is based on open standards and manufactured by multiple vendors. It is the most cost-effective and efficient architecture for health and genomic research. Excess blockchain hardware capacity could be shared with health researchers and facilitate faster discovery of new drugs and treatments.

Blockchain technology also addresses the interoperability challenges within the health IT ecosystem. Health IT systems would use Open APIs to integrate and exchange data with the health blockchain. Open APIs are based on industry best practices. They are easy to work with and would eliminate the need for the development of complex point-to-point data integrations between the different systems.

Blockchain would allow patients, the health-care community, and researchers to access one shared data source to obtain timely, accurate, and comprehensive patient health data. Blockchain data structures combined with data lakes can support a wide variety of health data sources including data from patients' mobile applications, wearable sensors, EMRs, documents, and images. The data structures are flexible, extendable, and would be able to accommodate the unforeseen data that will be available in the future.

Data from cheap mobile devices and wearable sensors is growing at an exponential rate. Distributed architectures based on commodity hardware provide cost-efficient high scalability. As more health data is added to the blockchain cost-efficient commodity hardware can be easily added to handle the increased load. Another advantage of blockchain distributed architecture is built-in fault tolerance and disaster recovery. Data is distributed across many servers in many different locations. There is no single point of failure and it is unlikely a disaster would impact all locations at the same time.

Blockchain works with standard algorithms and protocols for cryptography and data encryption. These technologies have been heavily analyzed and accepted as secure and are widely used across all industries and many government agencies.

HEALTHCARE ADVANTAGES OF HEALTHCARE BLOCKCHAIN

Blockchain technology offers many advantages to medical researchers, health-care providers, caregivers, and individuals. Creation of a single storage location for all health data, tracking personalized data in real time, and the security to set data access permissions at a granular level would serve research as well as personalized medicine.

Health researchers require broad and comprehensive data sets in order to advance the understanding of diseases, accelerate biomedical discovery, fast track the development of drugs and design customized individual treatment plans based on patient genetics, lifecycle, and environment. The shared data environment provided by Blockchain would deliver a broad diverse data set by including patients from different ethnic and socioeconomic backgrounds and from various geographical environments. As blockchain collects health data across a patient's lifetime, it offers data ideal for longitudinal studies.

A health-care blockchain would expand the acquisition of health data to include data from populations of people who are currently underserved by the medical community or who do not typically participate in research. The shared data environment provided by Blockchain makes it easier to engage "hard-to-reach" populations and develop results more representative of the general public.

Blockchain data structures would work well for gathering data from wearable sensors and mobile applications and, thus, would contribute significant information on the risks versus benefits of treatments as well as patient reported outcomes. Furthermore, combining health data from mobile applications and wearable sensors with data from traditional EMRs and genomics will offer medical researchers increased capabilities to classify individuals into subpopulations that respond well to a specific treatment or who are more susceptible to a particular disease. Daily, personalized health data will likely engage a patient more in their own healthcare and improve patient compliance. Moreover, the ability for physicians to obtain more frequent data (i.e., daily blood pressures or blood sugar levels versus only when a patient appears for an appointment) would improve individualized care with specialized treatment plans based on outcomes/treatment efficacy.

Blockchain would ensure continuous availability and access to real-time data. Real-time access to data would improve clinical care coordination and improve clinical care in emergency medical situations. Real-time data would also allow researchers and public-health resources to rapidly detect, isolate and drive change for environmental conditions that impact public health. For example, epidemics could be detected earlier and contained.

The real-time availability of mobile applications and wearable sensor data from the blockchain would facilitate continuous, 24 hour-a-day monitoring of high-risk patients and drive the innovation of "smart" applications that would notify caregivers and health providers if a patient reached a critical threshold for action. Care teams could reach out to the patient and coordinate treatment options for early intervention.

A health-care blockchain would likely promote the development of a new breed of "smart" applications for health providers that would mine the latest medical research and develop personalized treatment paths. The health provider and patient would have access to the same information and would be able to engage in a collaborative, educated discussion about the best-case treatment options based on research rather than intuition.

Blockchain technology addresses interoperability challenges, is based on open standards, provides a shared distributed view of health data, and will achieve widespread acceptance and deployment throughout all industries.

Utilization of the proposed health blockchain described in this chapter has the potential to engage millions of individuals, health-care providers, health-care entities, and medical researchers to share vast amounts of genetic, diet, lifestyle, environmental, and health data with guaranteed security and privacy protection. The acquisition, storage, and sharing of this data would lay a scientific foundation for the advancement of medical research and precision medicine, help identify and develop new ways to treat and prevent disease and test whether or not mobile devices engage individuals more in their healthcare for improved health and disease prevention.

Blockchain technology definitely has a place in the health IT ecosystem, and the ONC should strongly consider basing their interoperability strategy on blockchain and using blockchain to promote the advancement of precision medicine.

Chapter 7 | **The Internet of Things**

Within the next ten years, it is predicted that half of all healthcare will be delivered virtually, with providers paid based on their teamwork and quality. It is expected that 24x7 diagnostics monitoring from phones, wearables, and even implantables has a dramatic growth in sensing technologies from the hospital to the home. The integration of device data (inpatient, outpatient, and home- or mobile-based) into medical records will be a major push for the foreseeable future. In large part because of widespread wastefulness in service delivery and the need for virtual care models, The McKinsey Global Institute forecasts that 40 percent of the global economic impact of the Internet of Things (IoT) revolution will occur in healthcare, more than any other sector. Mobile healthcare devices will be used to track everything from fitness goals to surgical rehab faster, more convenient, and at reduced costs. Two distinct factors have the potential to make dramatic changes in U.S. healthcare:

- Consumer engagement
- Payment for outcomes

These are crucial to meeting the needs brought by shifts in demographics.

Emerging 21st-century health-care platforms require titanic shifts in thinking, business models, and infrastructure. The old "mainframe health" paradigm (i.e., centralized, hospital-centric, expert-driven, reactive, costly) is giving way to a new "personal

This chapter includes text excerpted from "The Internet of Things and Healthcare Policy Principles," U.S. Senate Special Committee on Aging, July 25, 2014. Reviewed June 2021.

health" paradigm (i.e., distributed, data-rich, preventive, home- and consumer-centric, and efficiency-driven).

ECONOMIC IMPACT OF IoT APPLICATION
Population Aging
A shift from younger to the older population. Only three years from now, the human population will hit a crossover point for the first time in history. There will be more people over 65 years of age than under 5 years of age. "No other force is likely to shape the future of national economic health, public finances, and policymaking than the irreversible rate at which the world's population is aging," according to Standard & Poors. By 2030, China will have more people over 60 years of age than the total current U.S. population.

Chronic Diseases
A shift from predominantly infectious disease threats to predominantly chronic diseases, often exacerbated by lifestyle. Population aging increases the number of patients with heart disease, cancer, diabetes, lung and kidney disorders, Alzheimer, and overweight. These issues hinder productivity and are expensive and difficult to treat, requiring behavior changes. Today, 63 percent of the world's deaths are from noncommunicable diseases (NCDs) (noninfectious; not transmitted by humans). Low- to middle-income countries now carry roughly 80 percent of the burden of diseases, such as cardiovascular disease (CVD), diabetes, cancer, and chronic respiratory diseases.

Global Shortage of Health-Care Workers
The United States alone is projected to face a shortage of 124,000 physicians by the year 2025, yet this pales in comparison with the needs in Asia and Africa.

Inefficiency of Health-Care Sector
On top of demographic and workforce problems, the health-care sector is dramatically inefficient. Even if health-care services were

delivered efficiently, it would be extraordinarily difficult for a short-age of medical professionals to care for greater numbers of sicker people over the next several decades. Yet by all accounts, there are hundreds of billions of dollars in wasteful spending that need to be squeezed out of health-care systems worldwide.

Rise of Internet Culture

With the rise of the Internet culture, there is a shift from passive to active patients. Patients and families are more engaged and dig-itally monitored by a growing array of apps and devices. The Intel Healthcare Innovation Barometer, an eight-nation, 12,000-adult survey on 2013, revealed:

- 80 percent are optimistic about healthcare through innovation and technology.
- 70 percent are willing to see a doctor via video conference for nonurgent appointments.
- 70 percent are receptive to using toilet sensors, prescription bottle sensors, or swallowed health monitors.
- 50 percent believe the traditional hospital will be obsolete in the future and would trust a test they personally administered as much or more than if performed by a doctor.

Healthcare Tools

Health apps, social networks, and collaboration tools are grow-ing rapidly. Enterprise and consumer health apps will continue to proliferate, shake out. Parks Associates indicates that 28 percent of U.S. broadband households have used some type of virtual care communication tool, and estimates the figure will grow to 65 per-cent by 2018.

EMERGING IoT HEALTHCARE CATEGORIES

Three categories are emerging for IoT healthcare: Person to Person, Person to Computer, and Person as a Computer.

Person to Person

Dulcie Madden of Mimo developed an infant monitor that sends parents real-time information on their baby's breathing, skin temperature, sleeping position, and activity level. Mimo sends the baby's sleep data straight to her parents' smartphones.

Person to Computer

Vigilant, a Swiss company, has developed a smart insulin injection tracker to help diabetic patients manage their health. The injection tracker, called "Bee+," is an electronic cap that fits most insulin pens on the market. It wirelessly transmits a diabetic's insulin injection data to a smartphone app.

Person as Computer

Myo uses the electrical activity in your muscles to wirelessly control your computer, phone, and other favorite digital technologies. With a wave of your hand, Myo will transform how you interact with your digital world.

POLICY PRINCIPLES

The potential for IoT and consumer engagement to dramatically improve health status/outcomes is limited by policies defined by face-to-face transactions. The shift is beginning and the Congress and the Administration is urged to embrace new health-care models by tackling difficult policy decisions.

Require Data Standards for Connectivity and Interoperability

- IoT in healthcare has the potential to aggregate data from patient records, wearable sensors, labs, diet, the environment, and social networking in real time, but only if the data can be analyzed. This takes standardized data formats. Policymakers should strengthen current requirements for data exchange among EHR's and the emerging IoT devices/solutions.

Regulate Smartly/Do Not De-innovate

The regulation of software as a medical device has created confusion and missteps for health IT entrepreneurs. Today, Congress, regulators, and industry are collaborating to find the best regulatory framework through initiatives, such as the U.S. Food and Drug Administration Safety Innovation Act (FDASIA) to better define what attributes of technology are subject to the U.S. Food and Drug Administration (FDA) device regulation.

Regulatory pathways should be refined to reflect health technologies that are not medical devices. This will require alternative frameworks to ensure functionality and safety.

Rethink Reimbursement

- IoT provides a new platform for capturing daily biometric data that shows trends and changes in health status in real time. However, this rich and actionable data is not being used today because our health systems are unprepared to incorporate the data into the fee for service payments, or shared savings models. Even the Accountable Care Organizations which have incentives to offer innovative services, are restricted by outdated Medicare regulations which dictate that payment for virtual services is only for patients living in rural areas (20 percent of U.S.), and will not pay for services at home and certainly not "on the go."
- Healthcare IoT solutions poised to change access and outcomes for chronically ill patients are now delayed not by technology, but by the lack of payment where virtual care is substituted and enhanced over face-to-face visits.

Capture Patient Generated Health Data (PGHD) as a Vital Part of the Patient Record

- The $27B investment made by the U.S. government in electronic medical records has spurred unparalleled adoption rates – 78 percent of physicians and 66 percent of our nation's qualifying hospitals have been certified.

Yet, the real-time data from sensors, tablets, smartphones, and peripherals are not captured in the electronic health record (EHR). Physicians can now diagnose a patient's medical condition from daily feeds provided by IoT devices noting changes in environment, diet, exercise, and medications, giving more accurate and longitudinal data rather than through readings from occasional office visits. The U.S. Department of Health and Human Services (HHS) should address the issues of liability and data overload associated with PGHD and then recommend best practices for all future EHR regulations, including PGHD.

Privacy and Security Required for IoT Solutions

- According to the Office of Civil Rights in HHS, 199 PHI breaches were reported in 2013 affecting 7 million patient records. The need for security today in HIPAA-covered entities is pervasive and as health information transfers between consumer and enterprise devices, message-level data encryption, API management, and data tokenization will become essential. HHS should continue to work with the healthcare industry to achieve agreement on a universally accepted health IT security standard or principles that can be enforceable and agree on criteria that deem organizations "HIPAA Security Rule Compliant."

Part 2 | Technology and Preventive Healthcare

Chapter 8 | **Types of Telemedicine Technology**

Chapter Contents

Section 8.1 | **Real-Time Telehealth**

This section contains text excerpted from the following sources: Text beginning with the heading "What Is CVT?" is excerpted from "Clinical Video Telehealth (CVT)," U.S. Department of Veterans Affairs (VA), March 8, 2012. Reviewed June 2021; Text under the heading "What Are the Components of CVT?" is excerpted from "VHA Clinical Video Telehealth Technology: Fact Sheet," U.S. Department of Veterans Affairs (VA), March 3, 2017. Reviewed June 2021; Text under the heading "Clinical Video Telehealth Usage" is excerpted from "Department of Veterans Affairs (VA): A Primer on Telehealth," Congressional Research Service (CRS), July 26, 2019.

WHAT IS CVT?

Clinical video telehealth (CVT) uses video conferencing technology to conveniently, securely, and quickly provide veterans with access to health-care services from remote facilities. CVT instantly connects a veteran in one location with a health-care provider in a different location. This connection allows for real-time interaction between patient and provider. Specialty equipment (such as a high-resolution portable camera) provides a safe, reliable, and accurate way for providers to assess a patient and manage their treatment without physically being in the same location.

WHAT IS CVT LIKE TO USE?

Clinical video telehealth appointments feel a lot like traditional face-to-face appointments. When you come to your scheduled appointment, a staff member will escort you to the CVT equipped room. The television monitor and cameras will be set up so that you and your provider can both see and hear each other clearly. When your visit is over, you will let the staff know, take care of any business or follow-up appointment scheduling, and then go about your day.

WHY SHOULD YOU USE CVT?

Clinical video telehealth helps you access the best healthcare without having to make long trips to go see a specialist in person. Using advanced technology, the doctors can provide you with the care you need by CVT as effectively as they can with a traditional face-to-face appointment.

WHAT ARE THE COMPONENTS OF CVT?

A clinical video telehealth system has six major components, and compatible clinical video telehealth systems are required on both ends of the video call:

CODEC

The Coder-Decoder (CODEC) compresses (codes) the two-way audio and video streams so that they can be sent over the communications link, then decodes incoming signals from the far side. CODECs can be dedicated hardware "boxes" running proprietary software or can be based on a personal computer.

Video Camera

The CVT system camera and Webcam for computers are specially designed for videoconferencing applications. Some offer pan (side to side) and tilt (up and down) controls so that the user can easily point the camera at the appropriate subject. It also offers control of the zoom for a wider or tighter angle of view. The CVT systems provide multiple camera connections to facilitate additional specialized diagnostic cameras. Many systems allow control of the camera on the far end of the connection. This is especially useful because the consultant has direct control over the view so the consultant can frame the subject as needed. Far end camera control has become standard on newer systems.

Video Monitor

Each CVT system has at least one video monitor. Systems with a dedicated CODEC most often use a standard video monitor. Computer-based CODECs generally use a computer monitor, although some newer systems use a combination of one video monitor and one computer monitor for data display.

Microphone

Each end has at least one microphone to pick up the sound for transmission to the far end.

Speakers

Speakers allow the user to hear the sound from the far end.

Accessories

The CVT system accessories are available for virtually any specialized application. Some key accessories often used in telehealth applications include document cameras to share electrocardiograms (ECGs), x-rays, graphs, and other static materials. Diagnostic peripherals adapted for use with videoconferencing equipment include dermascope, ENT scope, digital stethoscope, still camera, etc.

CLINICAL VIDEO TELEHEALTH USAGE

The clinical video telehealth (CVT) modality allows a VA provider who is not located in the same location as a veteran patient to view, diagnose, monitor, and treat medical conditions of the veteran patient in real time. The CVT modality functions by allowing the VA provider and the veteran patient to see each other via an interactive live video technology. Telehealth episodes of care via the CVT modality transpire between different VA sites of care, such as from a VA medical center (VAMC) to a veteran patient's home or from a veteran patient's home to a VA provider's home office. From FY2009 to FY2018, the VA has provided 5.7 million telehealth encounters via the CVT modality to 2.1 million veteran patients.

In FY2018, the VA provided 1,074,422 telehealth episodes of care to 393,370 veteran patients through the CVT modality. According to the VA, the telehealth service that veteran patients accessed the most via the CVT modality is telemental health, which refers to the delivery of a mental-health service via telehealth. Figure 8.1 illustrates the percentage of veterans who received telehealth services and the number of telehealth encounters that transpired via the CVT modality, for each of the fiscal years FY2009–FY2018.

The upward trends in both the percentage of veterans who received telehealth services and the number of telehealth encounters that transpired via the CVT program seem to illustrate that veteran patients are increasingly interested in receiving VA telehealth

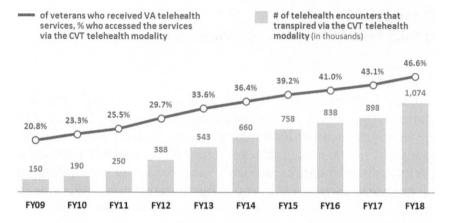

Figure 8.1. Distribution of Services That Transpired via the Clinical Video Telehealth (CVT) Modality for Those Veterans Who Received Telehealth Services, FY2009–FY2018. *(Source: Figure prepared by CRS based on data from an email that CRS received from the Veterans Health Administration of the U.S. Department of Veterans Affairs (VA), January 14, 2019.)*

Note: A single veteran could have received more than one telehealth service via the CVT modality.

services via this modality. Veteran patients' interest in the CVT program might stem from it being well established and publicized. The program is the VA's oldest method of telehealth delivery. Additionally, veterans have been able to access telemental healthcare services via the CVT modality since the VA started providing telehealth services.

Section 8.2 | **Store-and-Forward Telehealth**

This section includes text excerpted from "Store-and-Forward Telehealth," U.S. Department of Veterans Affairs (VA), June 3, 2015. Reviewed June 2021.

You have probably heard the expression that a picture is worth a thousand words? In some areas of healthcare pictures can be worth thousands of clinic visits. Three areas of healthcare where this is becoming commonplace in VA are radiology, dermatology, and checking for the effects of diabetes on the retina in the back of the eye.

Store-and-forward telehealth involves the acquisition and storing of clinical information (e.g., data, image, sound, video) that is then forwarded to (or retrieved by) another site for clinical evaluation. For many years, local and regional Store-and-forward Telehealth programs have been providing consultation to VHA sites in need of specialty expertise. The Veterans Health Administration's (VHA) first national Store-and-Forward Telehealth program was a primary care-based model that screens veterans with diabetes for retinopathy using teleretinal imaging that expedite referral for treatment and provide health information.

TELEDERMATOLOGY
Dermatology (skin) problems are common and often a source of discomfort and concern to patients. The diagnosis of a skin problem can often be made from a digital picture if it is sent to a skin specialist (dermatologist) to see. A report with recommendations for treatment can then be sent back to a patient's primary care, or other, physician. The recommendation may be for treatment in the form of a medication or maybe a referral to a dermatology clinic for a more detailed assessment. VA is using TeleDermatology to improve access to skincare for veteran patients who live in remote and other areas to save having to travel to a dermatology clinic.

TELERETINAL IMAGING
Diabetes can cause problems with the blood vessels in the back of the eye (retina), especially if the diabetes is poorly controlled. A special camera is available that can take pictures of the retina of the eye without needing to put drops in the eye to widen the pupil of the eye. The picture that is taken is then sent to an eye care specialist to review and a report is sent back to the patient's primary care physician who then follows up if treatment to prevent blindness is required. This investigation does not replace a full eye exam and is not suitable for people who already have complications of diabetes

but makes it does mean that those at risk of eye problems from diabetes can be assessed easily and conveniently in a local clinic.

The ability to acquire, store and then forward digital images for reporting is a crucial area of care coordination development within VHA. VA's computerized patient record called "VistA" has a component called "VistA Imaging." It enables the communication of clinical images throughout VA.

Chapter 9 | Digital Innovations in Preventive Medicine

Chapter Contents

Section 9.1 | Sensors

This section includes text excerpted from "Sensors," National Institute of Biomedical Imaging and Bioengineering (NIBIB), October 2016. Reviewed June 2021.

WHAT ARE SENSORS?

In medicine and biotechnology, sensors are tools that detect specific biological, chemical, or physical processes and then transmit or report this data. Some sensors work outside the body while others are designed to be implanted within the body.

Some monitoring devices consist of multiple sensors that measure a number of physical or biological parameters. Other devices may be multifunctional, incorporating sensors and then delivering a drug or intervention based on the sensor data obtained. Sensors may also be components in systems that process clinical samples, such as increasingly common "lab-on-a-chip" devices.

Sensors help health-care providers and patients monitor health conditions and ensure that they can make informed decisions about treatment. Sensors are also often used to monitor the safety of medicines, food, environmental conditions, and other substances that may be encountered.

HOW ARE SENSORS USED IN CURRENT MEDICAL PRACTICE?

Many different types of sensors are already used in healthcare, including self-care at home. Thermometers translate the expansion of a fluid or bending of a metal strip in response to heat into a number corresponding to body temperature. Paper-based home pregnancy tests contain a substance that changes color in the presence of hormones indicating pregnancy. In hospitals and other provider-based settings, you can find more complex types of sensors such as pulse oximeters (also known as "blood-oxygen monitors"), which measure changes in the body's absorption of special types of light to provide information on a patient's heart rate and the amount of oxygen in the blood.

HOW MIGHT NOVEL SENSORS IMPROVE MEDICAL CARE OR BIOMEDICAL RESEARCH?

Advances in technology, engineering, and materials science have opened the door for increasingly sophisticated sensors to be used in medical research. A group of NIBIB-funded researchers developed a compact, wireless, implantable brain sensor that can record and transmit brain activity data. Building on previously developed brain-computer interfaces that used wired connections, this new sensor may someday lead to unobtrusive, thought-controlled prosthetics and other assistive devices for people with amputated limbs, paralysis, or other movement impairments.

Researchers at the National Institute of Biomedical Imaging and Bioengineering (NIBIB) aim to improve existing sensors through a variety of means, such as making fluorescent probes easier to see and increasing the capabilities, and enhancing efficiency of individual sensors.

Some scientists are exploring biological sensors, which rely on substances that occur naturally in the body, or artificial compounds that mimic natural substances, to capture molecules that are important to measure in the body. Biosensors may provide insights into disease processes that are hard to detect directly, such as dysfunctions in brain chemistry that are thought to play a role in many mental disorders.

For example, one method for studying chemical processes in real time uses engineered cells that can be "programmed" with receptors that latch onto specific brain chemicals. The resulting chain of activity causes a protein within the cell to change color that researchers can detect with a certain type of laser microscope. The biosensors remain active in the brain for several days, allowing scientists to study changes in brain chemistry over time, which may help inform efforts to improve drug treatments for mental disorders.

While many advanced sensors are not practical for routine medical care, they allow researchers to study the basic foundations of disease in more detail than previously possible, and to develop new technologies that could dramatically improve the quality of life of people with severe disabilities.

WHAT TECHNOLOGIES ARE NIBIB-FUNDED RESEARCHERS DEVELOPING WITH SENSORS?

Sensors play key roles in all aspects of healthcare – prevention, diagnosis, disease monitoring, treatment monitoring – and the range of research involving sensors is equally broad. In addition to health-related applications, the NIBIB funds studies to test new materials and technologies for building sensors, to develop new sensors that can advance medical research, and to promote healthy independent living through home-based and wearable sensors.

New Materials and Technologies

Good health requires not only protecting our bodies but safeguarding things we put into our bodies as well. The NIBIB-funded researchers developed a sensor using a thin membrane made from a special kind of plastic. The researchers loaded the membrane with a compound that creates a voltage difference across the membrane in the presence of osteopathia striata with cranial sclerosis (OSCS), a potentially deadly contaminant sometimes found in preparations of the commonly used blood thinner heparin. OSCS is inherently highly charged and interacts with the compound-loaded membrane without the need to apply an external electrical current. By measuring the voltage, scientists can quickly identify OSCS-contaminated samples before the heparin is administered to a patient. The reaction between OSCS and the membrane is also reversible, so the sensors can be used repeatedly.

Another NIBIB grant supported research to develop an instrument to detect and monitor levels of vapor phase hydrogen peroxide (VPHP). VPHP is much stronger than the type of hydrogen peroxide commonly used in first aid care but has a similar use: to disinfect and sterilize pharmaceutical manufacturing equipment and facilities. After sterilization procedures, manufacturers have to ensure VPHP levels are reduced back to a minimum to protect workers and product quality. The researchers developed a sensor that uses a new type of highly efficient and extremely sensitive laser to continuously monitor VPHP levels throughout the sterilization process. The sensor can also detect how much VPHP has been absorbed by packaging and other materials within the facility, such as sterile isolators or other protective barriers.

Advancing Medical Research

Many illnesses develop and progress as a result of faulty regulation or dysfunction of a range of hormones, neurotransmitters, or other important body chemicals. Tracking such chemical activity is key to unraveling disease processes, but current sensors are generally limited in the number of chemicals that can be analyzed at one time or require those chemicals to be labeled first, thus greatly increasing the time, cost, and complexity of sensing. The NIBIB-funded researchers seek to improve on biosensors in a variety of ways, such as creating novel types of coatings that improve sensor sensitivity, selectivity, and stability; and developing a fluorescence-based strategy for detecting proteins in living organisms and in real time.

Healthy Independent Living

Environmental and mobile sensors are already a part of many people's everyday lives. For example, faucets that automatically start when you place your hands under them and shut off when you are done washing. Lights that turn themselves on when you enter a room. Wearable bands that track your daily activity, perhaps even coordinating with your smartphone to allow you to track data over time or share your information with others. The NIBIB supports initiatives to develop improved sensor and related information technologies for home and mobile use that will sustain wellness and facilitate coordinated management of chronic diseases. For example, one research team is working to improve the ability of "smart homes" to make sense of real-time sensor data and to recognize changes in a resident's activity patterns that may signal changes in well-being, such as a fall or disrupted meal schedule.

WHAT ARE IMPORTANT AREAS FOR FUTURE RESEARCH ON SENSORS?

The types of sensors being developed and studied currently may play key roles in expanding and greatly changing the delivery of healthcare. One area, in particular, that may benefit from sensor research is point-of-care (POC) technologies.

Point of care refers to the place where patients receive healthcare, which may be anywhere from primary care offices or community clinics to emergency rooms or even patients' own homes. POC research seeks to address barriers to healthcare that have arisen from the concentration of services in highly specialized medical centers and labs. POC technologies may allow providers to diagnose and treat a particular health condition in a single visit, so patients do not need to make additional appointments or wait for test results.

Besides funding studies seeking to improve the manufacturing process for low-cost POC technologies, the NIBIB-funded efforts are already underway to develop cost-effective POC solutions for detecting a range of medical conditions, including H5N1 influenza and allergies, and other autoimmune diseases. Miniature, implantable sensors could continuously monitor a person's health status, providing more accurate information than conventional disease screening and a clearer sense of when a doctor's visit is needed. Integrating compact, wireless sensing technologies into medical devices or chronic treatments such as long-term oxygen therapy may help lower treatment costs and be easier for patients to use. Such technologies may also be compatible with mobile devices, allowing for remote monitoring and assessments in real time.

Some of the challenges to sensor research include simplifying and automating the preparation of patient samples to be used at the point of care (POC) and overcoming the body's natural rejection response to implantable or minimally invasive sensors.

Section 9.2 | **Body Area Networks**

This section contains text excerpted from the following sources: Text in this section begins with excerpts from "Visualization of Body Area Networks," National Institute of Standards and Technology (NIST), September 21, 2016. Reviewed June 2021; Text beginning with the heading "What Are the Issues with BANs?" is excerpted from "Implant Communications in Body Area Networks," National Institute of Standards and Technology (NIST), November 15, 2019.

The term body area network (BAN) refers to a network intended to be used in or around the human body. While this is an emerging field, networks of medical sensors are anticipated to be a primary application. Such sensors would either be attached to or implanted in the human body and would communicate wirelessly both within the body and to devices outside the body.

For this technology to develop, a greater understanding of radio frequency (RF) propagation through the human body is needed.

MODELING AND VISUALIZATION OF BANs

Because experimentation on human subjects is currently not feasible, RF propagation through the human body is being modeled in software with a 3D full-wave electromagnetic field simulator. The 3D human body model includes frequency dependent dielectric properties of 300+ parts in a male human body. The data produced by this simulation software is then brought into a 3D immersive visualization system, which enables researchers to study the modeled RF propagation through direct interactions with the data.

IMMERSIVE VISUALIZATION SYSTEM

The immersive system includes several important components: three orthogonal screens that provide the visual display, the motion-tracked stereoscopic glasses, and a hand-held motion-tracked input device. The screens are large projection video displays that are placed edge-to-edge in a corner configuration. These three screens are used to display a single 3D stereo scene. The scene is updated based on the position of the user as determined by the motion tracker. This allows the system to present to the user a 3D virtual world within which the user can move and interact with the virtual objects. The main interaction device is a hand-held three button motion-tracked wand with a joystick.

This virtual environment allows for more natural interaction between experts with different backgrounds such as engineering and medical sciences. The researchers can look at data representations at any scale and position, move through data, change orientation, and control the elements of the virtual world using a variety of interaction techniques including measurement and analysis.

For example, interactive tools for probing the 3D data fields had been implemented. One tool enables the researcher to move the motion-tracked wand through the virtual scene, yielding a continuously updated display of the value of the data field at the position of the wand. Another tool enables the user to interactively stretch a line segment through virtual body, and to generate graphs of the 3D data fields along that path. It was found these to be effective tools in getting quantitative information from the 3D scene and in gaining insight into RF propagation through the human body.

WHAT ARE THE ISSUES WITH BANs?

There are no standards for short-range, wireless communication to/from an implant (or a sensor) located inside (or on the surface) of a human body. Developing such communication protocols is a difficult task since there are currently no models/data available to characterize the propagation from implanted devices. As physical experiments are nearly impossible, intricate simulation models are the only option to study this problem. Also, RF coexistence and interoperability of such body area sensors with other wireless technologies need to be thoroughly evaluated to determine their effectiveness for practical applications.

WHAT IS BEING DONE TO ADDRESS THE ISSUES?

Building a 3D immersive visualization platform to observe RF propagation from implant devices and investigating appropriate 3D data visualization schemes for various RF-related quantities. Obtaining path loss versus distance information between an implant and a body-surface node or between two implants.

Investigating the possibility of driving a statistical channel model for Medical Implant Communications Service (MICS) operation and incorporate the results into the channel modeling standard document. Studying coexistence or interoperability issues with other wireless systems and technologies.

Section 9.3 | Wireless Medical Devices

This section contains text excerpted from the following sources: Text in this section begins with excerpts from "Wireless Medical Devices," U.S. Food and Drug Administration (FDA), September 4, 2018; Text under the heading "Wireless Medical Telemetry Systems" is excerpted from "Wireless Medical Telemetry Systems," U.S. Food and Drug Administration (FDA), September 4, 2018; Text beginning with the heading "Radio Frequency Identification" is excerpted from "Radio Frequency Identification (RFID)," U.S. Food and Drug Administration (FDA), September 17, 2018.

Radio frequency (RF) wireless medical devices perform at least one function that utilizes wireless RF communication such as Wi-Fi, Bluetooth, and cellular/mobile phone to support health-care delivery. Examples of functions that can utilize wireless technology include controlling and programming a medical device, monitoring patients remotely, or transferring patient data from the medical device to another platform such as a cell phone. As RF wireless technology continues to evolve, this technology will increasingly be incorporated into the design of medical devices.

Examples of areas that utilize RF wireless technology include:
- Wireless medical telemetry
- Radio frequency identification (RFID)

BENEFITS AND RISKS

Incorporation of wireless technology in medical devices can have many benefits, including increasing patient mobility by eliminating wires that tether a patient to a medical bed, providing health-care professionals the ability to remotely program devices, and providing the ability of physicians to remotely access and monitor patient data regardless of the location of the patient or physician (hospital, home, office, etc.). These benefits can greatly impact patient outcomes by allowing physicians access to real-time data on patients without the physician physically being in the hospital and allowing real-time adjustment of patient treatment. Remote monitoring can also help special populations such as seniors, through home monitoring of chronic diseases so that changes can be detected earlier before more serious consequences occur.

INFORMATION FOR PATIENTS

The use of RF wireless technology can translate to advances in healthcare, and patients should be informed about the safe and effective use of these devices in the course of daily life.

Because the airways are shared, the functioning of your wireless medical device may be affected (such as data loss or disruption) by other wireless devices near you. As with any medical device, if you have problems or questions, please consult the information provided by the manufacturer or contact your health-care provider.

INFORMATION FOR HEALTH-CARE FACILITIES: RISK MANAGEMENT

Most well-designed and maintained RF wireless medical devices perform adequately. However, the increasingly crowded RF environment and competition from nonmedical wireless technology users could impact the performance of RF wireless medical devices. The FDA recommends that health-care facilities develop appropriate processes and procedures to assess and manage risks associated with the integration of RF wireless technology into medical systems.

Health-care facilities should also consider the following:
- Selection of wireless technology
- Quality of service
- Coexistence
- Security
- Electromagnetic compatibility (EMC)

In addition, the FDA recommends that health-care facilities periodically consult the Federal Communications Commission (FCC) website (www.fcc.gov) for new specifications and updated information that may affect their wireless infrastructure.

RF WIRELESS COEXISTENCE CHALLENGES

All wireless technologies face challenges coexisting in the same space. For example, devices operating under FCC Part 15 rules must accept any interference from primary users of the frequency band. (**Note:** FCC Part 15 is applicable to certain types of low-power, nonlicensed radio transmitters and certain types of electronic equipment that emit RF energy unintentionally.)

WIRELESS MEDICAL TELEMETRY SYSTEMS

Wireless medical telemetry is generally used to monitor a patient's vital signs (e.g., pulse, and respiration) using radio frequency (RF) communication. These devices have the advantage of allowing patient movement without restricting patients to a bedside monitor with a hard-wired connection.

RADIO FREQUENCY IDENTIFICATION

Radio frequency identification (RFID) refers to a wireless system that comprises of two components: tags and readers. The reader is a device that has one or more antennas that emit radio waves and receive signals back from the RFID tag. Tags, which use radio waves to communicate their identity and other information to nearby readers, can be passive or active. Passive RFID tags are powered by the reader and do not have a battery. Active RFID tags are powered by batteries.

Radio frequency identification tags can store a range of information from one serial number to several pages of data. Readers can be mobile so that they can be carried by hand, or they can be mounted on a post or overhead. Reader systems can also be built into the architecture of a cabinet, room, or building.

USES OF RADIO FREQUENCY IDENTIFICATION

Radio frequency identification systems use radio waves at several different frequencies to transfer data. In healthcare and hospital settings, RFID technologies include the following applications:
- Inventory control
- Equipment tracking

- Out-of-bed detection and fall detection
- Personnel tracking
- Ensuring that patients receive the correct medications and medical devices
- Preventing the distribution of counterfeit drugs and medical devices
- Monitoring patients
- Providing data for electronic medical records systems

The FDA is not aware of any adverse events associated with RFID. However, there is concern about the potential hazard of electromagnetic interference (EMI) to electronic medical devices from radio frequency transmitters like RFID. EMI is a degradation of the performance of equipment or systems (such as medical devices) caused by an electromagnetic disturbance.

Section 9.4 | Wearables and Safety

This section contains text excerpted from the following sources: Text in this section begins with excerpts from "Wearable Technologies for Improved Safety and Health on Construction Sites," National Institute for Occupational Safety and Health (NIOSH), Centers for Disease Control and Prevention (CDC), November 18, 2019; Text beginning with the heading "Categorization of Wearables" is excerpted from "Safety Concerns Associated with Wearable Technology Products," U.S. Consumer Product Safety Commission (CPSC), April 1, 2020.

Wearable technologies are an increasingly popular consumer electronics for a variety of applications at home and at work. In general, these devices include accessories and clothing that incorporate advanced electronic technologies, often with smartphone or Internet of Things (IoT) connectivity. While wearables are increasingly being used to improve health and well-being by aiding in personal fitness, innovative applications for monitoring occupational safety and health risk factors are becoming more common. Many of these devices have reached the market while others are still in development. As more wearables become available, they have the potential to positively impact and alter the landscape of society and work.

CATEGORIZATION OF WEARABLES

Wearables categorized are by their functions, product types, and potential hazards. A specific function may be incorporated into various product types. Evaluating the function of wearables is the first step in identifying potential product hazards. The categorization scheme includes products for data collection and storage, communication and repulsion, monitoring and alerting performance enhancement, and neural stimulation.

Some products included in the following categorization scheme may be considered medical devices, and thus, are not under the CPSC's jurisdiction. It is noted that, to date, no products have been categorically excluded from the CPSC jurisdiction, and jurisdictional determinations must be made on a product-by-product basis, typically determined by a manufacturer's marketing claims, health risk associated with the product, and other factors.

Product Functions, Types, and Potential Hazards

All are aware of incidents and recalls associated with wearable technology. Several fitness trackers and smartwatches have been recalled due to skin irritation. Fitness trackers and wireless headphones have been recalled due to overheating batteries. Skin irritation and overheating batteries comprise the majority of known incidents with skin irritation being the most predominant. There have been a few incidents where sharp edges were reported on the smartwatch/fitness tracker bands.

To focus efforts on addressing the potential safety hazards to consumers, it is important for designers and manufacturers to understand the function and potential hazards associated with each type of wearable. Potential hazards associated with a wearable are influenced largely by where and how consumers wear or apply the product to the body, and the functions and the types of technologies manufacturers use to carry out the intended purpose of the product. The product-type categories organize products by their proximity and level of interaction with the body. These categories include accessories, articles, patches, imbeds, and inserts. In addition to categorizing wearable by product type, the potential hazards associated with the intended use of each type of product are identified. These hazards include chemical, electrical, and electro-magnetic field-light, radio frequency, sonic, thermal, and vibration.

ACCESSORIES

Consumers wear accessories on the body that are loosely attached and easily removed. Data collection is a primary function of most wearable accessories. Fitness trackers, for example, have become immensely popular for measuring fitness-related data, such as heart rate, distance traveled, and calories burned. Other examples of wearable accessories include alerting devices, such as wristbands that provide a warning when the user is exposed to potentially harmful levels of ultraviolet radiation (UV) from the sun. Consumers can typically transmit information from wearable accessories to a cellular phone, computer, or other data storage device. Wearable accessories may use nonionizing radiation, such as radio frequencies, which are less energetic than devices providing cellular phone transmission. Although the acute energy potentially transferred to the body from nonionizing radiation is typically relatively low, wearable accessories may be worn directly on the skin for extended periods of time.

Additionally, given the prolonged dermal exposure and typical uses, the materials in these products may leach during physical activity, as the user sweats and the product rubs against the user's skin, resulting in irritation, rashes, or allergic reactions. Also, there are concerns about the dermal uptake of compounds that may cause systemic toxicity, as well as the potential for electrical com-ponents to heat up and cause consumers mild discomfort or burns.

ARTICLES

A wearable article is any fabric, clothing, or textile that contains electronic technology and is worn on the body. Examples of arti-cles include coats, jackets, dresses, skirts, and pants. It is antici-pated that biomonitoring is one of the primary functions of these products. Similar to wearable accessories, many wearable articles collect information on physiologic functions, such as heart rate and neurologic activity.

Relative to accessories, articles commonly allow manufacturers a larger surface area for embedded sensors and sampling, affording these products higher measurement accuracy and increased variety of data measured. It is anticipated that the ability of articles to be more precise in measuring data may be of particular importance in athletics. For example, sensors can monitor and assess physical performance, in addition to protecting athletes, by providing a warning when an athlete exceeds an overexertion threshold.

The human skin is the largest organ in the body and provides protection to our internal organs. Light-emitting fabrics use light to enhance the "style" of a piece of clothing, and some manufacturers market light-emitting fabrics for therapeutic applications. Consumers wearing light-emitting fabrics may experience irritation or burns of the skin, if the light emitted is too intense for sensitive populations.

In general, there are concerns that irritation, thermal burns, and allergic reactions may occur with many materials, especially as the fibers begin to wear from friction and from being laundered. As the materials degrade, performance and impact on the skin may change, releasing chemicals or particles bound in the fiber matrix more easily, resulting in greater chemical exposure to the wearer.

PATCH

Wearable patches are applied directly to the skin, fingernails, or toenails permanently or semipermanently (such as "tattoos"), and incorporate electronic circuitry. A common use of patches is for identification purposes. For example, amusement parks may use semi-permanent patches for managing access to rides or areas. Other applications include health and fitness, including physiological monitoring or delivery of health supplements or drugs. In the past, some patches have delivered compounds to the body, such as nicotine; however, new "smart" patches can include biomonitoring. Patches are attached directly to the skin, and in some cases, they are intended to be attached for long-term use. Given these factors, the likelihood of exposure to any potentially harmful materials could be greater, compared to other wearable products.

IMBED

Consumers apply imbed wearables beneath their skin, such as subdermal radio frequency products for identification and entry. Although the term "imbed" is commonly used interchangeably with "insert," the two are distinguished, based on application of the device under the skin, versus into an existing body portal (e.g., oral placement). There are concerns that the subdermal placement of imbeds allows even greater exposure to chemicals, relative to products placed on the skin, due, in part, to long-term use and access to the bloodstream, where potentially harmful compounds can circulate to targets within the body for physiologic effects. Furthermore, the insertion and removal of an imbed may increase infection opportunities. There are also concerns that if imbeds contain batteries or another source of energy, the products could cause burns or other harm to surrounding tissue.

INSERT

Insert wearables are placed into existing body orifices, such as the ears or mouth. Consumers have used inserts for many years; hearing aids are one example. Even with this well-known insert, technological innovations have vastly improved hearing aid performance and enhanced their capabilities. Hearing aids are now being marketed to consumers without impaired hearing. For example, "augmented hearing" or "hearable" products allow users to enhance and control their sense of hearing, including blocking out user-determined background noise. There are also concerns that consumer exposure to sound, electric, electromagnetic, and chemical product properties may be hazardous when in contact with sensitive body areas or during the process of insertion or removal.

DATA SECURITY

Many wearables connect to the Internet, and, likely unbeknownst to users, can have the same vulnerabilities for data security as with other connected products. "Data Security," as used in an Internet of Things (IoT) product, concerns all of the data stored in, or moving in or out of a connected product, which could include those impacting the safety of the product. This includes:

- Operational instructions (software)
- Consumer-originated data (biometrics, settings and preferences, multiple-user identification)
- Environmental metrics (e.g., location, temperature, atmosphere, energy)
- Manufacturing/product data (e.g., serial numbers across products)

Section 9.5 | Remote Patient Monitoring

This section contains text excerpted from the following sources: Text in this section begins with excerpts from "MDPC Comments to FTC on Connectivity of Devices," Federal Trade Commission (FTC), June 1, 2013. Reviewed June 2021; Text beginning with the heading "Telehealth and Remote Patient Monitoring" is excerpted from "Securing Telehealth Remote Patient Monitoring Ecosystem," National Cybersecurity Center of Excellence (NCCoE), National Institute of Standards and Technology (NIST), November 2020.

Remote patient monitoring (RPM) technologies can be effective in managing chronic disease and postacute care. They can also be used to alert caregivers to situations requiring immediate attention. Many medical devices on the market today come with remote communication abilities embedded or available as optional attachments. For example, many implanted cardiac devices (pacemakers, cardioverter defibrillators, etc.) allow for data to be transmitted to the manufacturer and then made accessible to the patient's health-care provider through a web interface. Some devices passively collect this data before transmitting it to the manufacturer (e.g., a wireless peripheral in the patient's home automatically receives information from the device) while others require some action by the patient (e.g., holding a wand near the body to upload information from the implanted device to a peripheral). The data may then be transmitted over an analog phone line, Global System for Mobile Communications (GSM) network, or via an Internet service provider (ISP).

Some remote patient monitoring technologies can be connected to multiple peripheral devices (e.g., blood pressure cuff, scale, glucose monitor, pulse oximeter, pedometer, etc.). The connections between the communicator and the peripheral devices may be wired or wireless. Any number of wireless transmission protocols or technologies may be used (e.g., Bluetooth™, Zigbee™, WiFi™, WiMax™, RFID, etc.).

As indicated, typically a web interface enables the patient's health-care provider to view, print, and/or download information transmitted to the manufacturer from the remote patient monitoring technology. The health-care provider may be able to configure periodic reports to be automatically transmitted. In addition, acute events may trigger an alert to the health-care provider via e-mail, fax, text message, or phone. Patients may be able to access some or all of the data related to them via patient-directed websites.

Security of data generated or transmitted by remote patient monitoring technologies is a priority. Manufacturers' websites typically employ firewalls and encryption to protect patient data. Users must register and are provided, or prompted to create, access credentials (username, password, etc.). With respect to the medical devices themselves, security requirements based on the risks must be incorporated into device design. For devices that employ wireless communication, the wireless signal could be subject to interception of data, and there is the potential for external interference (intentional or otherwise) which could impact device performance. For manufacturers, these security risks must be managed while keeping in mind design limitations. For example, implanted medical devices may require emergency access modes that bypass a subset of security features.

The Medical Device Privacy Consortium (MDPC) launched a new working group on medical device product security. The MDPC's product security working group aims to advance industry dialogue and information sharing on how to protect medical devices from security threats and address related privacy concerns. The working group intends to monitor, analyze, and influence global standards and guidelines on medical device product security and develop practical tools that can be used to enhance product security. Further, the working group intends to liaise with other medical device industry stakeholders to gather and share intelligence regarding industry-wide efforts related to product security.

At the regulatory level, both the U.S. Food and Drug Administration (FDA) medical device regulations and regulations promulgated by the U.S. Department of Health and Human Services (HHS) Office for Civil Rights (OCR) under the Health Insurance Portability and Accountability Act (HIPAA) can be relevant to remote patient monitoring privacy and security. As part of the FDA's premarket approval (PMA) process for Class III medical devices, the FDA considers various risks, which can include information security risks. Recommendations concerning the FDA's consideration of information security risks were recently the subject of a report by the U.S. Government Accountability Office. When patches are necessary to update the software on a medical device in response to a security vulnerability, the patch must undergo a thorough assessment and testing before it can be released. As the FDA explains in its guidance for industry on software validation:

- When changes are made to a software system, either during initial development or during postrelease maintenance, sufficient regression analysis, and testing should be conducted to demonstrate that portions of the software not involved in the change were not adversely impacted. This is in addition to testing that evaluates the correctness of the implemented change(s).

- The specific validation effort necessary for each software change is determined by the type of change, the development products affected, and the impact of those products on the operation of the software. Careful and complete documentation of the design structure and interrelationships of various modules, interfaces, etc., can limit the validation effort needed when a change is made. The level of effort needed to fully validate a change is also dependent upon the degree to which validation of the original software was documented and archived.

In addition to validation of the patch itself, in limited circumstances (e.g., where the patch could make the device less safe or effective), changes to medical device software can require FDA clearance or approval. Because there is a complex regulatory structure already covering prescription medical devices, the MDPC believes that any further regulatory initiatives relating to such devices should be led by the FDA.

Remote patient monitoring services can trigger a HIPAA business associate relationship between the service provider and the covered health-care provider. Under changes to the HIPAA regulations that became effective in March 2013, HIPAA business associates must comply with the Security Rule and many provisions of the Privacy Rule in their performance of the covered function or service.

TELEHEALTH AND REMOTE PATIENT MONITORING

Telehealth RPM solutions enable patients with chronic or recurring conditions to receive continuous monitoring and treatment from care providers while in their homes. Telehealth remote patient monitoring, which integrates video conferencing and biometric data collection, allows health-care provider teams to obtain vital information from patients where in-person interactions may not be convenient or feasible.

CHALLENGES IN TELEHEALTH AND REMOTE PATIENT MONITORING

Health-care facilities commonly use patient monitoring systems to capture biometric data and enable clinicians to make informed decisions in delivering patient care. Telehealth remote patient monitoring extends that capability by deploying biometric devices to the patient home and allowing for longitudinal data capture for patients with recurring or chronic conditions. Deploying health-care equipment to a patient's home, however, carries privacy and cybersecurity risk. Patient home environments may not offer the same level of privacy, cybersecurity, or physical access controls as may be found in a clinical setting. As telehealth use increases, it is important to ensure the confidentiality, integrity, and availability of patient data in support of the care and safety of patients.

APPROACH TOWARDS TELEHEALTH AND REMOTE PATIENT MONITORING

This project demonstrates how an organization may implement a solution to enhance privacy and secure their telehealth RPM ecosystem. The reference architecture includes technical and process controls to implement:

- An RPM reference architecture
- Biometric data communication across three domains that consist of the patient home, telehealth platform providers, and the Health Delivery Organization (HDO)
- A risk assessment assuring the measures and outcomes that were determined from the risk assessment activity

BENEFITS OF TELEHEALTH AND REMOTE PATIENT MONITORING

The potential business benefits of enacting appropriate privacy and security controls to a Telehealth RPM ecosystem include:

- Assure the confidentiality, integrity, and availability of an RPM solution
- Enhance patient privacy
- Limit HDO risk when implementing an RPM solution

Section 9.6 | Continuous Glucose Monitoring

This section contains text excerpted from the following sources: Text beginning with the heading "What Is Continuous Glucose Monitoring?" is excerpted from "Continuous Glucose Monitoring," National Institute of Diabetes and Digestive and Kidney Diseases (NIDDK), June 2017. Reviewed June 2021; Text under the heading "Blood Glucose Monitoring Devices" is excerpted from "Blood Glucose Monitoring Devices," U.S. Food and Drug Administration (FDA), April 4, 2019; Text under the heading "The FDA Approval for Continuous Glucose Monitoring System" is excerpted from "FDA Approves First Continuous Glucose Monitoring System for Adults Not Requiring Blood Sample Calibration," U.S. Food and Drug Administration (FDA), March 23, 2018.

WHAT IS CONTINUOUS GLUCOSE MONITORING?

Continuous glucose monitoring (CGM) automatically tracks blood glucose levels, also called "blood sugar," throughout the day and

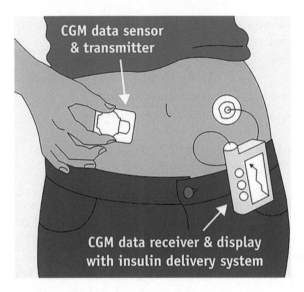

Figure 9.1. CGM Sensor

night. You can see your glucose level anytime at a glance. You can also review how your glucose changes over a few hours or days to see trends. Seeing glucose levels in real time can help you make more informed decisions throughout the day about how to balance your food, physical activity, and medicines.

HOW DOES A CONTINUOUS GLUCOSE MONITOR WORK?

A CGM works through a tiny sensor inserted under your skin, usually on your belly or arm. The sensor measures your interstitial glucose level, which is the glucose found in the fluid between the cells. The sensor tests glucose every few minutes. A transmitter wirelessly sends the information to a monitor.

The monitor may be part of an insulin pump or a separate device, which you might carry in a pocket or purse. Some CGMs send information directly to a smartphone or tablet.

SPECIAL FEATURES OF A CGM

Continuous glucose monitorings are always on and recording glucose levels – whether you are showering, working, exercising, or sleeping. Many CGMs have special features that work with information from your glucose readings:

- An alarm can sound when your glucose level goes too low or too high.
- You can note your meals, physical activity, and medicines in a CGM device, too, alongside your glucose levels.
- You can download data to a computer or smart device to more easily see your glucose trends.

Some models can send information right away to a second person's smartphone – perhaps a parent, partner, or caregiver. For example, if a child's glucose drops dangerously low overnight, the CGM could be set to wake a parent in the next room.

A CGM model is approved for treatment decisions, the Dexcom G5 Mobile. That means you can make changes to your diabetes care plan based on CGM results alone. With other models, you must first confirm a CGM reading with a finger-stick blood glucose test before you take insulin or treat hypoglycemia.

SPECIAL REQUIREMENTS NEEDED TO USE A CGM

Twice a day, you may need to check the CGM itself. You will test a drop of blood on a standard glucose meter. The glucose reading should be similar on both devices.

You will also need to replace the CGM sensor every 3 to 7 days, depending on the model.

For safety, it is important to take action when a CGM alarm sounds about high or low blood glucose. You should follow your treatment plan to bring your glucose into the target range, or get help.

WHO CAN USE A CGM?

Most people who use CGMs have type 1 diabetes. Research is underway to learn how CGMs might help people with type 2 diabetes.

CGMs are approved for use by adults and children with a doctor's prescription. Some models may be used for children as young

as 2 years of age. Your doctor may recommend a CGM if you or your child:
- Are on intensive insulin therapy, also called "tight blood sugar control"
- Have hypoglycemia unawareness
- Often have high or low blood glucose

Your doctor may suggest using a CGM system all the time or only for a few days to help adjust your diabetes care plan.

WHAT ARE THE BENEFITS OF A CGM?

Compared with a standard blood glucose meter, using a CGM system can help you:
- Better manage your glucose levels every day
- Have fewer low blood glucose emergencies
- Need fewer finger sticks

A graphic on the CGM screen shows whether your glucose is rising or dropping – and how quickly – so you can choose the best way to reach your target glucose level.

Over time, good management of glucose greatly helps people with diabetes stay healthy and prevent complications of the disease. People who gain the largest benefit from a CGM are those who use it every day or nearly every day.

WHAT ARE THE LIMITS OF A CGM?

Researchers are working to make CGMs more accurate and easier to use. But, you still need a finger-stick glucose test twice a day to check the accuracy of your CGM against a standard blood glucose meter.

With most CGM models, you cannot yet rely on the CGM alone to make treatment decisions. For example, before changing your insulin dose, you must first confirm a CGM reading by doing a finger-stick glucose test.

A CGM system is more expensive than using a standard glucose meter. Check with your health insurance plan or Medicare NIH to see whether the costs will be covered.

WHAT IS AN ARTIFICIAL PANCREAS?

A CGM is one part of the "artificial pancreas" systems that are beginning to reach people with diabetes.

The National Institute of Diabetes and Digestive and Kidney Diseases (NIDDK) has played an important role in developing artificial pancreas technology. An artificial pancreas replaces manual blood glucose testing and the use of insulin shots. A single system monitors blood glucose levels around the clock and provides insulin or both insulin and a second hormone, glucagon, automatically. The system can also be monitored remotely, for example, by parents or medical staff.

In 2016, the U.S. Food and Drug Administration (FDA) approved a type of artificial pancreas system called a "hybrid closed-loop system." This system tests your glucose level every five minutes throughout the day and night through a CGM, and automatically gives you the right amount of basal insulin, long-acting insulin, through a separate insulin pump. You will still need to test your blood with a glucose meter a few times a day. And you will manually adjust the amount of insulin the pump delivers at mealtimes and when you need a correction dose.

The hybrid closed-loop system may free you from some of the daily tasks needed to keep your blood glucose stable – or help you sleep through the night without the need to wake and test your glucose or take medicine. Talk with your health-care provider about whether this system might be right for you.

BLOOD GLUCOSE MONITORING DEVICES
What Is Glucose?

Glucose is a sugar that your body uses as a source of energy. Unless you have diabetes, your body regulates the amount of glucose in your blood. People with diabetes may need special diets and medications to control blood glucose.

What Does This Test Do?

This is a test system for use at home or in health-care settings to measure the amount of sugar (glucose) in your blood.

What Type of Test Is This?

This is a quantitative test, which means that you will find out the amount of glucose present in your blood sample.

Why Should You Take This Test?

You should take this test if you have diabetes and you need to monitor your blood sugar (glucose) levels. You and your doctor can use the results to:

- Determine your daily adjustments in treatment.
- Know if you have dangerously high or low levels of glucose.
- Understand how your diet and exercise change your glucose levels.

The Diabetes Control and Complications Trial (1993) showed that good glucose control using home monitors led to fewer disease complications.

How Often Should You Test Your Glucose?

Follow your doctor's recommendations about how often you test your glucose. You may need to test yourself several times each day to determine adjustments in your diet or treatment.

What Should Your Glucose Levels Be?

According to the American Diabetes Association, the blood glucose levels for an adult without diabetes are below 100 mg/dL before meals and fasting and are less than 140 mg/dL two hours after meals.

People with diabetes should consult their doctor or health-care provider to set appropriate blood glucose goals. You should treat your low or high blood glucose as recommended by your health-care provider.

How Accurate Is This Test?

The accuracy of this test depends on many factors including:

- The quality of your meter
- The quality of your test strips
  - Always use new test strips that are authorized for sale in the United States. The FDA has issued a safety communication warning about the risks of using previously owned test strips or test strips that are not authorized for sale in the United States.
- How well you perform the test. For example, you should wash and dry your hands before testing and closely follow the instructions for operating your meter.
- Your hematocrit (the amount of red blood cells in the blood). If you are severely dehydrated or anemic, your test results may be less accurate. Your health-care provider can tell you if your hematocrit is low or high, and can discuss with you how it may affect your glucose testing.
- Interfering substances. (Some substances, such as Vitamin C, Tylenol, and uric acid, may interfere with your glucose testing.) Check the instructions for your meter and test strips to find out what substances may affect the testing accuracy.
- Altitude, temperature, and humidity. (High altitude, low and high temperatures, and humidity can cause unpredictable effects on glucose results.) Check the meter manual and test strip package insert for more information.
- Store and handle the meter and strips according to manufacturer's instructions. It is important to store test strip vials closed.

How Do You Take This Test?

Before you test your blood glucose, you must read and understand the instructions for your meter. In general, you prick your finger with a lancet to get a drop of blood. Then you place the blood on a disposable "test strip" that is inserted into your meter. The test strip contains chemicals that react with glucose. Some meters measure the amount of electricity that passes through the test strip. Others measure how much light reflects from it. In the U.S., meters report results in milligrams of glucose per deciliter of blood, or mg/dl.

You can get information about your meter and test strips from several different sources, including the toll-free number in the manual that comes with your meter or on the manufacturer's website. If you have an urgent problem, always contact your health-care provider or a local emergency room for advice.

How Do You Choose a Glucose Meter?

There are many different types of meters available for purchase that differ in several ways, including:
- Accuracy
- Amount of blood needed for each test
- How easy it is to use
- Pain associated with using the product
- Testing speed
- Overall size
- Ability to store test results in memory
- Likelihood of interferences
- Ability to transmit data to a computer
- Cost of the meter
- Cost of the test strips used
- Doctor's recommendation
- Technical support provided by the manufacturer
- Special features such as automatic timing, error codes, large display screen, or spoken instructions or results

Talk to your health-care provider about the right glucose meter for you, and how to use it.

How can you check your meter's performance? There are three ways to make sure your meter works properly:
1. Use liquid control solutions:
   - Every time you open a new container of test strips
   - Occasionally as you use the container of test strips
   - If you drop the meter
   - Whenever you get unusual results

- To test a liquid control solution, you test a drop of these solutions just like you test a drop of your blood. The value you get should match the value written on the test strip vial label.

2. Use electronic checks. Every time you turn on your meter, it does an electronic check. If it detects a problem it will give you an error code. Look in your meter's manual to see what the error codes mean and how to fix the problem. If you are unsure if your meter is working properly, call the toll-free number in your meter's manual, or contact your health-care provider.

3. Compare your meter with a blood glucose test performed in a laboratory. Take your meter with you to your next appointment with your health-care provider. Ask your provider to watch your testing technique to make sure you are using the meter correctly. Ask your health-care provider to have your blood tested with a laboratory method. If the values you obtain on your glucose meter match the laboratory values, then your meter is working well and you are using good technique.

What Should You Do If Your Meter Malfunctions?

If your meter malfunctions, you should tell your health-care provider and contact the company that made your meter and strips.

Can You Test Blood Glucose from Sites Other than Your Fingers?

Some meters allow you to test blood from sites other than the fingertip. Examples of such alternative sampling sites are your palm, upper arm, forearm, thigh, or calf. Alternative site testing (AST) should not be performed at times when your blood glucose may be changing rapidly, as these alternative sampling sites may provide inaccurate results at those times. You should use only blood from your fingertip to test if any of the following applies:

- You have just taken insulin
- You think your blood sugar is low

- You are not aware of symptoms when you become hypoglycemic
- The results do not agree with the way you feel
- You have just eaten
- You have just exercised
- You are ill
- You are under stress

Also, you should never use results from an alternative sampling site to calibrate a continuous glucose monitor (CGM), or in insulin dosing calculations.

THE FDA APPROVAL FOR CONTINUOUS GLUCOSE MONITORING SYSTEM

The U.S. Food and Drug Administration (FDA) on September 27, 2017, approved the FreeStyle Libre Flash Glucose Monitoring System, the first continuous glucose monitoring system that can be used by adult patients to make diabetes treatment decisions without calibration using a blood sample from the fingertip (often referred to as a "fingerstick").

The system reduces the need for fingerstick testing by using a small sensor wire inserted below the skin's surface that continuously measures and monitors glucose levels. Users can determine glucose levels by waving a dedicated, mobile reader above the sensor wire to determine if glucose levels are too high (hyperglycemia) or too low (hypoglycemia), and how glucose levels are changing. It is intended for use in people 18 years of age and older with diabetes; after a 12-hour start-up period, it can be worn for up to 10 days.

"The FDA is always interested in new technologies that can help make the care of people living with chronic conditions, such as diabetes, easier and more manageable," said Donald St. Pierre, acting director of the Office of In Vitro Diagnostics and Radiological Health and deputy director of new product evaluation in the FDA's Center for Devices and Radiological Health. "This system allows people with diabetes to avoid the additional step of fingerstick calibration, which can sometimes be painful, but still provides necessary information for treating their diabetes – with a wave of the mobile reader."

People with diabetes must regularly test and monitor their blood sugar to make sure it is at an appropriate level, which is often done multiple times per day by taking a fingerstick sample and testing it with a blood glucose meter. Typically patients use results of a traditional fingerstick test to make diabetes treatment decisions; however, fingerstick testing is not needed to inform appropriate care choices or to calibrate glucose levels with this system.

According to the Centers for Disease Control and Prevention (CDC), more than 29 million people in the U.S. have diabetes. People with diabetes either do not make enough insulin (type 1 diabetes) or cannot use insulin properly (type 2 diabetes). When the body does not have enough insulin or cannot use it effectively, sugar builds up in the blood. High blood sugar levels can lead to heart disease; stroke; blindness; kidney failure; and amputation of toes, feet, or legs.

The FDA evaluated data from a clinical study of individuals 18 years of age and older with diabetes and reviewed the device's performance by comparing readings obtained by the FreeStyle Libre Glucose Monitoring System to those obtained by an established laboratory method used for analysis of blood glucose.

Risks associated with use of the system may include hypoglycemia or hyperglycemia in cases where information provided by the device is inaccurate and used to make treatment decisions, as well as mild skin irritations around the insertion site. It does not provide real-time alerts or alarms in the absence of a user-initiated action; for example, it cannot alert users to low blood glucose levels while they are asleep.

The FreeStyle Libre Flash Glucose Monitoring System is manufactured by Abbott Diabetes Care Inc.

The FDA, an agency within the U.S. Department of Health and Human Services (HHS), promotes and protects public health by, among other things, assuring the safety, effectiveness, and security of human and veterinary drugs, vaccines, and other biological products for human use, and medical devices. The agency also is responsible for the safety and security of our nation's food supply, cosmetics, dietary supplements, products that give off electronic radiation, and for regulating tobacco products.

Section 9.7 | **Mobile Medical Applications**

This section contains text excerpted from the following sources: Text in this section begins with excerpts from "Device Software Functions including Mobile Medical Applications," U.S. Food and Drug Administration (FDA), November 5, 2019; Text under the heading "Examples of Mobile Apps That Are Not Medical Devices" is excerpted from "Examples of Mobile Apps That Are Not Medical Devices," U.S. Food and Drug Administration (FDA), July 24, 2018.

The widespread adoption and use of software technologies is opening new and innovative ways to improve health and health-care delivery.

Software functions that meet the definition of a device may be deployed on mobile platforms, other general-purpose computing platforms, or in the function or control of a hardware device. The FDA's policies are independent of the platform on which they might run, are function-specific, and apply across platforms. The term "software functions" includes mobile applications (apps).

Mobile apps can help people manage their own health and wellness, promote healthy living, and gain access to useful information when and where they need it. These tools are being adopted almost as quickly as they can be developed. According to industry estimates in 2017, 325,000 health-care applications were available on smartphones, which equates to an expected 3.7 billion mobile health application downloads that year by smartphone users worldwide. Users include health-care professionals, consumers, and patients.

The FDA encourages the development of mobile medical apps (MMAs) that improve healthcare and provide consumers and health-care professionals with valuable health information. The FDA also has a public-health responsibility to oversee the safety and effectiveness of medical devices – including mobile medical apps.

The Policy for Device Software Functions and Mobile Medical Applications Guidance (www.fda.gov/regulatory-information/search-fda-guidance-documents/policy-device-software-functions-and-mobile-medical-applications), first issued in 2013 as "Mobile Medical Applications" (MMA guidance) and updated in 2015 and 2019, explains the agency's oversight of device software functions, including mobile medical apps, as devices and our focus only on the software that presents a greater risk to patients if it does not work as intended and on software that causes smartphones, computers, or other mobile platforms to impact the functionality or performance of traditional medical devices. In 2019, the FDA updated the guidance to reflect changes to the device definition in accordance with Section 3060 of the 21st Century Cures Act, which created a function-specific definition for device. The functions excluded from the device definition are independent of the platform on which they might run.

WHAT ARE MOBILE MEDICAL APPS?

Mobile apps are software programs that run on smartphones and other mobile communication devices. They can also be accessories that attach to a smartphone or other mobile communication devices or a combination of accessories and software.

Mobile medical apps are medical devices that are mobile apps, meet the definition of a medical device, and are an accessory to a regulated medical device or transform a mobile platform into a regulated medical device.

Consumers can use both mobile medical apps and mobile apps to manage their own health and wellness, such as to monitor their caloric intake for healthy weight maintenance. For example, the National Institutes of Health's LactMed app provides nursing mothers with information about the effects of medicines on breast milk and nursing infants.

Other apps aim to help health-care professionals improve and facilitate patient care. The Radiation Emergency Medical Management (REMM) app gives health-care providers guidance on diagnosing and treating radiation injuries. Some mobile medical apps can diagnose cancer or heart rhythm abnormalities, or function as the "central command" for a glucose meter used by an insulin-dependent diabetic patient.

HOW DOES THE FDA REGULATE DEVICE SOFTWARE FUNCTIONS?

The FDA applies the same risk-based approach to device software functions as the agency uses to assure safety and effectiveness for other medical devices. The guidance document provides examples of how the FDA might regulate certain moderate-risk (Class II) and high-risk (Class III) device software functions. The guidance also provides examples of software functions that:

- Are not medical devices
- Are medical devices, but for which the FDA intends to exercise enforcement discretion
- Are medical devices and are the focus of FDA oversight

DEVICE SOFTWARE FUNCTIONS THAT ARE THE FOCUS OF THE FDA OVERSIGHT

The FDA is taking a tailored, risk-based approach that focuses on the subset of software functions that meet the regulatory definition of "device." Software functions span a wide range of health functions. While some software carries minimal risk, those that can pose a greater risk to patients will require the FDA review.

SOFTWARE FUNCTIONS FOR WHICH THE FDA INTENDS TO EXERCISE ENFORCEMENT DISCRETION

For many software functions that meet the regulatory definition of a "device" but pose minimal risk to patients and consumers, the FDA will exercise enforcement discretion and will not expect manufacturers to submit premarket review applications or to register and list their software with the FDA. This includes device software functions that:

- Help patients/users self-manage their disease or condition without providing specific treatment suggestions; or
- Automate simple tasks for health-care providers.

DOES THE FDA REGULATE MOBILE DEVICES, SUCH AS SMARTPHONES OR TABLETS, AND MOBILE APP STORES?

The FDA's mobile medical apps policy does not regulate the sale or general consumer use of smartphones or tablets. The FDA's mobile medical apps policy does not consider entities that exclusively distribute mobile apps, such as the owners and operators of the "iTunes App Store" or the "Google Play Store," to be medical device manufacturers. The FDA's mobile medical apps policy does not consider mobile platform manufacturers to be medical device manufacturers just because their mobile platform could be used to run a mobile medical app regulated by the FDA.

EXAMPLES OF MOBILE APPS THAT ARE NOT MEDICAL DEVICES

This list provides examples of mobile app functionalities to illustrate the types of mobile apps that could be used in a health-care environment, in clinical care, or patient management, but are not considered medical devices. Because these mobile apps are not considered medical devices, the FDA does not regulate them. The FDA understands that there may be other unique and innovative mobile apps that may not be covered in this list that may also constitute health-care related mobile apps. This list is not exhaustive; it is only intended to provide clarity and assistance in identifying when a mobile app is not considered to be a medical device.

Appendix A in the guidance includes examples of mobile app functionalities not considered medical devices at the time the guidance was finalized.

- Mobile apps that are intended to provide access to electronic "copies" (e.g., e-books, audio books) of medical textbooks or other reference materials with generic text search capabilities. Examples include mobile apps that are:
  - Medical dictionaries
  - Electronic copies of medical textbooks or literature articles such as the Physician's Desk Reference or *Diagnostic and Statistical Manual of Mental Disorders* (*DSM*)
  - Library of clinical descriptions for diseases and conditions
  - Encyclopedia of first-aid or emergency care information
  - Medical abbreviations and definitions
  - Translations of medical terms across multiple languages

- Mobile apps that are intended for health-care providers to use as educational tools for medical training or to reinforce training previously received. These may have more functionality than providing an electronic copy of text (e.g., videos, interactive diagrams). Examples include mobile apps that are:
  - Medical flash cards with medical images, pictures, graphs, etc.
  - Question/Answer quiz apps
  - Interactive anatomy diagrams or videos
  - Surgical training videos
  - Medical board certification or recertification preparation apps
  - Games that simulate various cardiac arrest scenarios to train health professionals in advanced CPR skills
  - Digital education tools, quizzes, games, and questionnaires that help engage patients to actively participate in their general health and wellness (calorie consumption, benefits of physical activity)
- Mobile apps that are intended for general patient education and facilitate patient access to commonly used reference information. These apps can be patient-specific (i.e., filters information to patient-specific characteristics), but are intended for increased patient awareness, education, and empowerment, and ultimately support patient-centered healthcare. Examples include mobile apps that:
  - Provide a portal for health-care providers to distribute educational information (e.g., interactive diagrams, useful links and resources) to their patients regarding their disease, condition, treatment or up-coming procedure
  - Help guide patients to ask appropriate questions to their physician relevant to their particular disease, condition, or concern
  - Provide information about gluten-free food products or restaurants

- Help match patients with potentially appropriate clinical trials and facilitate communication between the patient and clinical trial investigators
- Provide tutorials or training videos on how to administer first-aid or CPR
- Allow users to input pill shape, color or imprint and displays pictures and names of pills that match this description
- Find the closest medical facilities and doctors to the user's location
- Provide lists of emergency hotlines and physician/nurse advice lines
- Provide and compare costs of drugs and medical products at pharmacies in the user's location
- Provide access to education materials using digital media to help patients cope with stress
- Mobile apps that automate general office operations in a health-care setting. Examples include mobile apps that:
  - Determine billing codes such as ICD-9 (international statistical classification of diseases)
  - Enable insurance claims data collection and processing and other apps that are similarly administrative in nature
  - Analyze insurance claims for fraud or abuse
  - Perform medical business accounting functions or track and trend billable hours and procedures
  - Generate reminders for scheduled medical appointments or blood donation appointments
  - Help patients track, review and pay medical claims and bills online
  - Manage shifts for doctors
  - Manage or schedule hospital rooms or bed spaces
  - Provide wait times and electronic check-in for hospital emergency rooms and urgent care facilities
  - Allow health-care providers or staff in health-care setting to process payments (e.g., a HIPAA compliant app)

- Track or perform patient satisfaction survey after an encounter or a clinical visit
- Mobile apps that are generic aids or general purpose products. Examples include mobile apps that:
  - Use the mobile platform as a magnifying glass (but are not specifically intended for medical purposes[1])
  - Use the mobile platform for recording audio, note-taking, replaying audio with amplification, or other similar functionalities
  - Allow patients or health-care providers to interact through e-mail, web-based platforms, video or other communication mechanisms (but are not specifically intended for medical purposes)
  - Provide maps and turn-by-turn directions to medical facilities
  - Allow health-care providers to communicate in a secure and protected method (e.g., HIPAA compliant)
  - Use the mobile platform to translate unintelligible speech for better clarity

Note: These apps are not considered devices because they are not intended for use in the diagnosis of disease or other conditions, or in the cure, mitigation, treatment, or prevention of disease.

[1] *Medical purpose magnifiers are regulated either under 21 CFR 886.5840 – Magnifying spectacles ("devices that consist of spectacle frames with convex lenses intended to be worn by a patient who has impaired vision to enlarge images"), or under 21 CFR 886.5540 – Low-vision magnifiers ("a device that consists of a magnifying lens intended for use by a patient who has impaired vision. The device may be held in the hand or attached to spectacles").*

Chapter 10 | Medical Device Data Systems

Medical device data systems (MDDS) are hardware or software products intended to transfer, store, convert formats, and display medical device data. An MDDS does not modify the data or modify the display of the data, and it does not by itself control the functions or parameters of any other medical device. MDDS may or may not be intended for active patient monitoring.

Per section 520(o)(1)(D) of the U.S. Federal Food, Drug, and Cosmetic Act (FD&C Act):

- Software functions that are solely intended to transfer, store, convert formats, and display medical device data or medical imaging data, are not devices and are not subject to the U.S. Food and Drug Administration (FDA) regulatory requirements applicable to devices. The FDA describes these software functions as "nondevice-MDDS."
- Hardware functions that are solely intended to transfer, store, convert formats, and display medical device data or results are "device-MDDS."

Examples of nondevice-MDDS include software functions that:
- Store patient data, such as blood pressure readings, for review at a later time

This chapter contains text excerpted from the following sources: Text in this chapter begins with excerpts from "Medical Device Data Systems," U.S. Food and Drug Administration (FDA), September 26, 2019; Text under the heading "Medical Device Data Systems" is excerpted from "Medical Device Data Systems, Medical Image Storage Devices, and Medical Image Communications Devices," U.S. Food and Drug Administration (FDA), September 26, 2019.

- Convert digital data generated by a pulse oximeter into a format that can be printed
- Display a previously stored electrocardiogram for a particular patient

MEDICAL DEVICE DATA SYSTEMS AND THE FDA

The FDA recognizes that the progression to digital health offers the potential for better, more efficient patient care and improved health outcomes. To achieve this goal requires that many medical devices be interoperable with other types of medical devices and with various types of health information technology. The foundation for such inter-communication is hardware and software, typically referred to as "medical device data systems" (MDDS) that transfer, store, convert formats, and display medical device data or medical imaging data.

On February 15, 2011, the FDA issued a regulation down-classifying MDDS from Class III (high-risk) to Class I (low-risk) ("MDDS regulation"). Since down-classifying MDDS, the FDA has gained additional experience with these types of technologies and has determined that these devices pose a low risk to the public. On February 9, 2015, the FDA issued a guidance document to inform manufacturers, distributors, and other entities that the Agency does not intend to enforce compliance with the regulatory controls that apply to MDDS, medical image storage devices, and medical image communications devices, due to the low risk they pose to patients and the importance they play in advancing digital health.

Since the issuance of the guidance document in 2015 (www.fda. gov/media/88572/download), section 3060(a) of the 21st Century Cures Act (Cures Act) amended section 520 of the FD&C Act on December 13, 2016, removing certain software functions from the definition of device in section 201(h) of the FD&C Act. Pursuant to section 520(o)(1)(D) of the FD&C Act, software functions that are solely intended to transfer, store, convert formats, and display medical device data or medical imaging data, unless the software function is intended to interpret or analyze clinical laboratory test or other device data, results, and findings, are not devices and are not subject to the FDA laws and regulations applicable to devices.

The definition of MDDS in 21 CFR 880.6310 is currently inconsistent with the definition of device as amended pursuant to the Cures Act. The FDA intends to amend the regulation to be consistent with the amended device definition. The FDA's current thinking on the definition of MDDS is reflected in this guidance.

Hardware products that are intended to transfer, store, convert formats, and display medical device data and results remain devices under section 201(h) of the FD&C Act. The FDA does not intend to enforce compliance with the regulatory controls for such devices, provided that the hardware function is limited to assisting the following software functions: electronic transfer, storage, conversion of formats, or display of medical device data.

Chapter 11 | Medical Device Interoperability

In February 2019, the Networking and Information Technology Research and Development (NITRD) Program's Health Information Technology Research and Development Interagency Working Group (HITRD IWG) issued a request for information (RFI) to collect input from industry, academia, and nongovernmental organizations on new approaches to solve the interoperability issues between medical devices, data, and platforms. On July 17, 2019, the group followed up with an in-person Listening Session that included 76 representatives from the device, standards, academic, and medical communities, and the government.

Both the RFI and the Listening Session were focused on the interoperability of medical and consumer health devices, applications, and platforms, including the ability to submit data to the electronic health record (EHR). The challenge is that devices, applications, and platforms can deliver more real-time data than the current EHR environment can technically support. This is an important issue because patient-centric device interoperability is necessary to enable a new generation of applications, safety interlocks, closed-loop device control, and other innovative patient-care solutions.

EXCHANGE AND SEMANTICS OF DATA AND METADATA

To enable the reliable and usable exchange of data and metadata, information-sharing networks require the consistent use

This chapter includes text excerpted from "The Interoperability of Medical Devices, Data, and Platforms to Enhance Patient Care," Networking and Information Technology Research and Development (NITRD), March 2020.

111

of standards (e.g., for semantics) and a common set of rules for exchange. Needs for below factors are emphasized:

- An ontological framework to allow for all relevant data to be interoperable or at least for users to understand safety implications. Current terminologies are diverse, ambiguous, ill defined, and lacking such a framework.
- A common understanding of the data represented for stakeholders and data users. Semantic standardization is necessary but often lacks the necessary detail (e.g., Is the blood glucose value taken when fasting or at various times during the day?).
- Metadata that describes measurement context and patient variables (e.g., the signal averaging time, body site, patient position, environmental conditions, concomitant technical alarms, and how often data are transmitted from the device) to create and implement advanced analytics typically achieved by a co-located expert clinician. Interaction between medical devices in real time and with EHR data is severely limited by the absence of device metadata.
- A standardized device interface for all devices that are deemed interoperable. Data that is traditionally displayed to a medical device operator should go through a standardized device interface so as not to disrupt intellectual property. Such a system will require versatility and integration of nonmedical device data. Alternatively, the community could consider other approaches (e.g., the DataStream model) to provide prespecified, interoperable data necessary for use in new systems, without giving users additional access to all the device or system data being generated.
- Interoperability that occurs across the entire data lifecycle both in and across different settings, such as: within a clinic or hospital, between remote monitoring products, outpatient and emergency-care devices, and medical equipment management and maintenance.

112

- Clear definitions of who owns the data (e.g., device manufacturer, health-care provider, patient) versus who can access the data for purposes of interoperability.
- Methods to support the middleware required for interoperability. This could include licensing and subscriptions if a clear commercial benefit does not otherwise exist.
- A community forum for stakeholders to define use cases, models, and verification activities, and to enable improvements through problem sharing.
- Benchmarks should be developed to establish ground truth for interoperability.

ACCESS TO CONTROL OF DEVICES

There is value in the automation of health-care processes to enhance patient care and safety. The advantages of closed-loop systems (i.e., where machines interact and control functions in an automated system) and medical devices that exchange information (e.g., to stabilize a patient without human intervention)require functional medical device interoperability. Currently, this level of closed-loop control is only available as a vertically integrated solution from a single manufacturer. The need for below factors are emphasized:

- A clearance pipeline for interoperable devices, such as the FDA 510K certification. This pipeline could have separate streams for hardware, software, and updates.
- Postlaunch maintenance of interoperability and identification and management of emergent behaviors are needed to identify undesirable consequences and establish mechanisms to provide feedback.
- Policy and protocols to support safety investigations (as in other industries) that span regulatory agencies.
- Access and control of both pre- and post-market data to protect manufacturers' intellectual property but also to ensure data are not reverse engineered by competitors to identify proprietary information.

- A legal construct for information sharing to support safety, security, and reliability. For example, if a patient is injured while a set of interoperable devices is being used to support their care, robust systems will be needed to perform root-cause analysis. There is a lack of clarity on the distribution of responsibilities when groups of interoperable devices are incorporated into broader IT systems.
- Platforms to provide supporting functionality to enable application development without recreating the sensor/actuator infrastructure. This can promote innovation by enabling the evaluation of new technologies and decreasing time to market.

INCENTIVES

The current business models of medical device manufacturers and EHR vendors lack enough incentives to drive interoperable or semi-interoperable solutions. In fact, many stakeholders see open communication between devices as a threat to their market share. The use of government incentive programs, such as the 2009 Health Information Technology for Economic and Clinical Health Act were mentioned. An incentive strategy should consider:

- Learning from business models and standards adopted by other industries that have achieved interoperability. For example, before cell phone service became interoperable, network providers had to move between service zones.
- Educating stakeholders about the benefits of data interoperability to improve care for patients and reduce costs for insurers and purchasers of insurance.
- Adopting a flexible approach that encourages the adoption of data field and format standards, such as Fast Healthcare Interoperability Resources, while avoiding strict mandates that fail to keep pace with innovation.
- Adding value to industry stakeholders, such as a reduced timeframe for premarket approval and clearance.

- Highlighting examples and opportunities for different approaches by creating platforms, such as Challenge. gov (www.challenge.gov).
- Supporting innovative business models, such as tying adoption of interoperability standards to reimbursement and/or linking interoperable equipment to value-based care.
- Increasing innovation in small businesses by reducing perceived regulatory burden for clearance and supporting nontraditional funding approaches (Small Business Innovation Research, collaboration with another similar system).
- Coordinating standards across government agencies, including those who deliver healthcare.
- Leveraging "patent pools" like those the communications and information technology industries used to achieve interoperability.

MANAGEMENT AND MODERNIZATION OF STANDARDS

There was general agreement that data must be available where and when it is needed, in a reusable format that supports accurate identification of the device and patient. Current standards are either incomplete in their coverage of the total product lifecycle or they conflict with each other. Ways on how to develop interoperable system standards, and how manufacturers will readily adopt included:

- Establishing a common core of standards that allow proprietary improvements and are enforceable
- Solving questions of coverage, coordination, and harmonization
- Ensuring the privacy and security of patient information shared over devices complies with Health Insurance Portability and Accountability Act of 1996 regulations and other laws (federal, state, and local)
- Developing usable guidance and tools to support interoperability standards
- Disclosing standards to drive business including incentives for those who participate in standards development

- Setting new standards for control loop algorithms
- Creating an accelerator for adoption of standards (e.g., the DaVinci Project) to drive interoperability
- Establishing standards for compliant interface and data formats, communication, metadata common core, and for safety with a focus on error reduction
- Considering payment for those who participate in developing the standards
- Ensuring standards are readily updatable and are acceptable across relevant sectors
- Eliminating interference between medical devices and consumer devices
- Making clear standards and certifications available to buyers at each phase

INFRASTRUCTURE, TOOLS, PLATFORMS, TESTBEDS, AND USE CASES

Improved infrastructure and tools will enhance the development of interoperability of medical devices and their governance. These include reference architectures and open platforms, use cases, testbeds, test procedures, and implementation guides. Implementation guides are essential for users to understand system requirements and identify hazardous situations, and they should be complemented by robust test capabilities and procedures. For example, the provider-payer interoperability industry uses implementation guides to connect EHRs and billing management systems. Once created, implementation guides can greatly reduce the time and effort of implementing individual interoperability activities. However, creating these guides is a time-consuming process; they must be developed, tested, and then formalized by a respected governance and standards body.

Real-life, end-to-end use cases are also necessary to allow the interoperability ecosystem to identify gaps prior to full implementation, evaluate the developed processes and standards, and pilot new areas. Standards developers and promoters must start with, and continually work from, compelling, real-life use cases that reflect the needs, concerns, and constraints of potential standards adopters and allow stakeholders to get a clear sense of the direct benefits (e.g., for clinical care, business, or clinical research).

CATALYST FOR INTEROPERABILITY

Even though medical device interoperability has been a focus of government and industry for the past decade, it seems that little progress has been made. RFI and Listening Session participants noted that catalysts are needed to drive the advancement and adoption of interoperable systems. These catalysts must highlight the safety and cost benefits of better measurements, avoidable errors, and enhanced security and privacy. Potential catalysts include:

- Leveraging current health-care system concerns, such as clinician burnout, efforts to contain health-care costs, consumer health technology used outside the health-care system, low productivity, and high capital and operating costs.
- Engaging patient safety organizations to support interoperability standards.
- Teaming with Medicare and top health-care providers (e.g., both government and for-profit providers) to be early adopters.
- Presenting interoperability as the path forward for data privacy in the 21st century.
- Educating the public (including lawmakers) on the socioeconomic benefits of medical device interoperability.

Finally, future medical devices, data, and platforms, which include standards for interoperability, cybersecurity, and control, will support semiautonomous and fully autonomous medical care systems that improve patient safety and quality of care. To realize this vision of device interoperability requires an open, extensible architecture as a conceptual framework for innovation, supported by implementation guides, data and metadata standards, and test suites for conformance and compliance testing.

Chapter 12 | **Clinical Decision Support**

WHAT IS CLINICAL DECISION SUPPORT?

Clinical decision support (CDS) provides clinicians, staff, patients, or other individuals with knowledge and person-specific information, intelligently filtered or presented at appropriate times, to enhance health and healthcare. The CDS encompasses a variety of tools to enhance decision-making in the clinical workflow. These tools include computerized alerts and reminders to care providers and patients; clinical guidelines; condition-specific order sets; focused patient data reports and summaries; documentation templates; diagnostic support, and contextually relevant reference information, among other tools.

WHY CLINICAL DECISION SUPPORT?

The CDS has a number of important benefits, including:
- Increased quality of care and enhanced health outcomes
- Avoidance of errors and adverse events
- Improved efficiency, cost-benefit, and provider and patient satisfaction

The CDS is a sophisticated health IT component. It requires computable biomedical knowledge, person-specific data, and a

This chapter contains text excerpted from the following sources: Text under the heading "What Is Clinical Decision Support?" is excerpted from "Clinical Decision Support," HealthIT.gov, Office of the National Coordinator for Health Information Technology (ONC), April 10, 2018; Text under the heading "How Can Clinical Decision Support Be Put into Action?" is excerpted from "Clinical Decision Support," Agency for Healthcare Research and Quality (AHRQ), U.S. Department of Health and Human Services (HHS), June 2019.

reasoning or inferencing mechanism that combines knowledge and data to generate and present helpful information to clinicians as care is being delivered. This information must be filtered, organized, and presented in a way that supports the current workflow, allowing the user to make an informed decision quickly and take action. Different types of CDS may be ideal for different processes of care in different settings.

Health information technologies designed to improve clinical decision-making are particularly attractive for their ability to address the growing information overload clinicians face and to provide a platform for integrating evidence-based knowledge into care delivery. The majority of CDS applications operate as components of comprehensive EHR systems, although stand-alone CDS systems are also used.

CLINICAL DECISION SUPPORT PROMOTES PATIENT SAFETY

The CDS can significantly impact improvements in quality, safety, efficiency, and effectiveness of healthcare. The Office of the National Coordinator for Health IT (ONC) supports efforts to develop, adopt, implement, and evaluate the use of the CDS to improve health-care decision-making.

The CDS aims to help the health-care industry create the technical infrastructure needed to allow health systems to share data with each other electronically to provide the most complete information possible into the CDS systems. Complete records allow the CDS systems to help with diagnoses and track for negative drug interactions by having a better view of a patient's whole health.

HOW CAN CLINICAL DECISION SUPPORT BE PUT INTO ACTION?

The CDS can be used on a variety of platforms (such as the Internet, personal computers, electronic medical record networks, handheld devices, or written materials). Planning for a new health information technology system to support electronically-based CDS includes a number of key steps, such as identifying the needs of users and what the system is expected to do, deciding whether to purchase a commercial system or build the system, designing the system for a clinic's specific needs, planning the implementation process, and determining how to evaluate how well the system has addressed the identified needs. In the case of CDS, issues around design and implementation of the system are often interconnected.

The Agency for Healthcare Research and Quality's (AHRQ) CDS Initiative includes a variety of research projects and outreach efforts to develop agreement in the health-care field around the use of the CDS to promote safe and effective healthcare. Each part of the initiative attempts to engage clinicians, provider organizations, guideline, and quality measurement developers, and IT professionals in the ongoing work to improve making health-care decisions using the CDS systems.

Chapter 13 | Big Data

Chapter Contents

Section 13.1 | Big Data in the Age of Genomics

This section includes text excerpted from "Public Health Approach to Big Data in the Age of Genomics: How Can We Separate Signal from Noise?" Centers for Disease Control and Prevention (CDC), April 26, 2021.

WHAT IS BIG DATA?

The term big data is used to describe massive volumes of both structured and unstructured data that is so large and complex it is difficult to process and analyze. Examples of big data include the following: diagnostic medical imaging, DNA sequencing, and other molecular technologies, environmental exposures, behavioral factors, financial transactions, geographic information, and social media information. Genome sequencing of humans and other organisms has been a leading contributor to big data, but other types of data are increasingly larger, more diverse, and more complex, exceeding the abilities of currently used approaches to store, manage, share, analyze, and interpret it effectively. We have all heard claims that big data will revolutionize everything, including health and healthcare. Some scientists even claim that "the scientific method itself is becoming obsolete" as giant computers and data analytic software sift through the digital world to provide predictive models for health and disease based on the information available.

There are several promising applications of big data in improving health involving the use of genome sequencing technologies. For example:

- Diagnosis of rare and mysterious diseases
- Improved classification of cancer-based on tumor genomes rather than anatomic locations
- Genomically-driven personalized cancer treatment (precision medicine)
- Using whole-genome sequencing to improved public-health detection and response to outbreaks of infectious diseases

Big data today is often more noise than signal! Sorting through all of the data to determine what is a real signal and what is noise does not always work as expected. For example, in 2013, when influenza hit the U.S. hard and early, Google attempted to monitor the outbreak using analysis of flu-related Internet searches, drastically overestimating peak flu levels, compared with traditional public-health surveillance efforts. Even more problematic could be the potential for many false alarms by mindless examination, on a large scale, leading to putative associations between big data points and disease outcomes. This process may falsely infer causality and could potentially lead to ineffective or harmful interventions. To appropriately analyze big data, the field of genomics requires the use of epidemiologic studies, animal models, and other work in addition to big data analysis. Big data's strength is in finding associations, but its weakness is in not showing whether these associations have meaning. Finding a signal is only the first step.

GENOMICS TO IMPROVE HEALTH AND PREVENT DISEASE
Epidemiologic Foundation
We need a strong epidemiologic foundation for studying big data in health and disease. The associations found using big data need to be studied and replicated in ways that confirm the findings and make them generalizable. The study of well-characterized and representative populations, such as the National Cancer Institute (NCI) sponsored cohort consortium that has been collecting information on more than four million people over multiple decades. Big data analysis is currently based on convenient samples of people or data available on the Internet. Both sources may be fraught with all sorts of biases, such as selection, confounding, and lack of generalizability. For more than a decade, the CDC has promoted an epidemiologic approach to the human genome, and now it is time to extend this approach to all big data.

Knowledge Integration
We need to develop a robust "knowledge integration" (KI) enterprise to make sense of big data. In a recent article titled "Knowledge Integration at the Center of Genomic Medicine," the definition of KI has been elaborated along with its three components: knowledge

management, knowledge synthesis, and knowledge translation in genomics. A similar evidence-based knowledge integration process applies to all big data beyond genomics. The CDC hopes that the recently launched NIH Biomedical Data to Knowledge (BD2K) awards will support the development of new approaches, software, tools, and training programs to improve access, analysis, synthesis, and interpretation of genomic big data and improve the ability to make and validate new discoveries.

Evidence-Based Medicine

We should embrace (and not run away from) principles of evidence-based medicine and population screening. Big data is literally a hypothesis-generating machine that could lead to interesting, robust, and predictive associations with health outcomes. However, even after these associations are established, evidence of utility (i.e., improved health outcomes and no evidence of harm) is still needed. Documenting the health-related utility of genomics and big data information may necessitate the use of randomized clinical trials and other experimental designs.

Translational Research

As with genomic medicine, we need a robust translational research agenda for big data that goes beyond the initial discovery (the bench to bedside model). In genomics, most published research is either basic scientific discoveries or preclinical research designed to develop health-related tests and interventions. What happens after that is really the research "road less traveled." In fact, less than 1 percent of published research deals with validation, implementation, policy, communication, and outcomes in the real world. Reaping the benefits of using big data for genomics research will require a more expanded translational research agenda beyond the initial discoveries.

Section 13.2 | **Big Data for Infectious Disease Surveillance**

This section includes text excerpted from "Focus: Big Data for Infectious Disease Surveillance, Modeling," Fogarty International Center (FIC), National Institutes of Health (NIH), February 2017. Reviewed June 2021.

Big data derived from electronic health records, social media, the Internet, and other digital sources have the potential to provide more timely and detailed information on infectious disease threats or outbreaks than traditional surveillance methods, but there are challenges to overcome.

Traditional infectious disease surveillance – typically based on laboratory tests and other epidemiological data collected by public-health institutions – is the gold standard. But, the authors note it can include time lags, is expensive to produce, and typically lacks the local resolution needed for accurate monitoring. Further, it can be cost-prohibitive in low-income countries. In contrast, big data streams from Internet queries, for example, are available in real time and can track disease activity locally, but have their own biases. Hybrid tools that combine traditional surveillance and big data sets may provide a way forward, the scientists suggest, serving to complement, rather than replace, existing methods.

"The ultimate goal is to be able to forecast the size, peak, or trajectory of an outbreak weeks or months in advance in order to better respond to infectious disease threats. Integrating big data in surveillance is a first step toward this long-term goal," says Fogarty senior scientist Dr. Cecile Viboud, coeditor of the supplement. "Now that we have demonstrated proof of concept by comparing data sets in high-income countries, we can examine these models in low-resource settings where traditional surveillance is sparse."

The researchers report on the opportunities and challenges associated with three types of data: medical encounter files, such as records from health-care facilities and insurance claim forms; crowdsourced data collected from volunteers who self-report symptoms in near real time (part of the "citizen science" movement); and data generated by the use of social media, the Internet and mobile phones, which may include self-reporting of health, behavior and travel information.

But, big data's potential must be tempered with caution, the authors say. Nontraditional data streams may lack key demographic identifiers such as age and sex, and the information they provide may underrepresent infants, children, and the elderly, as well as residents of developing countries. Furthermore, social media outlets may not always be stable sources of data, as they can disappear if there is a loss of interest or financing. Most importantly, any novel data stream must be validated against established infectious disease surveillance data and systems, the authors emphasize.

ENSURING DATA PRIVACY

Big data offer a "tantalizing opportunity" to provide more information for public-health surveillance, but its use for that purpose is decades behind other fields, such as climatology and marketing. Electronic health records with identifying information removed, for example, may be a resource to monitor infectious disease outcomes, vaccine uptake, and adverse drug reactions. Applying the data to surveillance has been slow, in part because of ethical concerns about patient privacy. There is also a scarcity of academic studies demonstrating how this type of data performs against traditional surveillance methods.

HARVESTING MEDICAL INSURANCE CLAIM DATA

Medical insurance claim forms, used in the United States and other countries, document the date and location of a doctor's office visit as well as a diagnosis code, which researchers say is useful in tracking disease outbreaks, especially in large populations. Working with anonymized claim form data made available for research, investigators found "excellent alignment" between claim data for flu-like illnesses and proven influenza activity reported by the Centers for Disease Control and Prevention (CDC). The body of influenza research suggests medical claims data should be harvested to generate timely, local data on acute infections, according to the researchers.

ENGAGING THE PUBLIC TO TRACK THE FLU

A European surveillance system that began collecting crowd-sourced data on influenza-like illnesses as part of a research project is now considered an adjunct to existing surveillance activities.

Influenzanet, the system uses standardized online surveys to gather information from volunteers who self-report their symptoms on a weekly basis. Data are analyzed in real time and national and regional results are posted on the website. Established in 2009, the tool is now being used by a number of European countries and is being expanded to collect information on Zika, salmonella, and other diseases.

In their review, the standardization of the technological and epidemiological framework makes it easier for countries to join Influenzanet and allows for coherent surveillance. The timeliness of the reporting and the inclusion of people who may not go to the doctor for treatment of the flu are other strengths.

Downsides include the potential for misreporting and the lack of validation by a physician or lab test. But, the authors point out Influenzanet estimates of illness incidence compare well with data from traditional surveillance methods.

AGGREGATING ANTIBIOTIC RESISTANCE DATA

Noting that antibiotic resistance is a growing concern around the world, U.S. and Canadian scientists developed an online platform to monitor it at the regional level. ResistanceOpen aggregates publicly available, online data from community health-care institutions as well as regional, national and international bodies and displays the information on a navigable map. An analysis of the resource found that the online information compared favorably with traditional reporting systems in the United States and Canada.

The scientists who developed ResistanceOpen aim to expand the database and say the platform could help fill the gap in antimicrobial resistance surveillance in many low- and middle-income countries. ResistanceOpen is an extension of HealthMap, a project that collects and analyzes disparate online data sources to track infectious disease outbreaks around the world. HealthMap has been supported by private and public partners including the NIH, the CDC, and the USAID.

DETECTING ADVERSE DRUG REACTIONS

In addition to improving infectious disease surveillance, nontraditional data streams from the Internet and social media have the potential to supplement traditional systems for reporting adverse drug reactions (ADRs). While consumers rarely use official ADR reporting systems, they do search the web for information about medications and share a word of possible adverse reactions on social media sites and online health forums.

Mining and analyzing Internet search logs and social media posts may detect ADR signals more quickly than traditional physician-based reporting systems, but there are challenges. One of the many ethical questions surrounding the use of these nontraditional sources is whether privately-held data should be accessible for public-health research.

COMPARING EPIDEMIC AND WEATHER FORECASTING

In a comparison of the relatively new field of epidemic forecasting to the better-established one of weather forecasting, the authors note the former is much more difficult given that there is less observational data for disease, and because human behavior has the potential to rapidly alter the course of an epidemic.

Internet data streams, such as search queries and social media posts, may aid epidemic forecasting by providing information in near real time and at a more local level. But, Internet data, the authors say, are less reliable than information collected from weather stations and the availability can vary because of limited Internet access in many developing countries.

HARNESSING SPATIAL BIG DATA

To determine where an outbreak originated or where future ones may occur, for example, epidemiologists need spatial data. Medical insurance claims, social media posts, and mobile phones have the potential to fill geographical information gaps. But, the authors point out, there are technical, practical, and ethical issues that must be addressed. They note possible solutions to protect privacy, such as masking individual-level information by aggregating collected data to larger spatial resolutions.

CONNECTING MOBILITY TO INFECTIOUS DISEASES

With appropriate safeguards to ensure anonymity, call data records from mobile phones may provide researchers "an unprecedented opportunity" to determine how travel affects disease transmission. Studies of malaria and rubella in Kenya showed how call data improved the understanding of the spatial transmission of those diseases. Because mobile phone data has biases young children are not likely to be represented, for example. The authors say more research is needed to determine if mobility patterns derived from call data records are representative of general travel patterns.

CULLING INFORMATION FROM INTERNET REPORTS

Online news articles and health bulletins from public-health agencies can also be manually dissected to model the sequence of transmission chains in an outbreak. The transmission dynamics and risk factors of the Ebola epidemic in West Africa and a Middle East Respiratory Syndrome outbreak in South Korea were elucidated by this approach. Internet findings were in line with traditional data, providing a proof of concept that this approach can be generalized and automated to a variety of online sources and generate information on disease transmission. This is particularly useful to improve situational awareness and guide public-health interventions during emerging infectious disease crises when traditional surveillance data are particularly scarce.

MANAGING EPIDEMIC SIMULATION DATA

Researchers also describe the benefits of a novel, publicly available epidemic simulation data management system, called "epiDMS," which provides storage and indexing services for large data simulation sets, as well as search functionality and data analysis to aid decision-makers during health-care emergencies.

Big Data

While the new hybrid models that combine traditional and digital disease surveillance methods show promise, the scientists agree there is still an overall scarcity of reliable surveillance information, especially compared to other fields, such as climatology, where the data sets are huge.

Chapter 14 | Screening and Detection Technologies

Chapter Contents

Section 14.1 | **Advanced Molecular Detection**

This section includes text excerpted from "Advanced Molecular Detection (AMD)," Centers for Disease Control and Prevention (CDC), January 8, 2021.

THE ADVANCED MOLECULAR DETECTION PROGRAM

The Centers for Disease Control and Prevention's (CDC) Advanced Molecular Detection (AMD) program is helping modernize the public-health system's disease-investigation capabilities by employing the latest technologies and improving AMD capacity throughout the nation.

Under the AMD program, the CDC has been working to build on the nation's existing public-health infrastructure by integrating the AMD technologies. These modern tools deliver a greater level of detailed information on infectious pathogens than older, slower, and less cost-effective methods. Since its inception in 2014, the AMD program has increased the availability of next-generation sequencing and other AMD technologies within the CDC and in state and local public-health systems.

The AMD program works with experts across the CDC to ensure the United States has the infrastructure, including technology, needed to protect Americans from infectious disease threats. The AMD office collaborates with other CDC programs to facilitate the development and pilot testing of next-generation diagnostic tests and protocols. Other programs throughout the CDC leverage these tools against a variety of infectious pathogens and help state and local public-health agencies tap into them, as well.

AMD Technologies

The AMD program is helping build and integrate laboratory, bioinformatics, and epidemiology technologies across the CDC and nationwide. Building capacity in all three areas is necessary for creating a 21st-century public-health detection and surveillance system to protect the United States from disease threats.

LABORATORY TECHNOLOGIES

AMD technologies include laboratory methods to extract and sequence the DNA of pathogens, including next-generation genomic sequencing (NGS) and whole genome sequencing (WGS). Sequencing technologies range from portable sequencers for field-based testing to benchtop and full-sized sequencers for laboratory use.

EPIDEMIOLOGY TECHNOLOGIES

Epidemiologists help detect where data from their traditional field investigations intersect with genomic data to pinpoint disease outbreaks and clusters of human illnesses. Through training in molecular epidemiology, the CDC is helping build on the existing epidemiology workforce, so they can use genomic data generated and analyzed through bioinformatics pipelines to help solve outbreak mysteries.

BIOINFORMATICS TECHNOLOGIES

Even though infectious pathogens are small, sequencing their DNA generates a tremendous amount of genomic data. To analyze those data, experts in bioinformatics use high-performance computing systems to devise programs, often called "pipelines." Once designed and validated, these pipelines can speed up the detection and characterization of pathogens. By uploading DNA sequence data into a specific pipeline, scientists can rapidly find out which species or strain of the pathogen is involved in an outbreak and specific characteristics that can be important for fighting it, such as whether it is resistant to antimicrobials.

THE OFFICE OF ADVANCED MOLECULAR DETECTION RESPONSIBILITIES

The CDC's Office of Advanced Molecular Detection (OAMD) works with experts across the CDC to ensure the U.S. has the infrastructure, including technology, needed to protect Americans from infectious disease threats. The OAMD collaborates with other CDC programs to facilitate the development and pilot testing of next-generation diagnostics and protocols. Other programs throughout CDC leverage these tools against a variety of infectious pathogens and help state and local public-health agencies tap into them as well. The responsibilities of AMD are:

- Building capacity and workforce
- Exploring new technologies
- Enhancing surveillance
- Developing faster tests
- Uncovering emerging threats
- Improving vaccines
- Tracking global health
- Mapping environmental threats
- Strengthening food safety
- Identifying vector-borne diseases
- Combating HAIs and AMR
- Battling human immunodeficiency virus (HIV) and sexually transmitted diseases (STDs)

HOW ADVANCED MOLECULAR DETECTION PROGRAM WORKS

For over 20 years, public-health laboratories have used a DNA fingerprinting technology called "Pulsed-Field Gel Electrophoresis" (PFGE). In recent years, a set of new technologies have revolutionized the ability to decode DNA. Whole-genome sequencing (WGS) gives a much more detailed DNA fingerprint. In public health, this is transforming how epidemiologists and laboratory scientists approach the detection and investigation of outbreaks. This allows public-health agencies across the United States to detect outbreaks sooner, including many outbreaks that had previously gone undetected.

In the United States through the federally-funded AMD Program, public-health agencies are applying next-generation sequencing in almost every area of infectious disease public health.

In food safety, the CDC is working with the FDA, USDA, NIH, and state and local public-health agencies to intervene more quickly in outbreaks and to better understand how to prevent pathogens from getting into the food system in the first place.

In flu, sequencing is enabling faster, more effective characterization of viruses to better understand how they emerge and to improve vaccines.

In viral hepatitis, sequencing has proven invaluable in investigating outbreaks.

These are but a few of the areas where the application of sequencing is improving public-health surveillance and outbreak response.

WHAT IS NEW IN THE ADVANCED MOLECULAR DETECTION PROGRAM

The Centers for Disease Control and Prevention (CDC) has issued seven awards as part of the SARS-CoV-2 Sequencing for Public Health Emergency Response, Epidemiology, and Surveillance (SPHERES) Initiative. The awards, totaling nearly $14.5 million over two years, are intended to fill knowledge gaps and promote innovation in the U.S. response to the COVID-19 pandemic. SPHERES builds upon six years of investment by the CDC's Advanced Molecular Detection program. This program integrates next-generation genomic sequencing technologies with bioinformatics and epidemiology expertise across the U.S. public-health system. The SPHERES collaboration, which currently includes scientists from nearly 200 public-health, academic, clinical, and nonprofit laboratories and institutions, aims to accelerate the application of SARS-CoV-2 genome sequencing for genomic epidemiology and pandemic response.

Section 14.2 | Liquid Biopsy to Detect, Track, and Treat Cancer

This section includes text excerpted from "Liquid Biopsy: Using DNA in Blood to Detect, Track, and Treat Cancer," National Cancer Institute (NCI), November 8, 2017. Reviewed June 2021.

When a patient has a suspicious lump or symptoms, one of the first things a doctor may do is perform a tissue biopsy – a procedure to collect cells for closer examination.

Examining the appearance of the cells under the microscope can determine if cancer is present, show what type of cancer it is, and give clues about the patient's prognosis. In addition, molecular analysis of a tissue biopsy sample can also reveal information that may help guide a personalized treatment strategy.

Although they are important for patient care, tissue biopsies – which may involve a large needle, an endoscope, or open surgery – can be invasive, risky, costly, and painful. And some patients may not be able to have a tissue biopsy due to the inaccessibility of their tumors or because they have other health conditions that prevent them from undergoing the procedure.

Because these factors make it difficult to perform repeated biopsies on a patient, these tests can be an impractical method to track tumors as they develop and change over time. Nevertheless, they remain the gold standard for detecting and obtaining information about cancer.

But, researchers have been exploring a new approach that could potentially complement or, in some cases, serve as an alternative to tissue biopsies. The approach, often called a "liquid biopsy," relies on analyzing bits of tumor material – molecules as well as whole cells – that are found in bodily fluids such as blood or urine.

Although there is a widespread belief that liquid biopsies could eventually have a significant impact on patient care, most researchers in the field agree that the science around the approach is still evolving and important questions remain unanswered.

"I think the major stumbling block for moving these liquid biopsy tests forward is there is not enough clinical verification and validation to know and feel comfortable that what we're detecting with them is clinically meaningful," said Lynn Sorbara, Ph.D., of National Cancer Institute's (NCI) Division of Cancer Prevention.

DIFFERENT TESTS FOR DIFFERENT TUMOR MOLECULES

More than 100 years ago, scientists discovered that tumors shed molecules and cells into bodily fluids. Much more recently, researchers have shown that analyzing these molecules and cells can reveal some of the same information that tissue biopsies provide.

Liquid biopsy research has recently expanded, generating an entirely new field of study. Both academic and industry researchers from diverse areas of expertise are working on many fronts to develop, refine, and establish clinical uses for liquid biopsy tests.

Different liquid biopsy tests analyze different kinds of tumor material, such as DNA, RNA, proteins, tiny vesicles called "exosomes," and whole cells. The tests detect these molecules or cells in various bodily fluids, including blood, urine, cerebrospinal fluid, or saliva. These body fluids are usually readily accessible, and in most cases the procedure for collecting a sample is less invasive and more easily repeatable than a tissue biopsy.

This feature gives liquid biopsies the potential to be used for several important applications for which tissue biopsies are not well suited, explained Miguel Ossandon, M.S., program manager for the Cancer Diagnosis Program in NCI's Division of Cancer Treatment and Diagnosis.

For example, liquid biopsies could be used to monitor cancer development, track a patient's response to treatment, or as a "surveillance" method for people who have completed treatment but are at high risk of their disease returning, he said.

"The variety of technologies emerging to enable a more precise and robust analysis of circulating molecules, cells, and everything in-between, certainly suggests that the exciting clinical potential for liquid biopsy approaches is more a question of 'when' rather than 'if'," said Tony Dickherber, Ph.D., director of NCI's Innovative Molecular Analysis Technologies Program.

There has been a recent surge of research related to liquid biopsy tests that analyze tumor DNA in blood, called "circulating tumor DNA" (ctDNA), and several ctDNA-based liquid biopsy tests are in clinical development.

USING TUMOR DNA TO DETECT CANCER EARLY

One potential application of ctDNA-based liquid biopsies is for detecting cancer at an early stage, when treatment may be most successful. In several studies, for example, liquid biopsy tests detected ctDNA in blood samples collected from patients months before they were diagnosed with cancer by traditional methods, such as imaging tests.

But, in these studies, the tests sometimes produced false-positive test results – that is, they detected cancerous DNA when no cancer actually developed.

Another concern is that these tests will detect early-stage tumors that will not grow much or will grow so slowly that they would never actually harm the patient.

Treating these slow-growing tumors could actually do more harm than good, and "the risk of overtreatment is a major concern with early cancer detection," Dr. Sorbara noted. "The idea of diagnosing somebody using liquid biopsy alone has not been validated yet. We're still at the early stages and have a long way to go," she continued.

Prospective cohort studies are needed to truly determine if the presence of ctDNA in a patient's blood can be used as an accurate marker for early-stage cancer, she added. For example, studies are needed to determine if the detection of ctDNA warrants treatment and if that treatment improves patient outcomes.

The NCI is supporting an initiative to advance the development and validation of liquid biopsy technologies that can detect early-stage cancers, distinguish cancer from benign conditions, and identify fast- and slow-growing cancers. A major aim of the initiative is to create a public–private partnership that brings engineering and clinical experts together to accomplish these goals.

Looking forward, Dr. Sorbara envisions that liquid biopsy tests may be used to screen for early-stage cancer in high-risk individuals, such as those with hereditary cancer syndromes.

Or, she continued, they could be used in tandem with other tests, such as an MRI. For example, a liquid biopsy test could be used as a routine prescreening method in healthy individuals to identify those who may have early-stage cancer and are candidates for other (possibly more costly or invasive) screening tests.

TUMOR DNA MAY AID PRECISION CANCER TREATMENT

There is also hope that ctDNA-based liquid biopsies may guide precision medicine treatment by identifying unique molecular characteristics of an individual's cancer. In several research studies, liquid biopsies have pinpointed ctDNA mutations that could potentially be used to determine the optimal treatment.

For example, researchers at UC San Diego Moores Cancer Center analyzed blood samples from 168 patients with different types of cancer, including brain, lung, and breast cancer. For 58 percent of the participants, the researchers identified at least one cancer-related ctDNA mutation. For most of these patients, a U.S. Food and Drug Administration (FDA)-approved drug was available to treat cancers with that particular mutation.

Other studies have demonstrated the feasibility of using ctDNA-based liquid biopsies on a large scale to identify DNA mutations in patients' cancers. For instance, investigators used Guardant360 – a commercially available test that analyzes 70 cancer-related genes in a blood sample – to identify mutations in the ctDNA of more than 15,000 patients. The investigators found that, for most patients, the genetic mutations identified by the liquid biopsy test were consistent with those identified by a tissue biopsy test.

In 2016, the FDA approved a liquid biopsy test, called the "cobas® EGFR Mutation Test" for the detection of EGFR gene mutations in ctDNA of patients with lung cancer. The purpose of the test is to identify patients who may be candidates for treatment with erlotinib® (Tarceva®) and osimeritinib® (Tagrisso®) – targeted therapies that attack cancer cells with EGFR mutations. Because the test may produce a false-negative test result, the FDA recommends a tissue biopsy if the liquid biopsy is negative (meaning it does not detect an EGFR mutation).

Many other liquid biopsy tests are commercially available but have not been rigorously tested by scientists. Clinicians and researchers are still determining the limitations of these tests and, more importantly, whether they provide clinical benefit to patients. For example, it is unknown whether using a liquid biopsy test to help select treatment improves patient outcomes.

MONITORING TREATMENT RESPONSE WITH TUMOR DNA

Because they are noninvasive and easily repeated, ctDNA-based liquid biopsies may be useful for monitoring patients' responses to therapy both during treatment and after it is completed. Clinicians are hopeful that tracking a patient's response to treatment may allow adjustments to be made in real time. In other words, the treatment could be stopped or adjusted if the test indicates it is not working.

Imaging techniques such as CT scans are currently used to track treatment response for patients with certain cancer types, but they are not sensitive enough to detect small changes in tumor size and they tend to be costly, explained Mark Roschewski, M.D., of NCI's Center for Cancer Research.

As a potential alternative, Dr. Roschewski and his colleagues tested the ability of a liquid biopsy test to track treatment responses in patients with lymphoma. They showed that changes in ctDNA correlated with positive responses to chemotherapy. Furthermore, they were able to use ctDNA patterns to detect when some patients' disease was coming back – months before it was possible to do so via CT scan.

"In our study, the liquid biopsy test was much more sensitive than imaging techniques," said Dr. Roschewski.

Likewise, other the NCI researchers correlated changes in ctDNA levels with patients' responses to immunotherapy treatment. They found that they could detect these changes within two weeks of the start of treatment. Having an early indicator of the treatment's efficacy could be very helpful because only a small proportion of patients typically respond to immunotherapy treatment, they explained.

"Liquid biopsy tests have the added advantage of providing molecular information about the cancer, which can change during and after treatment," said Brian Sorg, Ph.D., also of NCI's Division of Cancer Treatment and Diagnosis. This additional information could potentially help doctors track the development of drug resistance and make more personalized treatment decisions.

For example, although most patients with lung cancer initially respond to treatment with a class of drugs called "tyrosine kinase inhibitors," the majority develop drug resistance within one or two years of starting treatment.

In one study, a team of researchers analyzed mutations in ctDNA from patients with lung cancer that had become resistant to certain tyrosine kinase inhibitors. They detected a genetic mutation causing the drug resistance in ctDNA from 80 percent of participants.

A separate study will be needed to determine if the liquid biopsy test can identify patients whose tumors have this mutation and who are most likely to benefit from a different treatment, the researchers noted.

According to an expert review released by the American Society of Clinical Oncology (ASCO) and College of American Pathologists (CAP), most liquid biopsy tests are not yet ready for routine use in clinical cancer care. Based on an analysis of 77 liquid biopsy studies, the organizations concluded that most liquid biopsy tests designed to track treatment responses need more evidence to confirm that the tests correctly identify patients for whom a particular treatment is likely to be effective. The evidence on the validity of these tests is "still emerging," they wrote.

LIMITATIONS OF ctDNA-BASED LIQUID BIOPSIES

While there are many potential applications for ctDNA-based liquid biopsies, there are also several limitations.

Most cancer types lack well-established biomarkers (such as a specific DNA mutation) that allow scientists to identify and track the disease via ctDNA. For example, a biomarker commonly used to track advanced pancreatic cancer is considered unreliable for early detection of the disease.

"While the technology for detecting ctDNA in body fluids has improved dramatically, the knowledge required to identify appropriate biomarkers for many cancer types has not," said Dr. Dickherber.

And DNA mutations vary even among patients with the same cancer type, so although a particular mutation may be common for one type of cancer, many patients with that cancer type may not have it. This adds a layer of complexity to the challenge of identifying ctDNA biomarkers for every cancer type and stage.

One possible solution could involve combining tissue and liquid biopsies, said Ossandon. First, a tissue biopsy could be used to identify unique biomarkers for an individual's tumor, he explained, and then liquid biopsy tests could be used to track those biomarkers.

Another limitation is that ctDNA in the blood may not be truly representative of DNA in the actual tumor, and, therefore, may not be the best source of information for guiding clinical decisions. Tumors are heterogeneous – meaning DNA mutations vary between cancer cells in a single tumor – and it is not known whether ctDNA is released from the whole tumor or only certain parts of it, explained Dr. Sorg.

It is also unknown whether the mutations found in ctDNA are "driver" mutations – those that play an important role in the cancer's biology – said Dr. Sorbara. They may instead be "passenger" mutations, that is, changes that accompany the development of cancer but do not control its growth.

The ASCO and CAP review also found that the results of most liquid biopsy tests do not completely match results from tissue biopsies, calling into question the accuracy of these new tests. This discordance could be the result of biological differences (e.g., between blood and tissue samples) or limitations of the tests, the experts noted.

"Possibly the biggest unanswered question is whether liquid biopsy tests can improve patient survival," Dr. Roschewski said. Meaning, does using liquid biopsy tests to detect early-stage cancer, select treatment, or track disease progression ultimately extend patient survival or improve quality of life?

Many researchers, including the ASCO and CAP experts, agree that studies that prospectively analyze the effect of liquid biopsy tests on clinical outcome are needed.

Section 14.3 | DNA Microarray Technology

This section includes text excerpted from "DNA Microarray Technology Fact Sheet," National Human Genome Research Institute (NHGRI), August 15, 2020.

WHAT IS A DNA MICROARRAY?

Scientists know that a mutation – or alteration – in a particular gene's DNA may contribute to a certain disease. However, it can be very difficult to develop a test to detect these mutations, because most large

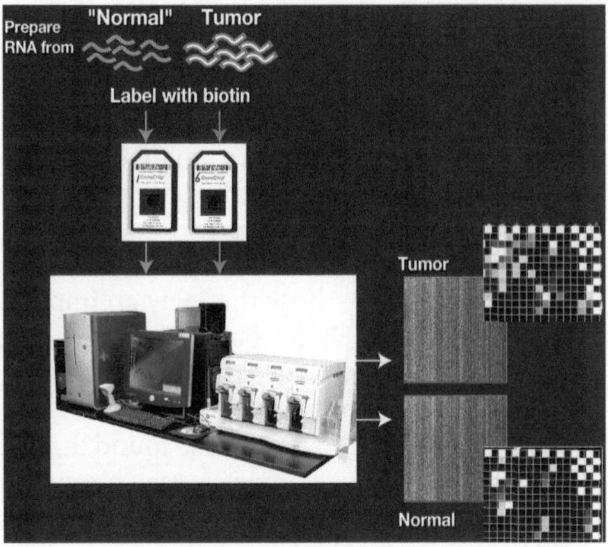

Figure 14.1. DNA Microarray Technology

genes have many regions where mutations can occur. For example, researchers believe that mutations in the genes *BRCA1* and *BRCA2* cause as many as 60 percent of all cases of hereditary breast and ovarian cancers. But, there is not one specific mutation responsible for all of these cases. Researchers have already discovered over 800 different mutations in *BRCA1* alone. The DNA microarray is a tool used to determine whether the DNA from a particular individual contains a mutation in genes, such as *BRCA1* and *BRCA2*. The chip consists of a small glass plate encased in plastic. Some companies manufacture microarrays using methods similar to those used to make computer microchips. On the surface, each chip contains thousands of short, synthetic, single-stranded DNA sequences, which together add up to the normal gene in question, and to variants (mutations) of that gene that have been found in the human population.

WHAT IS A DNA MICROARRAY USED FOR?

When they were first introduced, DNA microarrays were used only as a research tool. Scientists continue today to conduct large-scale population studies; for example, to determine how often individuals with a particular mutation actually develop breast cancer, or to identify the changes in gene sequences that are most often associated with particular diseases. This has become possible because, just as is the case for computer chips, very large numbers of 'features' can be put on microarray chips, representing a very large portion of the human genome.

Microarrays can also be used to study the extent to which certain genes are turned on or off in cells and tissues. In this case, instead of isolating DNA from the samples, RNA (which is a transcript of the DNA) is isolated and measured.

Today, DNA microarrays are used in clinical diagnostic tests for some diseases. Sometimes they are also used to determine which drugs might be best prescribed for particular individuals because genes determine how the bodies handle the chemistry related to those drugs. With the advent of new DNA sequencing technologies, some of the tests for which microarrays were used in the past now use DNA sequencing instead. But, microarray tests still tend to be less expensive than sequencing, so they may be used for very large studies, as well as for some clinical tests.

HOW DOES A DNA MICROARRAY WORK?

To determine whether an individual possesses a mutation for a particular disease, a scientist first obtains a sample of DNA from the patient's blood as well as a control sample – one that does not contain a mutation in the gene of interest.

The researcher then denatures the DNA in the samples – a process that separates the two complementary strands of DNA into single-stranded molecules. The next step is to cut the long strands of DNA into smaller, more manageable fragments and then label each fragment by attaching a fluorescent dye (There are other ways to do this, but this is one common method.) The individual's DNA is labeled with green dye and the control – or normal – DNA is labeled with red dye. Both sets of labeled DNA are then inserted into the chip and allowed to hybridize – or bind – to the synthetic DNA on the chip.

If the individual does not have a mutation for the gene, both the red and green samples will bind to the sequences on the chip

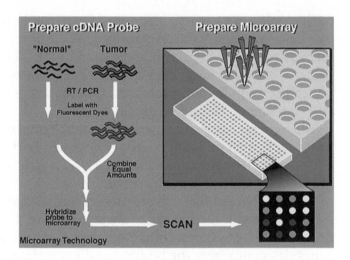

Figure 14.2. The Working of DNA Microarray

that represent the sequence without the mutation (the "normal" sequence).

If the individual does possess a mutation, the individual's DNA will not bind properly to the DNA sequences on the chip that represent the "normal" sequence but instead will bind to the sequence on the chip that represents the mutated DNA.

Section 14.4 | Genetic Testing

This section includes text excerpted from "Genetic Testing," Centers for Disease Control and Prevention (CDC), March 23, 2020.

WHAT IS GENETIC TESTING?

Genetic testing looks for changes, sometimes called "mutations" or "variants," in your DNA. Genetic testing is useful in many areas of medicine and can change the medical care you or your family member receives. For example, genetic testing can provide a diagnosis for a genetic condition, such as fragile X, or information about your risk to develop cancer. There are many different kinds of genetic tests. Genetic tests are done using a blood or spit sample and results are usually ready in a few weeks. Because we share DNA with our family members, if you are found to have a genetic change, your family members may have the same change. Genetic counseling before and after genetic testing can help make sure that you are the right person in your family to get a genetic test, you are getting the right genetic test, and that you understand your results.

REASONS FOR GENETIC TESTING
- To learn whether you have a genetic condition that runs in your family before you have symptoms
- To learn about the chance a current or future pregnancy will have a genetic condition
- To diagnose a genetic condition if you or your child has symptoms
- To understand and guide your cancer prevention or treatment plan

TYPES OF GENETIC TESTS
There are many different kinds of genetic tests. There is no single genetic test that can detect all genetic conditions. The approach to genetic testing is individualized based on your medical and family history and what condition you are being tested for.

Single Gene Testing
Single gene tests look for changes in only one gene. Single gene testing is done when your doctor believes you or your child have symptoms of a specific condition or syndrome. Some examples of this are Duchenne muscular dystrophy (DMD) or sickle cell disease (SCD). Single gene testing is also used when there is a known genetic mutation in a family.

Panel Testing
A panel genetic test looks for changes in many genes in one test. Genetic testing panels are usually grouped into categories based

on different kinds of medical concerns. Some examples of genetic panel tests are low muscle tone, short stature, or epilepsy. Panel genetic tests can also be grouped into genes that are all associated with higher risk of developing certain kinds of cancer, such as breast or colorectal (colon) cancer.

Large-Scale Genetic or Genomic Testing

There are two different kinds of large-scale genetic tests.

- Exome sequencing looks at all the genes in the DNA (whole exome) or just the genes that are related to medical conditions (clinical exome).
- Genome sequencing is the largest genetic test and looks at all of a person's DNA, not just the genes.

Exome and genome sequencing are ordered by doctors for people with complex medical histories. Large-scale genomic testing is also used in research to learn more about the genetic causes of conditions. Large-scale genetic tests can have findings unrelated to why the test was ordered in the first place (secondary findings). Examples of secondary findings are genes associated with a predisposition to cancer or rare heart conditions when you were looking for a genetic diagnosis to explain a child's developmental disabilities.

TESTING FOR CHANGES OTHER THAN GENE CHANGES

- **Chromosomes.** DNA is packaged into structures called "chromosomes." Some tests look for changes in chromosomes rather than gene changes. Examples of these tests are karyotype and chromosomal microarrays.
- **Gene expression.** Genes are expressed, or turned on, at different levels in different types of cells. Gene expression tests compare these levels between normal cells and diseased cells because knowing about the difference can provide important information for treating the disease. For example, these tests can be used to guide chemotherapy treatment for breast cancer.

TYPES OF GENETIC TEST RESULTS

- **Positive.** The test found a genetic change known to cause disease.
- **Negative.** The test did not find a genetic change known to cause disease. Sometimes a negative result occurs when the wrong test was ordered or there is not a genetic cause for that person's symptoms. A "true negative" is when there is a known genetic change in the family and the person tested did not inherit it. If your test results are negative and there is no known genetic change in your family, a negative test result may not give you a definite answer. This is because you might not have been tested for the genetic change that runs in your family.
- **Uncertain.** A variant of unknown or uncertain significance means there is not enough information about that genetic change to determine whether it is benign (normal) or pathogenic (disease-causing).

Section 14.5 | Sensitive Stroke Detection

This section includes text excerpted from "More Sensitive Stroke Detection," National Institutes of Health (NIH), August 20, 2015. Reviewed June 2021.

Researchers at the National Institute of Neurological Disorders and Stroke (NINDS) have found that magnetic resonance imaging (MRI) can provide a more sensitive diagnosis than computed tomography (CT) for the most common type of stroke, called "ischemic stroke."

The researchers studied more than 350 patients who arrived in the emergency room with suspected strokes to determine whether MRI or CT was better for rapid diagnosis. Doctors face an urgent need to swiftly distinguish between acute ischemic stroke, which is caused by clots in blood vessels, and hemorrhagic stroke, which is caused by bleeding into the brain because the two types of stroke are treated in very different ways.

Standard CT uses x-rays that are passed through the body at different angles and processed by a computer as cross-sectional images or slices of the internal structure of the body or organ. Standard MRI uses computer-generated radio waves and a powerful magnet to produce detailed slices or three-dimensional images of body structures and nerves. A contrast dye may be used in both imaging techniques to enhance the visibility of certain areas or tissues.

Results of the NINDS study showed that standard MRI is superior to standard CT in diagnosing acute stroke, particularly acute ischemic stroke. That is very good news for patients, says NINDS Deputy Director Walter J. Koroshetz, M.D., noting that brain injury from ischemic stroke often can be avoided if clot-busting therapy is administered within three hours of stroke onset.

Section 14.6 | Tool to Detect Cardiovascular Disease Risk

This section includes text excerpted from "New NIST Tool Aims to Improve Accuracy of Test to Determine Cardiovascular Disease Risk," National Institute of Standards and Technology (NIST), May 17, 2018.

Cardiovascular disease caused one out of three deaths in the United States in 2016, and for decades it has been the leading killer for both men and women. Hoping to reduce these numbers, researchers at the National Institute of Standards and Technology (NIST) have developed a new standard reference material (SRM) that can improve the results of a common blood test used to assess a person's risk of heart disease.

The blood test measures C-reactive protein (CRP), which is a marker for inflammation in the body. While the precise relationship between slightly elevated CRP levels and cardiovascular disease is still being determined, research suggests that inflammation in arteries can lead to plaque buildup, and then to heart attacks and strokes. Some studies indicate that high-sensitivity CRP (hsCRP) tests – which detect minute amounts of the protein in blood – may have advantages for predicting heart disease when cholesterol counts are normal.

The hsCRP test kits are made from antibodies that attach to CRP in a blood sample such as a lock and key to provide an accurate count of the protein. However, depending on their source and quality, some of these antibodies attach better than others, leading to variable results between batches and kit makers.

"We began developing a reference material for the hsCRP test when we recognized that a patient's test results might depend on which test kit was used," said Eric Kilpatrick, a biologist who has specialized in protein measurement at NIST for more than a decade. "Repeatable, reliable results, no matter when or where the blood test is performed, are critical to health, and without them, it is difficult for doctors to use hsCRP to decide treatment options and to follow a patient's progress accurately," he said.

The NIST's SRM 2924 (www-s.nist.gov/srmors/view_detail. cfm?srm=2924) C-Reactive Protein Solution provides a reference benchmark tool that manufacturers can use to ensure their kit test results are consistent from batch to batch by confirming that the antibodies going into the kits correctly bind CRP.

When the results of hsCRP tests can be traced to the NIST SRM, doctors can have greater trust in the test scores, and treat and advise their patients with confidence.

Researchers are continuing their quest for ultimate accuracy. "The gold standard for CRP will be an SRM in serum, the liquid component of blood," Kilpatrick said. That work will begin soon, and SRM 2924 is leading the way.

Standard reference materials are among the most widely used NIST products. The institute prepares, analyzes, and sells more than 1,200 carefully characterized materials used to check the accuracy of instruments and test procedures used in manufacturing, clinical chemistry, environmental monitoring, electronics, criminal forensics, and dozens of other fields.

Section 14.7 | **AI-Assisted Medical Devices**

This section includes text excerpted from "Artificial Intelligence and Machine Learning in Software as a Medical Device," U.S. Food and Drug Administration (FDA), January 12, 2021.

The U.S. Food and Drug Administration's (FDA) Center for Devices and Radiological Health (CDRH) is considering a total product lifecycle-based regulatory framework for these technologies that would allow for modifications to be made from real-world learning and adaptation while ensuring that the safety and effectiveness of the software as a medical device are maintained.

WHAT IS ARTIFICIAL INTELLIGENCE AND MACHINE LEARNING?

Artificial intelligence has been broadly defined as the science and engineering of making intelligent machines, especially intelligent computer programs. Artificial intelligence can use different techniques, including models based on statistical analysis of data, expert systems that primarily rely on if-then statements, and machine learning.

Machine learning is an artificial intelligence technique that can be used to design and train software algorithms to learn from and act on data. Software developers can use machine learning to create an algorithm that is 'locked' so that its function does not change, or 'adaptive' so its behavior can change over time based on new data.

Some real-world examples of artificial intelligence and machine learning technologies include:
- An imaging system that uses algorithms to give diagnostic information for skin cancer in patients
- A smart sensor device that estimates the probability of a heart attack

HOW ARE ARTIFICIAL INTELLIGENCE AND MACHINE LEARNING TRANSFORMING MEDICAL DEVICES?

Artificial intelligence (AI) and machine learning (ML) technologies have the potential to transform healthcare by deriving new and important insights from the vast amount of data generated during the delivery of healthcare every day. Medical device manufacturers are using these technologies to innovate their products to better assist health-care providers and improve patient care. One of the greatest benefits of AI/ML in software resides in its ability to learn from real-world use and experience, and its capability to improve its performance.

HOW IS THE FDA CONSIDERING REGULATION OF ARTIFICIAL INTELLIGENCE AND MACHINE LEARNING MEDICAL DEVICES?

Traditionally, the FDA reviews medical devices through an appropriate premarket pathway, such as premarket clearance (510(k)), De Novo classification, or premarket approval. The FDA may also review and clear modifications to medical devices, including software as a medical device, depending on the significance or risk posed to patients of that modification.

The FDA's traditional paradigm of medical device regulation was not designed for adaptive artificial intelligence and machine learning technologies. Under the FDA's current approach to software modifications, the FDA anticipates that many of this artificial intelligence and machine learning-driven software changes to a device may need a premarket review.

On April 2, 2019, the FDA published a discussion paper "Proposed Regulatory Framework for Modifications to Artificial Intelligence/Machine Learning (AI/ML)-Based Software as a Medical Device (SaMD) – Discussion Paper and Request for Feedback" (www.fda.gov/media/122535/download) that describes the FDA's foundation for a potential approach to premarket review for artificial intelligence and machine learning-driven software modifications.

The ideas described in the discussion paper leverage practices from the current premarket programs and rely on IMDRF's risk categorization principles, the FDA's benefit-risk framework, risk management principles described in the software modifications guidance, and the organization-based total product lifecycle approach (also envisioned in the Digital Health Software Precertification (Pre-Cert) Program).

In the framework described in the discussion paper, the FDA envisions a "predetermined change control plan" in premarket submissions. This plan would include the types of anticipated modifications – referred to as the "Software as a Medical Device Pre-Specifications" – and the associated methodology being used to implement those changes in a controlled manner that manages risks to patients – referred to as the "Algorithm Change Protocol."

In this potential approach, the FDA would expect a commitment from manufacturers on transparency and real-world performance monitoring for artificial intelligence and machine learning-based software as a medical device, as well as periodic updates to the FDA on what changes were implemented as part of the approved prespecifications and the algorithm change protocol.

Such a regulatory framework could enable the FDA and manufacturers to evaluate and monitor a software product from its premarket development to postmarket performance. This approach could allow for the FDA's regulatory oversight to embrace the iterative improvement power of artificial intelligence and machine learning-based software as a medical device while assuring patient safety.

As part of the AI/ML Action Plan, the FDA is highlighting its intention to develop an update to the proposed regulatory framework presented in the AI/ML-based SaMD discussion paper, including through the issuance of draft guidance on the predetermined change control plan.

Part 3 | Diagnostic Technology

Chapter 15 | Imaging Services

Chapter Contents

Section 15.1 | **Computed Tomography**

This section includes text excerpted from "Computed Tomography (CT)," U.S. Food and Drug Administration (FDA), June 14, 2019.

Computed tomography (CT), sometimes called "computerized tomography" or "computed axial tomography" (CAT), is a non-invasive medical examination or procedure that uses specialized x-ray equipment to produce cross-sectional images of the body. Each cross-sectional image represents a "slice" of the person being imaged, such as the slices in a loaf of bread. These cross-sectional images are used for a variety of diagnostic and therapeutic purposes.

CT scans can be performed on every region of the body for a variety of reasons (e.g., diagnostic, treatment planning, interventional, or screening). Most CT scans are performed as outpatient procedures.

HOW A CT SYSTEM WORKS

- A motorized table moves the patient through a circular opening in the CT imaging system.
- While the patient is inside the opening, an x-ray source and a detector assembly within the system rotate around the patient. A single rotation typically takes a second or less. During rotation, the x-ray source produces a narrow, fan-shaped beam of x-rays (see Figure 15.1) that passes through a section of the patient's body.
- Detectors in rows opposite the x-ray source register the x-rays that pass through the patient's body as a snapshot in the process of creating an image. Many different "snapshots" (at many angles through the patient) are collected during one complete rotation.
- For each rotation of the x-ray source and detector assembly, the image data are sent to a computer to reconstruct all of the individual "snapshots" into one or multiple cross-sectional images (slices) of the internal organs and tissues.

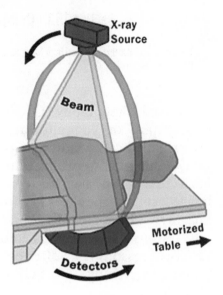

Figure 15.1. CT Fan Beam

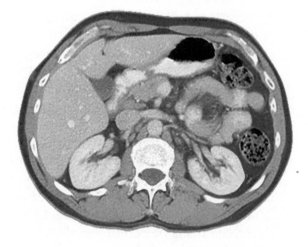

Figure 15.2. CT Image of the Abdomen

CT images of internal organs, bones, soft tissue, and blood vessels provide greater clarity and more details than conventional x-ray images, such as a chest x-ray (see Figures 15.2 and 15.3).

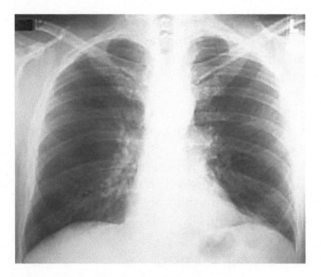

Figure 15.3. Image of a Conventional Chest X-ray

USES OF A CT SCAN

A CT is a valuable medical tool that can help a physician:
- Diagnose disease, trauma, or abnormality
- Plan and guide interventional or therapeutic procedures
- Monitor the effectiveness of therapy (e.g., cancer treatment)

BENEFITS AND RISKS OF A CT SCAN

When used appropriately, the benefits of a CT scan far exceed the risks. CT scans can provide detailed information to diagnose, plan treatment for, and evaluate many conditions in adults and children. Additionally, the detailed images provided by CT scans may eliminate the need for exploratory surgery.

Concerns about CT scans include the risks from exposure to ionizing radiation and possible reactions to the intravenous contrast agent, or dye, which may be used to improve visualization. Exposure to ionizing radiation may cause a small increase in a person's lifetime risk of developing cancer. Exposure to ionizing

165

radiation is of particular concern in pediatric patients because the cancer risk per unit dose of ionizing radiation is higher for younger patients than adults, and younger patients have a longer lifetime for the effects of radiation exposure to manifest as cancer.

However, in children and adults, the risk from a medically necessary imaging exam is quite small when compared to the benefit of accurate diagnosis or intervention. It is especially important to make sure that CT scans in children are performed with appropriate exposure factors, as use of exposure settings designed for adults can result in a larger radiation dose than necessary to produce a useful image for a pediatric patient.

INFORMATION FOR PATIENTS AND PARENTS

If a physician recommends a CT scan for you or your child, the U.S. Food and Drug Administration (FDA) encourages you to discuss the benefits and risks of the CT scan, as well as any past x-ray procedures you or your child have had, with your physician. A CT scan should always be performed if it is medically necessary and other exams using no or less radiation are unsuitable. At this time, the FDA does not see a benefit to whole-body scanning of individuals without symptoms.

INFORMATION FOR HEALTH-CARE PROVIDERS

The FDA has regulations covering the safety and effectiveness and radiation control of all x-ray imaging devices, including CT. Individual states and other federal agencies regulate the use of CT devices through recommendations and requirements for personnel qualifications, quality assurance and quality control programs, and facility accreditation.

Exam Justification: CT Screening Guidelines and Incidental Findings

The individual risk from a necessary imaging exam is quite small when compared to the benefit of aiding accurate diagnosis or intervention. However, the FDA recommends that health-care professionals and hospital administrators work to reduce radiation exposure to patients by following these steps:

- Discuss the rationale for the examination with the patient and/or parent to make sure there is a clear understanding of benefits and risks.
- Justify CT exams by:
  - Making sure the CT exam is necessary to answer a clinical question
  - Considering other examinations that use less or no radiation exposure, such as ultrasound or MRI, if appropriate
  - Checking the patient's medical imaging history to avoid duplicate examinations

These precautions are especially important with pediatric patients since children are more susceptible to radiation effects than adults.

In addition to referral (also called "appropriate use") criteria, screening guidelines are an important tool available to the referring physician to determine if a certain CT examination is justified.

Optimization: Facility Quality Assurance and Personnel Training

The imaging team (e.g., physician, radiologic technologist, and medical physicist) should use techniques and protocols that administer the lowest radiation dose that will yield an image quality adequate for diagnosis and intervention.

Section 15.2 | **Electrocardiogram**

This section includes text excerpted from "Electrocardiogram," MedlinePlus, National Institutes of Health (NIH), December 10, 2020.

WHAT IS AN ELECTROCARDIOGRAM TEST?

An electrocardiogram (EKG) test is a simple, painless procedure that measures electrical signals in your heart. Each time your heart beats, an electrical signal travels through the heart. An EKG can show if your heart is beating at a normal rate and strength. It also helps show the size and position of your heart's chambers. An abnormal EKG can be a sign of heart disease or damage.

WHAT IS IT USED FOR?

An EKG test is used to find and/or monitor various heart disorders. These include:

- Irregular heartbeat (known as "arrhythmia")
- Blocked arteries
- Heart damage
- Heart failure
- Heart attack. EKGs are often used in the ambulance, emergency room, or other hospital room to diagnose a suspected heart attack.

An EKG test is sometimes included in a routine exam for middle-aged and older adults, as they have a higher risk of heart disease than younger people.

WHY DO YOU NEED AN ELECTROCARDIOGRAM TEST?

You may need an EKG test if you have symptoms of a heart disorder. These include:

- Chest pain
- Rapid heartbeat
- Arrhythmia (it may feel like your heart has skipped a beat or is fluttering)
- Shortness of breath

- Dizziness
- Fatigue

You may also need this test if you:
- Have had a heart attack or other heart problems in the past
- Have a family history of heart disease
- **Are scheduled for surgery.** Your health-care provider may want to check your heart health before the procedure.
- **Have a pacemaker.** The EKG can show how well the device is working.
- **Are taking medicine for heart disease.** The EKG can show if your medicine is effective, or if you need to make changes in your treatment.

WHAT HAPPENS DURING AN ELECTROCARDIOGRAM TEST?

An EKG test may be done in a provider's office, outpatient clinic, or a hospital. During the procedure:
- You will lie on an exam table.
- A health-care provider will place several electrodes (small sensors that stick to the skin) on your arms, legs, and chest. The provider may need to shave or trim excess hair before placing the electrodes.
- The electrodes are attached by wires to a computer that records your heart's electrical activity.
- The activity will be displayed on the computer's monitor and/or printed out on paper.
- The procedure only takes about three minutes.

WILL YOU NEED TO DO ANYTHING TO PREPARE FOR THE TEST?

You do not need any special preparations for an EKG test.

ARE THERE ANY RISKS TO THE TEST?

There is very little risk to having an EKG. You may feel a little discomfort or skin irritation after the electrodes are removed. There is no risk of electric shock. The EKG does not send any electricity to your body. It only records electricity.

WHAT DO THE RESULTS MEAN?

Your health-care provider will check your EKG results for a consistent heartbeat and rhythm. If your results were not normal, it may mean you have one of the following disorders:

- Arrhythmia
- A heartbeat that is too fast or too slow
- Inadequate blood supply to the heart
- A bulge in the heart's walls. This bulge is known as an "aneurysm."
- Thickening of the heart's walls
- A heart attack (Results can show if you have had a heart attack in the past or if you are having an attack during the EKG.)

If you have questions about your results, talk to your health-care provider.

EKG VERSUS ECG

An electrocardiogram may be called an "EKG" or an "ECG." Both are correct and commonly used. EKG is based on the German spelling, elektrokardiogramm. EKG may be preferred over ECG to avoid confusion with an EEG, a test that measures brain waves.

Section 15.3 | Functional Near-Infrared Spectroscopy

This section includes text excerpted from "Functional Near-Infrared Spectroscopy (fNIRS) Cognitive Brain Monitor," NASA's Technology Transfer Program, National Aeronautics and Space Administration (NASA), October 1, 2015. Reviewed June 2021.

Innovators at the National Aeronautics and Space Administration's (NASA) Glenn Research Center have developed a Functional Near-Infrared Spectroscopy (fNIRS) Cognitive Brain Monitor with improved signal processing to obtain more accurate data. fNIRS has been used successfully to monitor cognitive states and activity, and Glenn's system can be used to continuously monitor brain function during safety-critical tasks, such as flying an airplane or driving a train. Using head-worn sensors, the technique employs near-infrared light and advanced signal processing to allow real-time, in-task monitoring. The system not only determines changes in cognitive state by tracking blood hemoglobin levels in the brain but also filters nonrelevant artifacts, such as the probes' own motion, rendering the collected data even more accurate. Glenn's novel use and refinement of fNIRS signals stands to improve safety in a wide variety of applications and environments.

BENEFITS OF fNIRS
- **Improved safety.** Continuous monitoring of brain activity during safety-critical tasks could prevent serious accidents
- **High accuracy.** Removing motion artifacts allows real-world data capture to approach laboratory quality
- **Portability.** The system features comfortable head-worn sensors and is compact enough to fit into smaller spaces

APPLICATION OF fNIRS
- Safety simulations, training, and monitoring for airline pilots, train and mass transit engineers, ship captains, truck drivers, crane, and other heavy-equipment operators, and air traffic controllers
- Military simulations and training
- In-home, real-time monitoring and feedback during patient rehabilitation for cognitive impairment or depression
- Replacement for or supplement to functional brain imaging

THE TECHNOLOGY
Functional near-infrared spectroscopy is an emerging hemody-namic neuroimaging brain-computer interface (BCI) technology

that indirectly measures neuronal activity in the brain's cortex via neurovascular coupling. fNIRS works by quantifying hemoglobin-concentration changes in the brain based on optical intensity measurements, measuring the same hemodynamic changes as functional magnetic resonance imaging (fMRI). With enough probes in enough locations, fNIRS can detect these hemodynamic activations across the subject's entire head, thus allowing the determination of cognitive state through the use of pattern classification. fNIRS systems offer low-power, low-cost, highly mobile alternatives for real-time monitoring in safety-critical situations.

Glenn's specific contribution to this field is the algorithms capable of removing motion artifacts (environment- or equipment-induced errors) from the device's head-worn optical sensors. In other words, Glenn's adaptive filter can determine the presence of a potential motion artifact based on a phase shift in the data measured; identify the artifact by examining the correlation between the phase shift and changes in hemoglobin concentration; and finally remove the artifact using Kalman filtering whenever changes in hemoglobin level and changes in the phase shift are not correlated. Glenn's breakthrough allows the advantages of fNIRS to be used for noninvasive real-time brain monitoring applications in motion-filled environments that could potentially save lives.

Section 15.4 | Magnetic Resonance Imaging

This section includes text excerpted from "MRI (Magnetic Resonance Imaging)," U.S. Food and Drug Administration (FDA), August 29, 2018.

Magnetic resonance imaging (MRI) is a medical imaging procedure for making images of the internal structures of the body. MRI scanners use strong magnetic fields and radio waves (radiofrequency energy) to make images. The signal in an MR image comes mainly from the protons in fat and water molecules in the body.

During an MRI exam, an electric current is passed through coiled wires to create a temporary magnetic field in a patient's body.

Radio waves are sent from and received by a transmitter/receiver in the machine, and these signals are used to make digital images of the scanned area of the body. A typical MRI scan last from 20 to 90 minutes, depending on the part of the body being imaged.

For some MRI exams, intravenous (IV) drugs, such as gadolinium-based contrast agents (GBCAs) are used to change the contrast of the MR image. Gadolinium-based contrast agents are rare earth metals that are usually given through an IV in the arm.

USES OF AN MRI

An MRI gives health-care providers useful information about a variety of conditions and diagnostic procedures including:
- Abnormalities of the brain and spinal cord
- Abnormalities in various parts of the body such as breast, prostate, and liver
- Injuries or abnormalities of the joints
- The structure and function of the heart (cardiac imaging)
- Areas of activation within the brain (functional MRI or fMRI)
- Blood flow through blood vessels and arteries (angiography)
- The chemical composition of tissues (spectroscopy)

In addition to these diagnostic uses, MRI may also be used to guide certain interventional procedures.

BENEFITS AND RISKS
Benefits

An MRI scanner can be used to take images of any part of the body (e.g., head, joints, abdomen, legs, etc.) in any imaging direction. MRI provides better soft tissue contrast than CT and can differentiate better between fat, water, muscle, and other soft tissue than CT. (CT is usually better at imaging bones.) These images provide information to physicians and can be useful in diagnosing a wide variety of diseases and conditions.

Risks

An MR image is made without using any ionizing radiation, so patients are not exposed to the harmful effects of ionizing radiation. But, while there are no known health hazards from temporary exposure to the MR environment, the MR environment involves a strong, static magnetic field, a magnetic field that changes with time (pulsed gradient field), and radiofrequency energy, each of which carry specific safety concerns:

- The strong, static magnetic field will attract magnetic objects (from small items such as keys and cell phones, to large, heavy items such as oxygen tanks and floor buffers) and may cause damage to the scanner or injury to the patient or medical professionals if those objects become projectiles. Careful screening of people and objects entering the MR environment is critical to ensure nothing enters the magnet area that may become a projectile.
- The magnetic fields that change with time create loud knocking noises which may harm hearing if adequate ear protection is not used. They may also cause peripheral muscle or nerve stimulation that may feel like a twitching sensation.
- The radiofrequency energy used during the MRI scan could lead to heating of the body. The potential for heating is greater during long MRI examinations.

The use of gadolinium-based contrast agents (GBCAs) also carries some risk, including side effects such as allergic reactions to the contrast agent.

Some patients find the inside of the MRI scanner to be uncomfortably small and may experience claustrophobia. Imaging in an open MRI scanner may be an option for some patients, but not all MRI systems can perform all examinations, so you should discuss these options with your doctor. Your doctor may also be able to prescribe medication to make the experience easier for you.

To produce good quality images, patients must generally remain very still throughout the entire MRI procedure. Infants, small children, and other patients who are unable to lay still may need to be sedated or anesthetized for the procedure. Sedation and anesthesia carry risks not specific to the MRI procedure, such as slowed or difficult breathing, and low blood pressure.

Adverse Events

Adverse events for MRI scans are very rare. Millions of MRI scans are performed in the U.S. every year, and the FDA receives around 300 adverse event reports for MRI scanners and coils each year from manufacturers, distributors, user facilities, and patients. The majority of these reports describe heating and/or burns (thermal injuries). Second-degree burns are the most commonly reported patient problem. Other reported problems include injuries from projectile events (objects being drawn toward the MRI scanner), crushed and pinched fingers from the patient table, patient falls, and hearing loss or a ringing in the ear (tinnitus). The FDA has also received reports concerning the inadequate display or quality of the MR images.

WHAT PATIENTS SHOULD KNOW BEFORE HAVING AN MRI EXAM

Before your MRI exam, you will likely be asked to fill out a screening questionnaire. The International Society for Magnetic Resonance in Medicine (ISMRM) has a sample patient screening form available on its website (www.ismrm.org/smrt/safety_page/PreScrnF.pdf). For your safety, answering the questionnaire accurately is extremely important. In particular, make sure you notify the MRI technologist or radiologist if you have any implanted medical devices, such as stents, knee or hip replacements, pacemakers, or drug pumps. Also be sure to tell the technologist if you have any tattoos or drug patches as these can cause skin irritation or burns during the exam. The medical team will need to make sure that these devices can safely enter the MR environment.

Some devices are MR Safe or MR Conditional, meaning that they can be safely used in the MR environment under specific conditions. If you have an implant card for your device, bring it with you to your MRI exam so that you can help the doctor or the MRI technologist identify what type of device you have.

The space where you will lay in an MRI scanner to have your images taken can be a tight fit for some people, especially larger individuals. If you believe that you will feel claustrophobic, tell the MRI technologist or your doctor.

The MRI scanner will make a lot of noise as it takes images. This is normal. You should be offered earplugs and/or headphones to make the noise sound less loud. You may also be able to listen to music through the headphones to make the MRI exam more enjoyable.

If your exam includes a contrast agent, the MRI technologist will place a small intravenous (IV) line in one of your arms. You may feel some coldness when the contrast agent is injected. Be sure to notify the technologist if you feel any pain or discomfort.

Remember, your doctor has referred you to have an MRI because she or he believes the scan will provide useful information. If you have any questions about your procedure, do not be afraid to ask.

Questions to Ask Your Doctor

- "What information will the MRI scan provide? How might this change my treatment options?"
- "Is there any reason why I shouldn't have an MRI scan?" (If you have any implanted devices (such as a pacemaker, stents, an insulin pump, or an artificial joint), be sure your doctor knows about them.)
- "Will my exam involve contrast agent? What additional information will, using the contrast agent provide?"

Questions to Ask the MRI Technologist

- "How long can I expect my scan to last?"
- "Can I listen to music during my MRI scan? Can I choose the music?"
- "Where is the call button I can use to let you know if there is a problem?"

Section 15.5 | **Mammogram**

This section contains text excerpted from the following sources: Text beginning with the heading "What Is a Mammogram?" is excerpted from "Mammograms," Office on Women's Health (OWH), U.S. Department of Health and Human Services (HHS), April 1, 2019; Text beginning with the heading "Facility Certifications" is excerpted from "Mammography: What You Need to Know," U.S. Food and Drug Administration (FDA), January 13, 2021.

WHAT IS A MAMMOGRAM?

A mammogram is a low-dose x-ray exam of the breasts to look for changes that are not normal. The results are recorded on x-ray film or directly into a computer for a doctor called a "radiologist" to examine.

A mammogram allows the doctor to have a closer look for changes in breast tissue that cannot be felt during a breast exam. It is used for women who have no breast complaints and for women who have breast symptoms, such as a change in the shape or size of a breast, a lump, nipple discharge, or pain. Breast changes occur in almost all women. In fact, most of these changes are not cancer and are called "benign," but only a doctor can know for sure. Breast changes can also happen monthly, due to your menstrual period.

WHAT IS THE BEST METHOD OF DETECTING BREAST CANCER AS EARLY AS POSSIBLE?

A high-quality mammogram plus a clinical breast exam, an exam done by your doctor, is the most effective way to detect breast cancer early. Finding breast cancer early greatly improves a woman's chances for successful treatment.

Like any test, mammograms have both benefits and limitations. For example, some cancers cannot be found by a mammogram, but they may be found in a clinical breast exam.

Checking your own breasts for lumps or other changes is called a "breast self-exam" (BSE). Studies so far have not shown that BSE alone helps reduce the number of deaths from breast cancer. BSE should not take the place of routine clinical breast exams and mammograms.

If you choose to do BSE, remember that breast changes can occur because of pregnancy, aging, menopause, menstrual cycles, or from taking birth control pills (BCPs) or other hormones. It is normal for breasts to feel a little lumpy and uneven. Also, it is common for breasts to be swollen and tender right before or during a menstrual period. If you notice any unusual changes in your breasts, contact your doctor.

HOW IS A MAMMOGRAM DONE?

You stand in front of a special x-ray machine. The person who takes the x-rays, called a "radiologic technician," places your breasts, one at a time, between an x-ray plate and a plastic plate. These plates are attached to the x-ray machine and compress the breasts to flatten them. This spreads the breast tissue out to obtain a clearer picture. You will feel pressure on your breast for a few seconds. It may cause you some discomfort; you might feel squeezed or pinched. This feeling only lasts for a few seconds, and the flatter your breast, the better the picture. Most often, two pictures are taken of each breast – one from the side and one from above. A screening mammogram takes about 20 minutes from start to finish.

ARE THERE DIFFERENT TYPES OF MAMMOGRAMS?

- Screening mammograms are done for women who have no symptoms of breast cancer. It usually involves two x-rays of each breast. Screening mammograms can detect lumps or tumors that cannot be felt. They can also find microcalcifications or tiny deposits of calcium in the breast, which sometimes mean that breast cancer is present.
- Diagnostic mammograms are used to check for breast cancer after a lump or other symptom or sign of breast cancer has been found. Signs of breast cancer may include pain, thickened skin on the breast, nipple discharge, or a change in breast size or shape. This type of mammogram also can be used to find out more about breast changes found on a screening mammogram or to view breast

tissue that is hard to see on a screening mammogram. A diagnostic mammogram takes longer than a screening mammogram because it involves more x-rays in order to obtain views of the breast from several angles. The technician can magnify a problem area to make a more detailed picture, which helps the doctor make a correct diagnosis.

A digital mammogram also uses x-rays to produce an image of the breast, but instead of storing the image directly on film, the image is stored directly on a computer. This allows the recorded image to be magnified for the doctor to take a closer look. Current research has not shown that digital images are better at showing cancer than x-ray film images in general. But, women with dense breasts who are pre- or peri-menopausal, or who are younger than 50 years of age, may benefit from having a digital rather than a film mammogram. Digital mammography may offer these benefits:

- Long-distance consultations with other doctors may be easier because the images can be shared by computer.
- Slight differences between normal and abnormal tissues may be more easily noted.
- The number of follow-up tests needed may be fewer.
- Fewer repeat images may be needed, reducing exposure to radiation.

WHAT CAN MAMMOGRAMS SHOW?

The radiologist will look at your x-rays for breast changes that do not look normal and for differences in each breast. She or he will compare your past mammograms with your most recent ones to check for changes. The doctor will also look for lumps and calcifications.

- **Lump or mass.** The size, shape, and edges of a lump sometimes can give doctors information about whether or not it may be cancer. On a mammogram, a growth that is benign often looks smooth and round with a clear, defined edge. Breast cancer often has a jagged outline and an irregular shape.

- **Calcification.** A calcification is a deposit of the mineral calcium in the breast tissue. Calcifications appear as small white spots on a mammogram. There are two types:
  - Macrocalcifications are large calcium deposits often caused by aging. These usually are not a sign of cancer.
  - Microcalcifications are tiny specks of calcium that may be found in an area of rapidly dividing cells.

If calcifications are grouped together in a certain way, it may be a sign of cancer. Depending on how many calcium specks you have, how big they are, and what they look like, your doctor may suggest that you have other tests. Calcium in the diet does not create calcium deposits, or calcifications, in the breast.

WHAT IF YOUR SCREENING MAMMOGRAM SHOWS A PROBLEM?

If you have a screening test result that suggests cancer, your doctor must find out whether it is due to cancer or to some other cause. Your doctor may ask about your personal and family medical history. You may have a physical exam. Your doctor also may order some of these tests:

- Diagnostic mammogram, to focus on a specific area of the breast
- Ultrasound, an imaging test that uses sound waves to create a picture of your breast. The pictures may show whether a lump is solid or filled with fluid. A cyst is a fluid-filled sac. Cysts are not cancer. But, a solid mass may be cancer. After the test, your doctor can store the pictures on video or print them out. This exam may be used along with a mammogram.
- Magnetic resonance imaging (MRI), which uses a powerful magnet linked to a computer. MRI makes detailed pictures of breast tissue. Your doctor can view these pictures on a monitor or print them on film. MRI may be used along with a mammogram.

- Biopsy, a test in which fluid or tissue is removed from your breast to help find out if there is cancer. Your doctor may refer you to a surgeon or to a doctor who is an expert in breast disease for a biopsy.

WHERE CAN YOU GET A HIGH-QUALITY MAMMOGRAM?

Women can get high-quality mammograms in breast clinics, hospital radiology departments, mobile vans, private radiology offices, and doctors' offices. The U.S. Food and Drug Administration (FDA) certifies mammography facilities that meet strict quality standards for their x-ray machines and staff and are inspected every year. You can ask your doctor or the staff at the mammography center about the FDA certification before making your appointment. A list of FDA-certified facilities can be found on the Internet.

Your doctor, local medical clinic, or local or state health department can tell you where to get no-cost or low-cost mammograms. You can also call the National Cancer Institute's Cancer Information Service toll free at 800-422-6237.

HOW DO YOU GET READY FOR YOUR MAMMOGRAM?

First, check with the place you are having the mammogram for any special instructions you may need to follow before you go. Here are some general guidelines to follow:

- If you are still having menstrual periods, try to avoid making your mammogram appointment during the week before your period. Your breasts will be less tender and swollen. The mammogram will hurt less and the picture will be better.
- If you have breast implants, be sure to tell your mammography facility that you have them when you make your appointment.
- Wear a shirt with shorts, pants, or a skirt. This way, you can undress from the waist up and leave your shorts, pants, or skirt on when you get your mammogram.

- Do not wear any deodorant, perfume, lotion, or powder under your arms or on your breasts on the day of your mammogram appointment. These things can make shadows show up on your mammogram.
- If you have had mammograms at another facility, have those x-ray films sent to the new facility so that they can be compared to the new films.

FACILITY CERTIFICATIONS

Mammograms continue to be the best primary tool for breast cancer screening. The FDA, along with some FDA-approved State certifying agencies, certify facilities to perform mammography. The FDA also clears and approves new mammography devices for sale in the United States.

Congress enacted the Mammography Quality Standards Act (MQSA) in 1992 to ensure all women have access to quality mammography for the detection of breast cancer in its early, most treatable stages. Always look for the MQSA certificate at the mammography facility, which is required to be displayed and indicates that the facility meets the national baseline standards for mammography.

To continue to protect women's health, the FDA is proposing updates to the mammography regulations to reflect advances in mammography technology and processes since the current regulations were published.

WHY IS FACILITY CERTIFICATION IMPORTANT?

Under the MQSA, mammography facilities must be certified by the FDA, or an FDA-approved state certifying agency, to provide mammography services. Certification is important because it indicates that a facility has met the MQSA requirements for practicing quality mammography. A high-quality mammogram can help detect breast cancer in its earliest, most treatable stages.

Each mammography facility is inspected every year. During the inspection, an FDA or FDA-trained inspector checks the facility's equipment, staff training qualifications, and quality control records. Each facility also undergoes an in-depth accreditation process every three years to be eligible for an MQSA certificate.

The certificate, which is required to be prominently displayed, shows that the facility has met the MQSA quality standards and may legally perform mammography. When you arrive for your mammogram, look for the certificate. If you do not see it, ask for where the certificate is in the facility.

WHAT ARE 3D MAMMOGRAMS?

New breast imaging equipment must receive the FDA's approval or clearance before being sold in the U.S. In recent years, the FDA has approved 3D advanced mammography devices that can create multiple cross-sectional images of the breast from x-rays taken from multiple angles. These devices provide informative images of the breast tissue and may be helpful in evaluating dense breast tissue.

Before granting approval, the FDA determined there was a reasonable assurance that the new 3D devices were safe and effective for their intended use. This determination was based on a review of clinical studies involving multiple radiologists and hundreds of cases. The FDA also sought input on the safety and effectiveness of the devices from a panel of non-FDA clinical and technical experts.

HOW WILL THE PROPOSED MQSA CHANGES (IF FINALIZED), HELP YOU?

If finalized, the proposed MQSA amendments would, among additional updates and changes:

- Better inform you and your health-care provider about your mammography results by providing specific information on breast density, an independent risk factor for breast cancer.
- Strengthen the FDA's ability to suspend or revoke the certificates of facilities that are noncompliant with the regulations.
- Require facilities to provide mammography personnel access to their own records of MQSA-qualifying training and experience upon their reasonable request, so they may continue to provide mammography services.

Section 15.6 | **Medical X-ray Imaging**

This section includes text excerpted from "Medical X-ray Imaging," U.S. Food and Drug Administration (FDA), September 28, 2020.

Medical imaging has led to improvements in the diagnosis and treatment of numerous medical conditions in children and adults.

There are many types – or modalities – of medical imaging procedures, each of which uses different technologies and techniques. Computed tomography (CT), fluoroscopy, and radiography ("conventional x-ray" including mammography) all use ionizing radiation to generate images of the body. Ionizing radiation is a form of radiation that has enough energy to potentially cause damage to DNA and may elevate a person's lifetime risk of developing cancer.

A CT, radiography, and fluoroscopy all work on the same basic principle: an x-ray beam is passed through the body where a portion of the x-rays are either absorbed or scattered by the internal structures, and the remaining x-ray pattern is transmitted to a detector (e.g., film or a computer screen) for recording or further processing by a computer. These exams differ in their purpose:

- **Radiography.** A single image is recorded for later evaluation. Mammography is a special type of radiography to image the internal structures of breasts.

- **Fluoroscopy.** A continuous x-ray image is displayed on a monitor, allowing for real-time monitoring of a procedure or passage of a contrast agent ("dye") through the body. Fluoroscopy can result in relatively high radiation doses, especially for complex interventional procedures (such as placing stents or other devices inside the body) which require fluoroscopy to be administered for a long period of time.

- **Computed tomography.** Many x-ray images are recorded as the detector moves around the patient's body. A computer reconstructs all the individual images into cross-sectional images or "slices" of internal organs and tissues. A CT exam involves a higher radiation dose than conventional radiography because the CT image is reconstructed from many individual x-ray projections.

BENEFITS AND RISKS
Benefits

The discovery of x-rays and the invention of CT represented major advances in medicine. X-ray imaging exams are recognized as a valuable medical tool for a wide variety of examinations and procedures. They are used to:

- Noninvasively and painlessly help to diagnose disease and monitor therapy.
- Support medical and surgical treatment planning.
- Guide medical personnel as they insert catheters, stents, or other devices inside the body, treat tumors, or remove blood clots or other blockages.

Risks

As in many aspects of medicine, there are risks associated with the use of x-ray imaging, which uses ionizing radiation to generate images of the body. Ionizing radiation is a form of radiation that has enough energy to potentially cause damage to DNA. Risks from exposure to ionizing radiation include:

- A small increase in the possibility that a person exposed to x-rays will develop cancer later in life.
- Tissue effects such as cataracts, skin reddening, and hair loss, which occur at relatively high levels of radiation exposure and are rare for many types of imaging exams. For example, the typical use of a CT scanner or conventional radiography equipment should not result in tissue effects, but the dose to the skin from some long, complex interventional fluoroscopy procedures might, in some circumstances, be high enough to result in such effects.

Another risk of x-ray imaging is possible reactions associated with an intravenously injected contrast agent, or "dye," that is sometimes used to improve visualization.

The risk of developing cancer from medical imaging radiation exposure is generally very small, and it depends on:

- **Radiation dose.** The lifetime risk of cancer increases the larger the dose and the more x-ray exams a patient undergoes.
- **Patient's age.** The lifetime risk of cancer is larger for a patient who receives x-rays at a younger age than for one who receives them at an older age.
- **Patient's sex.** Women are at a somewhat higher lifetime risk than men for developing radiation-associated cancer after receiving the same exposures at the same ages.
- **Body region.** Some organs are more radiosensitive than others.

The above statements are generalizations based on scientific analyses of large population data sets, such as survivors exposed to radiation from the atomic bomb. While specific individuals or cases may not fit into such generalizations, they are still useful in developing an overall approach to medical imaging radiation safety by identifying at-risk populations or higher-risk procedures.

Because radiation risks are dependent on exposure to radiation, an awareness of the typical radiation exposures involved in different imaging exams is useful for communication between the physician and patient.

The medical community has emphasized radiation dose reduction in CT because of the relatively high radiation dose for CT exams (as compared to radiography) and their increased use, as reported in the National Council on Radiation Protection and Measurements (NCRP) Report No. 160. Because tissue effects are extremely rare for typical use of many x-ray imaging devices (including CT), the primary radiation risk concern for most imaging studies is cancer; however, the long exposure times needed for complex interventional fluoroscopy exams and resulting high skin doses may result in tissue effects, even when the equipment is used appropriately.

Balancing Benefits and Risks

While the benefit of a clinically appropriate x-ray imaging exam generally far outweighs the risk, efforts should be made to minimize this risk by reducing unnecessary exposure to ionizing radiation. To help reduce risk to the patient, all exams using ionizing radiation should be performed only when necessary to answer a medical question, treat a disease, or guide a procedure. If there is a medical need for a particular imaging procedure and other exams using no or less radiation are less appropriate, then the benefits exceed the risks, and radiation risk considerations should not influence the physician's decision to perform the study or the patient's decision to have the procedure. However, the "As Low as Reasonably Achievable" (ALARA) principle should always be followed when choosing equipment settings to minimize radiation exposure to the patient.

- Patient factors are important to consider in this balance of benefits and risks. For example:
- Because younger patients are more sensitive to radiation, special care should be taken in reducing radiation exposure to pediatric patients for all types of x-ray imaging exams.
- Special care should also be taken in imaging pregnant patients due to possible effects of radiation exposure to the developing fetus.
- The benefit of possible disease detection should be carefully balanced against the risks of an imaging screening study on healthy, asymptomatic patients.

INFORMATION FOR PATIENTS

X-ray imaging (CT, fluoroscopy, and radiography) exams should be performed only after careful consideration of the patient's health needs. They should be performed only when the referring physician judges them to be necessary to answer a clinical question or to guide treatment of a disease. The clinical benefit of a medically appropriate x-ray imaging exam outweighs the small radiation risk. However, efforts should be made to help minimize this risk.

Questions to Ask Your Health-Care Provider

Patients and parents of children undergoing x-ray imaging exams should be well informed and prepared by:

- Keeping track of medical-imaging histories as part of a discussion with the referring physician when a new exam is recommended.
- Informing their physician if they are pregnant or think they might be pregnant.
- Asking the referring physician about the benefits and risks of imaging procedures, such as:
  - How will the results of the exam be used to evaluate my condition or guide my treatment (or that of my child)?
  - Are there alternative exams that do not use ionizing radiation that are equally useful?
- Asking the imaging facility:
  - If it uses techniques to reduce radiation dose, especially to sensitive populations such as children.
  - About any additional steps that may be necessary to perform the imaging study (e.g., administration of oral or intravenous contrast agent to improve visualization, sedation, or advanced preparation).
  - If the facility is accredited. (Accreditation may only be available for specific types of x-ray imaging such as CT.)

Section 15.7 | Nuclear Medicine

This section includes text excerpted from "Nuclear Medicine," National Institute of Biomedical Imaging and Bioengineering (NIBIB), July 2016. Reviewed June 2021.

WHAT IS NUCLEAR MEDICINE?

Nuclear medicine is a medical specialty that uses radioactive tracers (radiopharmaceuticals) to assess bodily functions and to diagnose and treat disease. Specially designed cameras allow doctors to track the path of these radioactive tracers. Single photon emission computed tomography (SPECT) and positron emission tomography (PET) scans are the two most common imaging modalities in nuclear medicine.

WHAT ARE RADIOACTIVE TRACERS?

Radioactive tracers are made up of carrier molecules that are bonded tightly to a radioactive atom. These carrier molecules vary greatly depending on the purpose of the scan. Some tracers employ molecules that interact with a specific protein or sugar in the body and can even employ the patient's own cells. For example, in cases where doctors need to know the exact source of intestinal bleeding, they may radiolabel (add radioactive atoms) to a sample of red blood cells taken from the patient. They then reinject the blood and use a SPECT scan to follow the path of the blood in the patient. Any accumulation of radioactivity in the intestines informs doctors of where the problem lies.

For most diagnostic studies in nuclear medicine, the radioactive tracer is administered to a patient by intravenous injection. However a radioactive tracer may also be administered by inhalation, by oral ingestion, or by direct injection into an organ. The mode of tracer administration will depend on the disease process that is to be studied.

Approved tracers are called "radiopharmaceuticals" since they must meet the U.S. Food and Drug Administration's (FDA) exacting standards for safety and appropriate performance for the approved clinical use. The nuclear medicine physician will select the tracer that will provide the most specific and reliable information for a patient's particular problem. The tracer that is used determines whether the patient receives a SPECT or PET scan.

WHAT IS SINGLE PHOTON EMISSION COMPUTED TOMOGRAPHY?

Single photon emission computed tomography imaging instruments provide three-dimensional (tomographic) images of the distribution of radioactive tracer molecules that have been introduced into the patient's body. The 3D images are computer generated from a large number of projection images of the body recorded at different angles. SPECT imagers have gamma camera detectors that can detect the gamma ray emissions from the tracers that have been injected into the patient. Gamma rays are a form of light that moves at a different wavelength than visible light. The cameras are mounted on a rotating gantry that allows the detectors to be moved in a tight circle around a patient who is lying motionless on a pallet.

WHAT IS POSITRON EMISSION TOMOGRAPHY?

Positron emission tomography scans also use radiopharmaceuticals to create three-dimensional images. The main difference between SPECT and PET scans is the type of radiotracers used. While SPECT scans measure gamma rays, the decay of the radiotracers used with PET scans produce small particles called "positrons." A positron is a particle with roughly the same mass as an electron but oppositely charged. These react with electrons in the body and when these two particles combine they annihilate each other. This annihilation produces a small amount of energy in the form of two photons that shoot off in opposite directions. The detectors in the PET scanner measure these photons and use this information to create images of internal organs.

WHAT ARE NUCLEAR MEDICINE SCANS USED FOR?

Single photon emission computed tomography scans are primarily used to diagnose and track the progression of heart disease, such as blocked coronary arteries. There are also radiotracers to detect disorders in bone, gall bladder disease, and intestinal bleeding. SPECT agents have recently become available for aiding in the diagnosis of Parkinson disease (PD) in the brain, and distinguishing this malady from other anatomically-related movement disorders and dementias.

The major purpose of PET scans is to detect cancer and monitor its progression, response to treatment, and to detect metastases. Glucose utilization depends on the intensity of cellular and tissue activity so it is greatly increased in rapidly dividing cancer cells. In fact, the degree of aggressiveness for most cancers is roughly paralleled by their rate of glucose utilization. In the last 15 years, slightly modified radiolabeled glucose molecules (F-18 labeled deoxyglucose or FDG) have been shown to be the best available tracer for detecting cancer and its metastatic spread in the body.

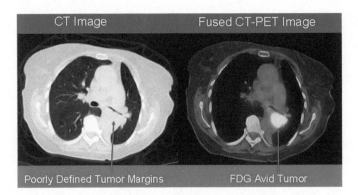

Figure 15.4. Fused CT-PET Scan

A combination instrument that produces both PET and CT scans of the same body regions in one examination (PET/CT scanner) has become the primary imaging tool for the staging of most cancers worldwide.

A PET probe was approved by the FDA to aid in the accurate diagnosis of Alzheimer disease (AD), which previously could be diagnosed with accuracy only after a patient's death. In the absence of this PET imaging test, AD can be difficult to distinguish from vascular dementia or other forms of dementia that affect older people.

ARE THERE RISKS?

The total radiation dose conferred to patients by the majority of radiopharmaceuticals used in diagnostic nuclear medicine studies is no more than what is conferred during routine chest x-rays or CT exams. There are legitimate concerns about possible cancer induction even by low levels of radiation exposure from cumulative medical imaging examinations, but this risk is accepted to be quite small in contrast to the expected benefit derived from a medically needed diagnostic imaging study.

Like radiologists, nuclear medicine physicians are strongly committed to keeping radiation exposure to patients as low as possible, giving the least amount of radiotracer needed to provide a diagnostically useful examination.

HOW ARE NIBIB-FUNDED RESEARCHERS ADVANCING NUCLEAR MEDICINE?

Research in nuclear medicine involves developing new radio tracers as well as technologies that will help physicians produce clearer pictures.

Developing New Tracers

A bacterial infection is a common complication of implanting a medical device into the body. With more patients receiving device implants than ever before, infections from implants are a growing problem. Currently, these types of infections are diagnosed based on physical exam results and microbial cultures. However, such techniques are only useful for detecting late stage infections, which usually have already become difficult to treat. Conversely, medical devices may be needlessly removed when doctors mistake inflammation that is a normal consequence of surgery with inflammation due to an infection.

The National Institute of Biomedical Imaging and Bioengineering (NIBIB) is supporting research to develop a new family of PET imaging contrast agents that are taken up specifically by bacterial cells, but not human cells. Such imaging agents would allow doctors to visualize early-stage bacterial infections so they can be easily treated, thereby reducing the number of implanted devices that are unnecessarily removed. They also have the potential to be used for diagnosing infections not associated with medical devices, for example, those affecting the heart or lungs.

Creating New Technology

A SPECT tracer is available for an accurate diagnosis of PD. However, the small region in the brain that must be imaged requires a dedicated brain SPECT imager with special gamma cameras to provide high resolution, which adds to the cost of the procedure. The NIBIB is supporting research to create an inexpensive adapter for the conventional SPECT imagers that most hospitals already have. The adapter would allow standard clinical SPECT cameras to provide the same high resolution that currently only dedicated SPECT brain imaging systems can produce. These improvements would make Parkinson diagnosis less costly and more widely available.

Section 15.8 | Optical Imaging

This section includes text excerpted from "Optical Imaging," National Institute of Biomedical Imaging and Bioengineering (NIBIB), December 2, 2020.

WHAT IS OPTICAL IMAGING?

Optical imaging uses light and special properties of photons to obtain detailed images of organs, tissues, cells and even molecules. The techniques offer minimally or noninvasive methods for looking inside the body.

WHAT ARE THE ADVANTAGES OF OPTICAL IMAGING?

Optical imaging significantly reduces patient exposure to harmful radiation by using nonionizing radiation, which includes visible, ultraviolet, and infrared light. Because it is much safer than techniques that require ionizing radiation, such as x-rays, optical imaging can be used for repeated procedures to monitor the progression of disease or the results of treatment.

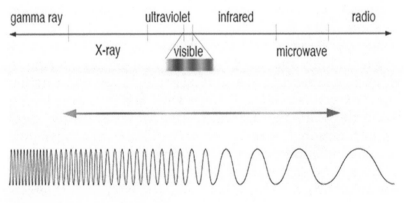

Figure 15.5. Electromagnetic Spectrum

Optical imaging is particularly useful for measuring multiple properties of soft tissue. Because of the wide variety of ways different soft tissues absorb and scatter light, optical imaging can measure metabolic changes that are early markers of abnormal functioning of organs and tissues.

Optical imaging can be combined with other imaging techniques, such as MRI or x-rays, to provide enhanced information for doctors monitoring complex diseases or researchers working on intricate experiments.

WHAT TYPES OF OPTICAL IMAGING ARE THERE AND WHAT ARE THEY USED FOR?

Endoscopy uses an endoscope, which is a flexible tube with a light source to illuminate an organ or tissue. An endoscope can be inserted through a patient's mouth and into the digestive cavity to find the cause of symptoms such as pain, difficulty swallowing, or gastrointestinal bleeding.

Optical coherence tomography (OCT) is a technique for obtaining sub-surface images such as diseased tissue just below the skin. Ophthalmologists use OCT to obtain detailed images from within the retina. Cardiologists also use it to help diagnose coronary artery disease.

Photoacoustic imaging delivers laser pulses to a patient's tissues; the pulses generate heat, expanding the tissues and enabling their structure to be imaged. The technique can help monitor blood vessel growth in tumors, detect skin melanomas, and track blood oxygenation in tissues.

Diffuse optical tomography (DOT) and Imaging (DOI) are noninvasive techniques that use light in the near-infrared region to measure tissue properties such as total hemoglobin concentration and blood oxygen saturation. Because DOT and DOI work well in soft tissue, the techniques are widely used for breast cancer imaging, brain functional imaging, stroke detection, photodynamic therapy, and radiation therapy monitoring.

Raman spectroscopy relies on Raman scattering of visible, near-infrared, or near-ultraviolet light. The laser light interacts with molecular vibrations in the material, with shifts in energy revealing the material's chemical properties. Applications include identifying chemical compounds and the structure of materials and crystals. During surgery, Raman gas analyzers are used to monitor the mixture of gases used for anesthesia.

Super-resolution microscopy encompasses a number of techniques to obtain very high-resolution images of individual cells. One example is photoactivated localization microscopy (PALM), which uses individual fluorescently marked molecules to create a super-resolution image comprised of a compilation of individual molecules in a cell or tissue.

WHAT ARE NIBIB-FUNDED RESEARCHERS DEVELOPING IN THE AREA OF OPTICAL IMAGING?

Novel optical imaging for more accurate glaucoma screening. Glaucoma is a leading cause of blindness. Early diagnosis and treatment can slow or stop progression to blindness, but the current test for elevated intraocular pressure is inadequate for detecting glaucoma at an early stage. Changes in the collagen fibers of the sclera (white of the eye) play a significant role in the disease process, potentially offering a reliable marker of early stage glaucoma. The National Institute of Biomedical Imaging and Bioengineering (NIBIB)-funded biomedical engineers are developing a novel optical imaging technique that can detect changes in the structure of the collagen fibers of the eye sclera. The technique employs a computational model that correlates specific changes in sclera proteins with early onset glaucoma. The new test will enable early initiation of vision-sparing treatment and continuous noninvasive monitoring of the response to treatment.

Assessing and treating neurological damage associated with cardiac arrest. Eighty to ninety percent of cardiac arrest (CA) survivors suffer significant neurological damage. Addressing these devastating effects has not been possible due to the need for imaging of rapid changes to blood flow and metabolism in the brain during CA and during emergency CPR. Engineers are developing an optical imaging system for critical real-time imaging that measures cerebral blood flow and metabolic functions such as oxygen consumption. Optical imaging will be paired with electroencephalography (EEG) to study neurological changes related to interrupted blood flow. The system will enable advanced study of brain injury during CA and CPR and offer real-time treatment options that can improve survival and outcome for CA patients.

Noninvasive imaging to monitor breast cancer chemotherapy. Bioengineers are developing noninvasive optical imaging techniques that can monitor tumor chemotherapy and rapidly identify the 20 percent of breast tumors that do not respond. Signals emitted from painless near-infrared light-based probes provide measurements of fat content, blood vessel formation, and oxygen levels, which indicate whether or not the chemotherapy has begun to shrink the tumor early in the course of treatment. Such information will allow physicians to stop chemotherapy and/or change treatment if the patient is not responding, enabling overall improved management of breast cancer treatment.

Section 15.9 | Ultrasound

This section includes text excerpted from "Ultrasound Imaging," U.S. Food and Drug Administration (FDA), September 28, 2020.

Ultrasound imaging (sonography) uses high-frequency sound waves to view inside the body. Because ultrasound images are captured in real-time, they can also show movement of the body's internal organs as well as blood flowing through the blood vessels. Unlike x-ray imaging, there is no ionizing radiation exposure associated with ultrasound imaging.

In an ultrasound exam, a transducer (probe) is placed directly on the skin or inside a body opening. A thin layer of gel is applied to the skin so that the ultrasound waves are transmitted from the transducer through the gel into the body.

The ultrasound image is produced based on the reflection of the waves off of the body structures. The strength (amplitude) of the sound signal and the time it takes for the wave to travel through the body provide the information necessary to produce an image.

USES OF ULTRASOUND IMAGING

Ultrasound imaging is a medical tool that can help a physician evaluate, diagnose and treat medical conditions. Common ultrasound imaging procedures include:

- Abdominal ultrasound (to visualize abdominal tissues and organs)
- Bone sonometry (to assess bone fragility)
- Breast ultrasound (to visualize breast tissue)
- Doppler fetal heart rate monitors (to listen to the fetal heartbeat)
- Doppler ultrasound (to visualize blood flow through a blood vessel, organs, or other structures)
- Echocardiogram (to view the heart)
- Fetal ultrasound (to view the fetus in pregnancy)
- Ultrasound-guided biopsies (to collect a sample of tissue)
- Ophthalmic ultrasound (to visualize ocular structures
- Ultrasound-guided needle placement (in blood vessels or other tissues of interest)

BENEFITS AND RISKS

Ultrasound imaging has been used for over 20 years and has an excellent safety record. It is based on nonionizing radiation, so it does not have the same risks as x-rays or other types of imaging systems that use ionizing radiation.

Although ultrasound imaging is generally considered safe when used prudently by appropriately trained health-care providers, ultrasound energy has the potential to produce biological effects on the body. Ultrasound waves can heat the tissues slightly. In some cases, it can also produce small pockets of gas in body fluids or tissues (cavitation). The long-term consequences of these effects are still unknown.

Because of the particular concern for effects on the fetus, organizations such as the American Institute of Ultrasound in Medicine (AIUM) have advocated prudent use of ultrasound imaging in pregnancy. Furthermore, the use of ultrasound solely for nonmedical purposes such as obtaining fetal 'keepsake' videos has been discouraged. Keepsake images or videos are reasonable if they are produced during a medically indicated exam, and if no additional exposure is required.

INFORMATION FOR PATIENTS INCLUDING EXPECTANT MOTHERS

For all medical imaging procedures, the U.S. Food and Drug Administration (FDA) recommends that patients talk to their health-care provider to understand the reason for the examination, the medical information that will be obtained, the potential risks, and how the results will be used to manage the medical condition or pregnancy. Because ultrasound is not based on ionizing radiation, it is particularly useful for women of child-bearing age when CT or other imaging methods would otherwise result in exposure to radiation.

Expectant Mothers

Ultrasound is the most widely used medical imaging method for viewing the fetus during pregnancy. Routine examinations are performed to assess and monitor the health status of the fetus and mother. Ultrasound examinations provide parents with a valuable opportunity to view and hear the heartbeat of the fetus, bond with the unborn baby, and capture images to share with family and friends.

In fetal ultrasound, three-dimensional (3D) ultrasound allows the visualization of some facial features and possibly other parts such as fingers and toes of the fetus. Four-dimensional (4D) ultrasound is 3D ultrasound in motion. While ultrasound is generally considered to be safe with very low risks, the risks may increase with unnecessary prolonged exposure to ultrasound energy, or when untrained users operate the device.

Expectant mothers should also be aware of concerns with purchasing over-the-counter (OTC) fetal heartbeat monitoring systems (also called "doptones"). These devices should only be used by trained health-care providers when medically necessary. Use of these devices by untrained persons could expose the fetus to prolonged and unsafe energy levels or could provide information that is interpreted incorrectly by the user.

Chapter 16 | Advances in Imaging

Chapter Contents

Section 16.1 | **Magnetic Resonance Elastography**

This section includes text excerpted from "Imaging a Brain Thinking, Using a New MRI Technique," National Institute of Biomedical Imaging and Bioengineering (NIBIB), August 13, 2019.

An international team of researchers with partial support from the National Institute of Biomedical Imaging and Bioengineering (NIBIB) developed a new magnetic resonance imaging (MRI) technique that can capture an image of a brain's thinking by measuring changes in tissue stiffness. The results show that brain function can be tracked on a time scale of 100 milliseconds – 60 times faster than previous methods. The technique could shed new light on altered neuronal activity in brain diseases.

The human brain responds almost immediately to stimuli, but noninvasive imaging techniques have not been able to keep pace with the brain. Currently, several noninvasive brain imaging methods measure brain function, but they all have limitations. Most commonly, clinicians and researchers use functional magnetic resonance imaging (fMRI) to measure brain activity via fluctuations in blood oxygen levels. However, a lot of vital brain activity information is lost using fMRI because blood oxygen levels take about six seconds to respond to a stimulus.

Since the mid-1990s, researchers have been able to generate maps of tissue stiffness using an MRI scanner, with a noninvasive technique called "magnetic resonance elastography" (MRE). Tissue stiffness cannot be measured directly, so instead researchers use MRE to measure the speed at which mechanical vibrations travel through tissue. Vibrations move faster through stiffer tissues, while vibrations travel through softer tissue more slowly; therefore, tissue stiffness can be determined. MRE is most commonly used to detect the hardening of liver tissue but has more recently been applied to other tissues such as the brain.

"This study has the potential to revolutionize the way scientists study brain diseases," says Krishna Kandarpa, M.D., Ph.D., director of research science and strategic directions at the NIBIB. "Developing a new MRI technique relies heavily on physics and engineering principles, which are areas in which the NIBIB investigators excel. The results would have been hard to achieve without the collaboration of this team of experts."

Sam Patz, Ph.D., a professor of radiology at Harvard Medical School and a physicist at Brigham and Women's Hospital Department of Radiology, explained that his initial plan was to use MRE in combination with another MRI method to study scar tissue in the lung. "I did not have experience with MRE, so I turned to my colleague who is a pioneer in MRE, Dr. Ralph Sinkus," said Patz.

Sinkus, a professor of biomedical engineering at King's College London and cocorresponding author of the Science Advances publication, helped Patz set up the MRE lung imaging experiments in his Boston lab. As the team was working on launching the lung experiments, they ran into numerous complications and decided it was easier to start with the mouse brain. Due to their exciting results, the team continued to study the mouse brain.

Patz and Sinkus were elated with the first MRE images of the mouse brain – they were of excellent quality. "We observed that the auditory cortex, which a mouse uses to hear, was a bit stiffer than other parts of the cortex. We searched for an answer but came up empty-handed," stated Patz. "We hypothesized that perhaps the auditory cortex had increased blood flow due to the noise from the MRI scanner. The idea was that the auditory cortex capillaries were under higher pressure when stimulated; similar to when you turn on a garden hose, the hose gets stiffer."

Patz followed up with experiments to confirm the hypothesis by blocking one, or both of a mouse's ear canals with a gel to mute the noise from the MRI scanner. "The results were dramatic," Patz exclaimed. "It was clear that removing the stimulus resulted in softer tissue, and that the variation in stiffness was real."

Initially, it took the researchers about 20 minutes to obtain one MRE scan. The team was concerned the long stimulus time would lead to a reduced response after prolonged or repeated exposures, a phenomenon named as "habituation."

Together Patz and Sinkus worked to create a new MRI protocol to reduce the need for a long stimulus time, to avoid habituation. The new method switches between "on" and "off" stimulus states that are created by an electrical impulse delivered to a mouse's hind limb every nine seconds. Two images of the mouse brain are generated that correspond to each stimulus state and are subtracted to show changes in tissue stiffness. Nine seconds allows enough time for the blood flow in the activated areas of the brain to respond.

At first, the team thought that the changes in tissue stiffness were due to the changes in blood supply, another manifestation of what traditional fMRI detects. So, they decided to switch between the two stimulus states much faster than the blood system could respond. Remarkably, the data exhibited the same robust change in stiffness after a one-second stimulus, and the researchers concluded the changes they had observed in the mice had nothing to do with blood flow.

After this result, colleagues urged the researchers to try even faster speeds. The published results show about a 10 percent change in stiffness even after the stimulus states were varied every 100 milliseconds. These results are the closest to real-time MRI brain imaging researchers have achieved to date.

Now, the group is moving on to perform a similar study in healthy human brains to establish a robust protocol. Preliminary results from human brains show alterations in tissue stiffness in times as short as 24 milliseconds.

Once the technology has been translated to human use, the pair will be able to investigate brain diseases. The technique could provide new ways of diagnosing and understanding brain activity variation in diseases, such as Alzheimer, dementia, epilepsy, or multiple sclerosis (MS).

Additionally, the technology may also be applied to cancer patients with large brain tumors. Sometimes a large tumor mass will block the blood flow that traditional fMRI detects, so it is not possible to obtain a good image. Since the new methods are not thought to rely on blood flow, they may be able to attain better images in these patients and help inform treatment strategies.

Section 16.2 | **Neuroimaging Technique to Predict Autism among High-Risk Infants**

This section includes text excerpted from "Neuroimaging Technique May Help Predict Autism among High-Risk Infants," National Institute of Mental Health (NIMH), June 16, 2017. Reviewed June 2021.

Functional connectivity magnetic resonance imaging (fcMRI) may predict which high-risk, 6-month-old infants will develop autism spectrum disorder (ASD) by 2 years of age, according to a study funded by the *Eunice Kennedy Shriver* National Institute of Child Health and Human Development (NICHD) and the National Institute of Mental Health (NIMH), two components of the National Institutes of Health. The study was published in the June 7, 2017, issue of *Science Translational Medicine.*

Autism affects roughly 1 out of every 68 children in the United States. Siblings of children diagnosed with autism are at higher risk of developing the disorder. Although early diagnosis and intervention can help improve outcomes for children with autism, there currently is no method to diagnose the disease before children show symptoms.

"Previous findings suggest that brain-related changes occur in autism before behavioral symptoms emerge," said Diana Bianchi, M.D., NICHD Director. "If future studies confirm these results, detecting brain differences may enable physicians to diagnose and treat autism earlier than they do today."

In the current study, a research team led by NIH-funded investigators at the University of North Carolina at Chapel Hill and Washington University School of Medicine in St. Louis focused on the brain's functional connectivity – how regions of the brain work together during different tasks and during rest. Using fcMRI, the researchers scanned 59 high-risk, 6-month-old infants while they slept naturally. The children were deemed high-risk because they have older siblings with autism. At 2 years of age, 11 of the 59 infants in this group were diagnosed with autism.

The researchers used a computer-based technology called "machine learning," which trains itself to look for differences that can separate the neuroimaging results into two groups – autism or nonautism – and predict future diagnoses. One analysis predicted each infant's future diagnosis by using the other 58 infants' data to train the computer program. This method identified 82 percent of the infants who would go on to have autism (9 out of 11), and it correctly identified all of the infants who did not develop autism. In another analysis that tested how well the results could apply to other cases, the computer program predicted diagnoses for groups of 10 infants, at an accuracy rate of 93 percent.

"Although the findings are early-stage, the study suggests that in the future, neuroimaging may be a useful tool to diagnose autism or help health-care providers evaluate a child's risk of developing the disorder," said Joshua Gordon, M.D., Ph.D., NIMH Director.

Overall, the team found 974 functional connections in the brains of 6-month-olds that were associated with autism-related behaviors. The authors propose that a single neuroimaging scan may accurately predict autism among high-risk infants, but caution that the findings need to be replicated in a larger group.

Section 16.3 | Metal-Free MRI Contrast Agent

This section includes text excerpted from "NIH-Funded Researchers Develop Metal-Free MRI Contrast Agent," National Institute of Biomedical Imaging and Bioengineering (NIBIB), October 6, 2017. Reviewed June 2021.

A team led by the National Institutes of Health-funded researchers at the Massachusetts Institute of Technology (MIT) and the University of Nebraska has developed a method to enhance a magnetic resonance imaging (MRI) contrast agent with safe-to-use, metal-free compounds. The researchers used organic molecules carried by synthetic nanoparticles. The nanoparticles illuminated tumor tissue in mice just as well as metal-based contrast agents.

"The ability to diagnose and monitor many diseases using MRI can be greatly enhanced with the use of contrast agents," said Shumin Wang, Ph.D., program director of the National Institute of Biomedical Imaging and Bioengineering (NIBIB) program in Magnetic Resonance Imaging. "The new metal-free contrast agents on the horizon are an exciting prospect that may be helpful for people who cannot tolerate metal-based MRI contrast agents, which are currently the only clinically available option for patients."

As with x-ray imaging, MRI is a noninvasive way to scan internal anatomy. While x-rays make bone visible, MRI scans mainly depict the soft tissues of the body. The MRI machine creates a magnetic field, pulling and then releasing spinning protons in the water molecules in the body. This releases energy that MRI sensors can detect and translate into an image of the tissue.

MRI contrast agents change the magnetic properties of water molecules and cause spinning protons to respond differently to the magnetic field created by an MRI magnet. These differences affect how different tissues appear on the MRI scans and can make certain tissues, such as tumors, more visible. Tumor tissue tends to draw in certain contrast agents so that it accumulates there temporarily making it possible for physicians to see the tumor clearly and monitor the disease progression.

All current MRI contrast agents are metal-based and have been used by radiologists for more than 30 years. Currently, gadolinium is the most commonly used metal in MRI contrast agents. Existing gadolinium agents are small molecules that, after a time, are cleared from the body relatively quickly through the kidneys. However, radiologists cannot use it with certain high-risk groups, primarily patients with kidney disease and those who have allergic reactions to it. While recent studies have shown that gadolinium from MRI procedures can be found in brain and bone tissue even years after its application, at this time the U.S. Food and Drug Administration (FDA) says the agent has not been proven to be harmful based on existing studies.

In their study, published July 12, 2017, in *ACS Central Science*, the researchers who developed this new organic-based contrast agent contend that a nonmetal alternative would most benefit patients who cannot currently tolerate the metal-based agents but its use could be broadened to all patients needing MRI contrast agents. This approach would minimize concerns about contrast agent accumulation as clinically viable, nanoparticle-based MRI contrast agents are developed.

The researchers developed the metal-free agent through a collaboration among research labs. The team from University of Nebraska, who design and produce a variety of organic radical molecules, shared their organic compound with MIT researchers who specialize in the synthesis of complex polymer architectures. Polymers are made from various types of molecules that assemble into shapes that affect how they interact within biological systems.

Jeremiah Johnson, Ph.D., is the Firmenich Career Development Associate Professor of Chemistry at MIT and senior author of the study. His team designed a polymer shape they call the bottle brush because of its resemblance to the kitchen tool. By configuring multiple bottle-brush polymers into a spherical shape, they produced a variation on the bottle brush polymer they called a "brush-arm star polymer" (BASP).

"This BASP nanostructure has useful features, including excellent scalability," Johnson said. Johnson's team previously published studies in which they described how BASPs can be designed with attached drug molecules and contrast agents, including the organic radical compound, nitroxide. "We had already been making our polymers with nitroxide attached," he said, "but this is the first time we were able to attach this new nitroxide molecule that works much better as an MRI contrast agent." The molecule was developed in the laboratory of coauthor Andrzej Rajca, Ph.D., the Charles Bessey Professor of Chemistry at the University of Nebraska, Lincoln.

The BASP polymer structure plays a key role in how the organic compound enhances imaging for tumor tissue and then is eliminated from the body. Nitroxides are normally broken down by chemicals in living systems before they can help to create MRI images. Putting them on BASP polymers protected them, allowing them to circulate in the bloodstream long enough to accumulate in mouse tumors, and to generate contrast in MRI scans. The researchers found that the nitroxide BASP nanoparticles are stable enough to last for up to 20 hours in mice, where they accumulated in the mouse tumors. They also showed that the particles are not harmful to mice, even at high doses.

Section 16.4 | **Virtual Colonoscopy**

This section includes text excerpted from "Virtual Colonoscopy," National Institute of Diabetes and Digestive and Kidney Diseases (NIDDK), August 2016. Reviewed June 2021.

WHAT IS VIRTUAL COLONOSCOPY?

Virtual colonoscopy is a procedure in which a radiologist uses x-rays and a computer to create images of your rectum and colon from outside the body. Virtual colonoscopy can show ulcers, polyps, and cancer. Virtual colonoscopy is also called "computerized tomography (CT) colonography."

HOW IS VIRTUAL COLONOSCOPY DIFFERENT FROM COLONOSCOPY?

Colonoscopy and virtual colonoscopy are different in several ways. Colonoscopy is a procedure in which a trained specialist uses a long, flexible, narrow tube with a light and tiny camera on one end, called a "colonoscope" or "scope," to look inside your rectum and colon. Virtual colonoscopy is an x-ray test, takes less time, and does not require a doctor to insert a scope into the entire length of your colon. Unlike colonoscopy, virtual colonoscopy does not require sedation or anesthesia.

However, virtual colonoscopy may not be as effective as colonoscopy at finding certain polyps. Also, doctors cannot remove polyps or treat certain other problems during virtual colonoscopy, as they can during colonoscopy. Your health insurance coverage for virtual colonoscopy and colonoscopy also may be different.

WHY DO DOCTORS USE VIRTUAL COLONOSCOPY?

Doctors mainly use a virtual colonoscopy to screen for polyps or cancer. Screening may find diseases at an early stage when a doctor has a better chance of curing the disease.

Occasionally, doctors may use virtual colonoscopy when colonoscopy is incomplete or not possible due to other medical reasons.

SCREENING FOR COLON AND RECTAL CANCER

Your doctor will recommend screening for colon and rectal cancer at 50 years of age if you do not have health problems or other factors that make you more likely to develop colon cancer.

Factors that make you more likely to develop colorectal cancer include:

- Someone in your family has had polyps or cancer of the colon or rectum
- A personal history of inflammatory bowel diseases (IBDs), such as ulcerative colitis or Crohn disease
- Other factors, such as if you weigh too much or smoke cigarettes

If you are more likely to develop colorectal cancer, your doctor may recommend screening at a younger age, and you may need to be tested more often.

If you are older than 75 years of age, talk with your doctor about whether you should be screened.

Government health insurance plans, such as Medicare, and private health insurance plans sometimes change whether and how often they pay for cancer screening tests. Check with your insurance plan to find out if and how often your insurance will cover a screening virtual colonoscopy.

PREPARING FOR A VIRTUAL COLONOSCOPY

To prepare for a virtual colonoscopy, you will need to change your diet, clean out your bowel, and drink a special liquid called "contrast medium." The contrast medium makes your rectum and colon easier to see in the x-rays.

You should also priorly talk with your doctor about any medical conditions you have and all prescribed and over-the-counter (OTC) medicines, vitamins, and supplements you take, including:

- Arthritis medicines
- Aspirin or medicines that contain aspirin
- Blood thinners
- Diabetes medicines

- Nonsteroidal anti-inflammatory drugs, such as ibuprofen or naproxen
- Vitamins that contain iron or iron supplements

X-rays may interfere with personal medical devices. Tell your doctor if you have any implanted medical devices, such as a pacemaker.

CLEANING OUT YOUR BOWEL

As in colonoscopy, a health-care professional will give you written bowel prep instructions to follow at home before the procedure. A health-care professional orders a bowel prep so that little or no stool is present in your intestine. A complete bowel prep lets you pass stool that is clear and liquid. Stool inside your colon can prevent the x-ray machine from taking clear images of the lining of your intestine.

You may need to follow a clear liquid diet the day before the procedure. The instructions will provide specific directions about when to start and stop the clear liquid diet. In most cases, you may drink or eat the following:
- Fat-free bouillon or broth
- Gelatin in flavors, such as lemon, lime, or orange
- Plain coffee or tea, without cream or milk
- Sports drinks in such flavors as lemon, lime, or orange
- Strained fruit juice, such as apple or white grape – doctors recommend avoiding orange juice and red or purple beverages
- Water

Your doctor will tell you how long before the procedure you should have nothing by mouth.

A health-care professional will ask you to follow the directions for a bowel prep before the procedure. The bowel prep will cause diarrhea, so you should stay close to a bathroom.

Different bowel preps may contain different combinations of laxatives – pills that you swallow or powders that you dissolve in water and other clear liquids, and enemas. Some people will need to drink a large amount, often a gallon, of liquid laxative over a scheduled amount of time – most often the night before the procedure.

You may find this part of the bowel prep difficult; however, completing the prep is very important. The images will not be clear if the prep is incomplete.

HOW DO HEALTH-CARE PROFESSIONALS PERFORM A VIRTUAL COLONOSCOPY?

A specially trained x-ray technician performs a virtual colonoscopy at an outpatient center or a hospital. You do not need anesthesia.

For the procedure, you will lie on a table while the technician inserts a thin tube through your anus and into your rectum. The tube inflates your large intestine with air for a better view. The table slides into a tunnel-shaped device where the technician takes the x-ray images. The technician may ask you to hold your breath several times during the procedure to steady the images. The technician will ask you to turn over on your side or stomach so she or he can take different images of the large intestine. The procedure lasts about 10 to 15 minutes.

WHAT TO EXPECT AFTER A VIRTUAL COLONOSCOPY?

After a virtual colonoscopy, you can expect to:
- Feel cramping or bloating during the first hour after the test
- Resume your regular activities right after the test
- Return to a normal diet

After the test, a radiologist looks at the images to find any problems and sends a report to your doctor. If the radiologist finds problems, your doctor may perform a colonoscopy the same day or at a later time.

RISKS OF A VIRTUAL COLONOSCOPY

Inflating the colon with air has a small risk of perforating the lining of the large intestine. The doctor may need to treat perforation with surgery.

If you have any of the following symptoms after a virtual colonoscopy, you should seek medical attention right away:

- Severe pain in your abdomen
- Fever
- Bloody bowel movements or bleeding from your anus
- Dizziness
- Weakness

Section 16.5 | Advanced Magnetic Imaging Methods

This section includes text excerpted from "Advanced Magnetic Imaging," National Institute of Standards and Technology (NIST), May 4, 2021.

ULTRA-LOW FIELD MAGNETIC RESONANCE IMAGING

Magnetic resonance imaging (MRI) systems are widely used for clinical diagnostics where imaging is typically done in high-field magnets ranging from 1.5 T to 7 T to achieve a manageable signal-to-noise ratio needed for short imaging times (few minutes) and high resolution (1 mm or less). Ultra-low field (ULF) MRI (100 µT) has several potential advantages: (a) narrower instrumentation line widths; (b) greater T1 contrast; (c) minimal susceptibility artifacts due to metallic implants or the presence of air; (d) air core B0, B1, Gx, Gy and Gz coils with relaxed uniformity and power requirements (100 ppm versus 0.1 ppm, less than1 kW versus 10 kW or more).

Instrumentation for the Development of Ultra-Low Field Magnetic Resonance Contrast Agents

Magnetic particle contrast agents can be used to improve the sensitivity of ULF MRI. An instrument with the primary purpose of characterizing new types of contrast agents is described for use in ULF MRI. Specifically, the design and performance of a noncryogenic ULF MRI system based on Faraday detection operating at 5300 Hz (124 µT). The instrument is based on a previously published design with novel modifications including a more efficient

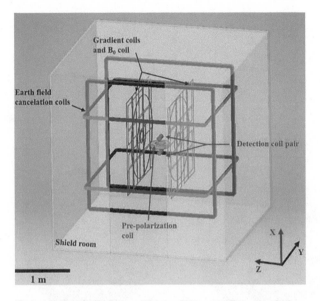

Figure 16.1. ULF MRI System Showing Differential Detection Coil on Either Side of the Shielded Prepolarization Coil

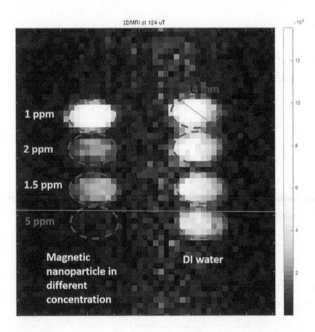

Figure 16.2. 2D Ultra-Low Field Magnetic Resonance Imaging

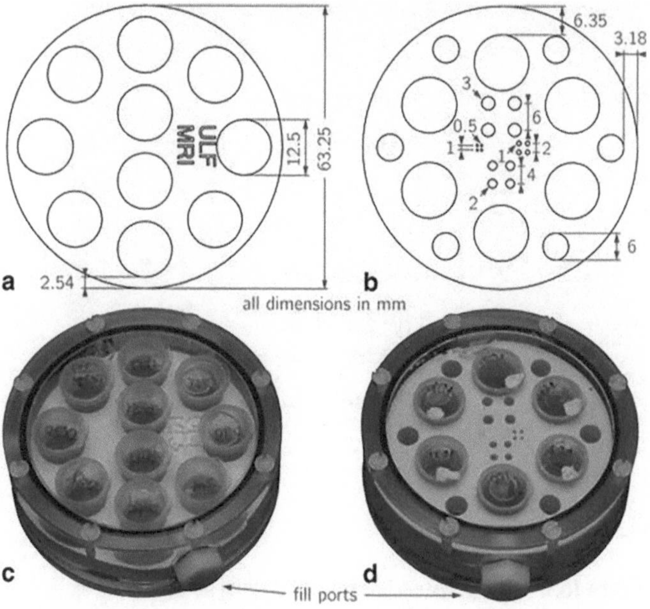

Figure 16.3. Schematics (a, b) and Photos (c, d) of ULF-MRI Phantoms

gradient coil design, differential Faraday coil pair of detectors, and a shielded prepolarization coil allowing for room temperature operation without the need for a SQUID detector (see Figure 16.1). Initial imaging results demonstrate an ability to observe vials ($\Phi=14$ mm) filled with DI water (Figure 16.2) and filled with different concentrations of magnetic particles (Figure 16.2), which are clearly identifiable in 2D ULF MRI.

Ultra-Low Field MRI Phantom

The prototype ULF-MRI phantom established a reference object for comparison of ULF-MRI scanners, as well as a quality control measure for any single site. T1 values of MnCl solutions demonstrated the expected linear increase in relaxation rate with increasing Mn concentration, and the longitudinal relaxivity in the μT regime matched previous literature results. Proton density measurements indicated a spatial dependence of signal intensity; mapping this variation with identical solutions allowed for spatial corrections.

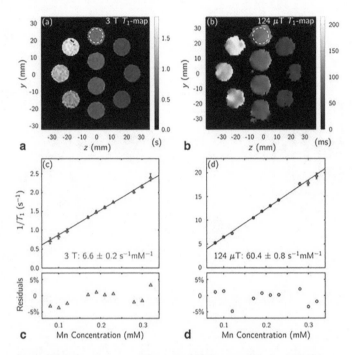

Figure 16.4. Comparison of 3 T and 124 T T1-Mapping Results of MnCL2 Solutions

Applying these corrections resulted in proton density measurements that exhibited excellent linearity. Finally, the resolution inset provided a means to characterize the resolving power of ULF-MRI, allowing for the determination of achievable resolution for a given scanner and pulse sequence.

DYNAMIC NUCLEAR POLARIZATION

Since its discovery in 1953, dynamic nuclear polarization (DNP) has provided a powerful means for enhancing the proton resonance signal. The majority of recent research effort has focused on high magnetic fields, leading to many transformative experiments. Initial research into solution DNP in low magnetic fields has also been very exciting, especially in light of models predicting the magnitude of DNP enhancement at very low magnetic fields could

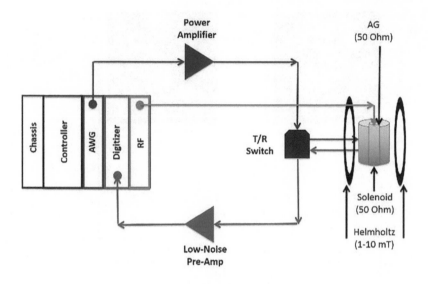

Figure 16.5. Digital Low Field DNP-NMR Instrument Diagram

be an order of magnitude greater than $\gamma e/\gamma H = 658x$ theoretical limit at high magnetic fields.

A Digital Low-Field Dynamic Nuclear Polarization Spectrometer

A digital DNP spectrometer with commercially available components designed was constructed to study the Overhauser (solution) effect at magnet fields from 230 μT–50 mT (10 kHz-2 MHz/NMR, 6.6 MHz-1.3 GHz/EPR). The system is based on PXI architecture. An embedded controller containing the CPU, hard drive, Ethernet, and peripheral ports removes the requirement of a separate PC. A magnetic resonance console and front panel GUI for single pulse NMR and DNP experiments were developed using commercial instrumentation control software. Single-pulse saturation recovery experiments to measure T1H can be carried out in the presence/absence of the radical to access the DNP leakage factor, f. The maximum frequency of operation for 1H with the current arbitrary waveform generator (AWG) card is 12.5 MHz. The operational range of this instrument could be extended to 0.3 T by simply

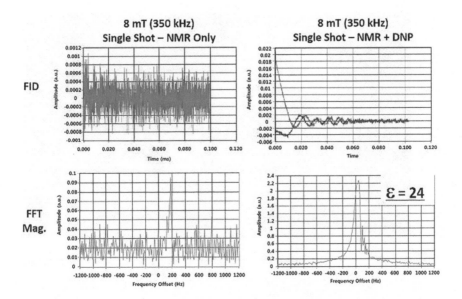

Figure 16.6. Comparison of the Single Shot Experiment with and without DNP Enhancement

replacing the current RF generator card with one where maximum output is in the 8-9 GHz region.

PORTABLE LOW-FIELD NUCLEAR MAGNETIC RESONANCE

There are many instances where the use of high magnetic field nuclear magnetic resonance (NMR) is either unnecessary or impractical due to cost and large instrument footprint. Low magnetic field NMR instruments are considerably less expensive to build or purchase, and can be made portable for application to a greater variety of materials in a wide variety of environments. In many cases, simple electromagnets or small permanent magnets are sufficient to generate the required fields. Magnetic fields less than 100 mT (4.26 MHz) are optimally suited for extremely heterogeneous mixtures containing both liquids and solids. Internal gradients created by differences in liquid/solid susceptibility scale with main field strength, and are smaller in the low field regime.

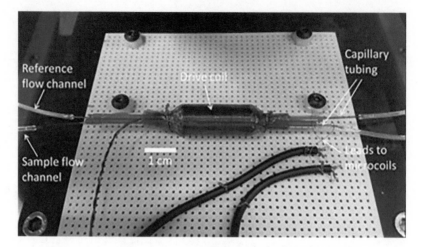

Figure 16.7. Microfluidic AC Susceptometer Breadboard Prototype

MAGNETIC PARTICLE IMAGING

A compact AC susceptometer was developed for real-time monitoring of the conversion of precursors to magnetic nanoparticles in batch or continuous flow reactors. The goal is to rapidly assess specific magnetic performance parameters that are relevant to the final intended use of the magnetic particle solution. Ideally, measurements on small sample aliquots (less than 1 μL) that are broadband and take a short time to perform (less than 1 s) are needed. Also, the physics package should be easily adaptable to the reactor as well as typical micropumps or syringes for fluid control.

Compact AC Susceptometer

A susceptometer measures the harmonic response of a magnetic nanoparticle solution when it is driven towards saturation. It is designed to benchmark the performance of the solution as a potential contrast agent for magnetic particle imaging (MPI) applications. Figure 16.7 shows the prototype physics package for the susceptometer where two nearly balanced micro pick-up coils (59 turns, 40-gauge copper wire) wrapped on silica capillary tubing (OD 661 μm, ID 532 μm) sit inside a common drive coil for low noise differential measurements. Figure 16.8 shows the differential

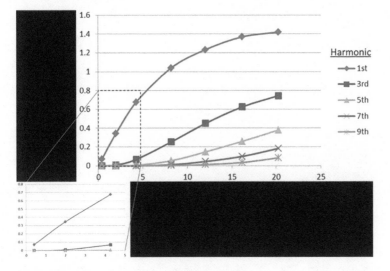

Figure 16.8. Harmonic Response of a Magnetic Fluid Measured as a Function of AC Field Magnitude

harmonic response voltage (Vrms = Vsample-Vref) between the sample and reference pick-up coils of a solution of magnetic ink (30 ± 15 nm particle diameter, $\chi i = 0.45$) as a function of the magnitude of a 10 KHz AC drive field.

Chapter 17 | Advanced Imaging in Laboratory Technology

Chapter Contents

Section 17.1 | **Live Cell Imaging**

This section contains text excerpted from the following sources: Text in this section begins with excerpts from "Live Cell Imaging of Induced Pluripotent Stem Cell Populations," National Institute of Standards and Technology (NIST), December 21, 2018; Text under the heading "Looking inside Living Cells" is excerpted from "Cool Videos: Looking inside Living Cells," National Institutes of Health (NIH), February 9, 2017. Reviewed June 2021.

Induced pluripotent stem cell (iPSC) populations are complex, dynamic, and heterogeneous. Individual cells within a population are constantly changing while maintaining the capacity to differentiate in numerous possible cell types. Sophisticated measurement tools are required to adequately describe and develop predictive models for complex cellular systems such as these. The technology to record live-cell images from cellular populations has been available for some time, but only recently has it become routine to derive quantitative data from these image sets using image analysis. The team then focuses on developing live cell imaging tools to monitor large numbers of single cells and to quantify changes in morphology and gene expression using fluorescence protein reporters.

IDENTIFICATION OF PROCESS CONTROL MEASUREMENTS

A critical component to the translation of iPSCs into therapeutic applications is to design principles for predictably and reproducibly culturing cells and efficiently differentiating them into cell types of interest. Live-cell imaging provides 'high-resolution' measurements to collect time-dependent data from large numbers of individual cells. This data is then used to discover lower resolution measurements, such as the activity of a biomarker at a single point in time, that can serve as critical process control points during the processing of pluripotent stem cells.

INTERPRETING BIOMARKERS

Cells are stochastic and dynamic and may interconvert between states and the expression of biomarkers can change over time. The predictive power of a biomarker or a set of biomarkers that indicates the differentiated state of a cell can be evaluated by examining the history of that cell by tracking forward and backward in time through a time-lapse image set.

PREDICTIVE MODELING

The fluctuations in promoter activity can be used in combination with appropriate models to predict rates of state change in cell populations. Similar mathematical models that can inform bio-processing decisions during scale-up will be critical to obtaining iPSC populations with a desired set of characteristics.

Over the past several years, tools were developed for measuring parameters related to size, shape, and intensity from single cells over time. Modeling tools were also developed for using temporal information to model the stochastic and deterministic components of gene expression.

These live-cell imaging tools are now applied to the study of stem cell pluripotency and differentiation. Induced pluripotent stem cell technologies are a powerful new tool for biomedical research and have the potential to revolutionize medicine.

LOOKING INSIDE LIVING CELLS

Cell biologists now possess an unprecedented set of laboratory tools to look inside living cells and study their inner workings. Many of these tools have only recently appeared, while others have deeper historical roots. Combining the best of the old with the best of the new, researchers now have the power to explore the biological underpinnings of life in ways never seen before.

That is the story of this video from the lab of Roberto Weigert, an intramural researcher with NIH's National Cancer Institute (NCI) and National Institute of Dental and Craniofacial Research (NIDCR). Weigert is a cell biologist who specializes in intravital microscopy (IVM), an extremely high-resolution imaging tool that traces its origins to the 19th century. What is unique about IVM is its phenomenal resolution that can be used in living animals, allowing researchers to watch biological processes unfold in organs under real physiological conditions and in real time.

However, the challenge has been that IVM is so high resolution that the most seemingly trivial movements, such as the animal's breathing or even a slight twitch, have a jarring visual effect that is somewhat like watching a series of major earthquakes. Weigert and his collaborators solved this problem by learning to better stabilize an organ of interest and minimize the motion artifacts. After accomplishing that, his group went on to maximize the optics of IVM, cracking the subcellular barrier about eight years ago to visualize the trafficking of molecules within the cell in nearly real time. He calls this high-resolution IVM approach Intravital SubCellular Microscopy (iSMIC).

That is where "new" enters the picture. New live cell-imaging probes, such as green fluorescent protein, have allowed Weigert and his colleagues to tag molecules of interest with high specificity and then trace their subcellular movements in a living animal. Or by using gene editing tools, such as CRISPR/Cas9, they can generate animal models with fluorescently tagged proteins even faster to study the effects of genetic alterations, all with tremendous specificity and clarity seen in this video.

The resolution of IVM is also getting even better. Six years ago, Weigert's cellular movies were shot in two dimensions. Now, all of his movies are shot in 4D (three dimensions over time) using a special image-capture system, called a "resonance scanner," that averages 30 frames per second. New resonance scanners have arrived on the IVM market that can go up to 430 frames per second, producing an enormous volume of information about the cell and its inner workings.

Section 17.2 | Nonlinear Optical Imaging

This section includes text excerpted from "Broadband Coherent Anti-Stokes Raman Scattering (BCARS) Microscopy," National Institute of Standards and Technology (NIST), October 28, 2020.

There is a need for label-free chemical microscopy in medicine, biology, and materials science. Most of the latest methods use chemical labels that often disturb the distribution and nature of chemical components being investigated. The method enables noninvasive and rapid collection of Raman spectra for imaging.

Broadband coherent anti-Stokes Raman scattering can be used to track cell signaling processes and can provide functional readouts of cell differentiation, allowing researchers to obtain cell responses to biomaterials in real time and on a cell-by-cell basis.

Broadband coherent anti-Stokes Raman scattering can be used to acquire high-resolution chemical maps of pharmaceutical tablets, including information on the morphology of active ingredients, 10 to 100 times faster than spontaneous Raman scattering.

All researchers who use Raman imaging methods will benefit from our work, including biomedical researchers (and, potentially, clinicians), pharmaceutical industry scientists, geologists, and others.

APPROACH

Coherent Anti-Stokes Raman Scattering provides a signal that contains the Raman response of interest for performing label-free chemically sensitive microscopy. In CARS, a vibrational coherence is generated when a pair of photons (pump and Stokes) interact with the sample to excite a vibrationally resonant Raman mode at frequency $\omega vib = \omega pump - \omega Stokes$. A third (probe) photon is inelastically scattered off this coherent excitation, and anti-Stokes light ($\omega as = \omega pump - \omega Stokes + \omega probe$) is emitted from the sample.

The CARS signal has a frequency-independent nonresonant component and a frequency-dependent resonant component. The nonresonant component is entirely in phase with the driving field of the laser and gives no information about the chemical nature of the sample. The resonant component contains the chemical information and has a frequency-dependent amplitude. It is out of phase with respect to the driving electric field of the laser. The resonant component contains elements with the same bandshape as the spontaneous Raman signal.

A broadband vibrational spectrum at each laser shot is obtained by using broadband Stokes light. The Stokes light contains 3000 cm^{-1} of bandwidth.

The spectra obtained from CARS include a resonant and nonresonant component, which made it difficult to extract the Raman spectrum of interest. A deterministic mathematical approach was developed to extracting the resonant (Raman) signal based on a time-domain Kramers-Kronig (TDKK) transform. The TDKK treatment makes the CARS signal linear in analyte concentration and quantitative. Based on imaging of a polymer blend below, that even minor components can be detected and quantitatively accounted for when the CARS signal is transformed in this way.

This TDKK transform allows to take advantage of intrinsic heterodyne amplification of the weak resonant signal and allowed the NIST to be the first group to obtain a full fingerprint and CH-stretch vibrational spectra simultaneously in biological cells. The chemical signatures contained in the combined CH and fingerprint spectral region allow to discriminate differentiated cells from stem cells.

Section 17.3 | Surface Plasmon Resonance Imaging

This section contains text excerpted from the following sources: Text in this section begins with excerpts from "Surface Plasmon Resonance Microscopy: Achieving a Quantitative Optical Response," National Institute of Standards and Technology (NIST), September 8, 2016. Reviewed June 2021; Text under the heading "Label-Free Imaging of Cells by Surface Plasmon Resonance Imaging" is excerpted from "Label-Free Imaging of Cells and Their Extracellular Matrix by SPR Imaging," National Institute of Standards and Technology (NIST), March 10, 2020.

Surface plasmon resonance imaging (SPRI) allows real time label-free imaging based on the index of refraction and changes in the index of refraction at an interface. SPRI can be carried out on a microscope by launching light into a sample and collecting reflected light through a high numerical aperture microscope objective. The SPR microscope enables spatial resolution that approaches the diffraction limit and has a dynamic range that allows detection of subnanometer to submicrometer changes in the thickness of biological material at a surface. However, unambiguous quantitative interpretation of SPR changes using the microscope system could not be achieved using the Fresnel model because of polarization-dependent attenuation and optical aberration that occurs in the high numerical aperture objective. To overcome this problem, an optical model was applied to correct for polarization diattenuation and optical aberrations in the SPRI data and developed a procedure to calibrate reflectivity to the index of refraction values. The calibration and correction strategy was validated by comparing the known indices of refraction of bulk materials with SPRI data interpreted with the corrected Fresnel model. Subsequently, SPR microscopy was used to evaluate the index of refraction for a series of polymer microspheres in aqueous media and validated the quality of the measurement with quantitative phase microscopy.

LABEL-FREE IMAGING OF CELLS BY SURFACE PLASMON RESONANCE IMAGING

Cellular remodeling of their neighboring environment, extracellular matrix (ECM), is an important biological process from developmental biology, to wound healing, to diseases and cancers.

Surface plasmon resonance imaging (SPRI) has been developed as quantitative, label-free microscopy to image real-time observation of live cell engagement with the surface, and protein deposition and remodeling. The SPRI technique is an alternative to the commonly used fluorescence microscopy for examining cell-matrix interactions. This technique removes the requirement for modified biological molecules and transfected cells.

Researchers here have improved upon the spatial resolution of SPRI enabling the ability to visualize subcellular structures near the sensor surface. Along with quantitative interpretation of the images, essentially refractive index measurements, dry mass values of subcellular components can now be measured. For example, a smooth muscle cell has been measured to have a focal adhesion dry mass of 980 ng/cm2 and can deposit up to 120 ng/cm2 of protein around its periphery under normal growth conditions.

Research is underway to develop SPRI as an imaging biosensor that can visualize dry mass changes down to a single bacterium that is part of a bacterial biofilm. Measuring antibiotic drug response at an individual cell level in addition to the biofilm as a whole can provide insight and understanding of how biofilms contribute to antibiotic drug resistance.

Chapter 18 | **Point-of-Care Diagnostic Testing**

Point-of-care testing allows patient diagnoses in the physician's office, an ambulance, the home, the field, or in the hospital. The results of care are timely, and allow rapid treatment to the patient. Empowering clinicians to make decisions at the "point of care" has the potential to significantly impact health-care delivery and to address the challenges of health disparities. The success of a potential shift from curative medicine, to predictive, personalized, and preemptive medicine could rely on the development of portable diagnostic and monitoring devices for point-of-care testing.

POINT-OF-CARE DIAGNOSTIC TESTING IN THE PAST

- In the earliest days of medicine, healthcare was similar to point of care in that it was delivered in the patient's home through physician house visits.
- As medical discoveries were made and new technologies developed, care then shifted to specialized hospitals with an emphasis on curative medicine.
- Large centralized laboratories were established, with cost savings realized through the development of automated systems for the analysis of patient samples.
- Point-of-care devices were used on a limited basis in the hospital for rapid analysis in intensive care units and for simple home testing, such as with pregnancy test kits.

This chapter contains text excerpted from the following sources: Text in this chapter begins with excerpts from "Point-of-Care Diagnostic Testing," National Institutes of Health (NIH), June 30, 2018; Text beginning with the heading "Point-of-Care Testing during COVID-19" is excerpted from "Guidance for SARS-CoV-2 Point-of-Care and Rapid Testing," Centers for Disease Control and Prevention (CDC), June 14, 2021.

CURRENT POINT-OF-CARE DIAGNOSTIC TESTING DIAGNOSTIC STANDARDS

- The emphasis of care is shifting toward prevention and early detection of disease, as well as management of multiple chronic conditions.
- Point-of-care testing gives immediate results in nonlaboratory settings to support more patient-centered approaches to health-care delivery.
- The National Institutes of Health (NIH) supports the development of sensors and microsystems and low-cost imaging technologies for point-of-care testing. These instruments combine multiple analytical functions into self-contained, portable devices that can be used by nonspecialists to detect and diagnose disease, and can enable the selection of optimal therapies through patient screening and monitoring of a patient's response to a chosen treatment.
- Sensor technologies enable the rapid analysis of blood samples for several critical care assays, including blood chemistry, electrolytes, blood gases, and hematology.
- Biosensors are used clinically for toxicology and drug screens, measurement of blood cells and blood coagulation, bedside diagnosis of heart disease through detection of cardiac markers in the blood, and glucose self-testing.
- Current developments in point-of-care testing are addressing the challenges of diagnosis and treatment of cancer, stroke, and cardiac patients.
- Circulating tumor cells (CTCs) that spread, or metastasize, from a primary malignant tumor to distant organs are responsible for 90 percent of cancer-related deaths, a number that exceeds 500,000 every year in the United States alone. Early detection of cancer might be possible through the capture and analysis of CTCs. In addition, the ability to capture and analyze CTCs in peripheral blood may be used in the development of therapeutic strategies that can be tailored to the individual

patient and monitor an individual's responses to cancer therapies.
- Researchers supported by the National Institute of Biomedical Imaging and Bioengineering (NIBIB) have developed a unique microfluidic device capable of efficient separation of CTCs from whole blood. This technology has broad implications both for advancing cancer biology research and for the clinical management of cancer, including detection, diagnosis, and monitoring.

FUTURE OF POINT-OF-CARE DIAGNOSTIC TESTING

- With the development of miniaturized devices and wireless communication, the way in which doctors care for patients will change dramatically and the role patients take in their own healthcare will increase. Healthcare will become more personalized through tailoring of interventions to individual patients.
- The next decade will bring a new realm of precision and efficiency to the way information is transmitted and interpreted and thus the way medicine is practiced. In the future, clinicians may be able to improve the regulation of diet in infants with inborn errors of metabolism through bedside monitoring. Currently, the management of such diseases requires complex testing in a hospital setting. However, researchers are developing a chemical sensor, using a small sample of blood from a finger stick, which changes color in response to metabolic irregularities. When such abnormalities are found, the diet of the infant can be adjusted immediately to prevent adverse effects, such as mental retardation.
- Low-cost diagnostic imaging devices can be used at the point-of-patient care for disadvantaged and underserved populations in the United States as well as in the developing world. The development of low-cost imaging devices could make affordable diagnostic imaging more widely available, particularly in remote or rural

communities and small hospitals that do not have ready access to these technologies.

- A new method using an optical probe for cervical cancer detection and treatment could significantly lower the mortality rate worldwide. Combining a small optical imaging device with a treatment modality could provide both diagnosis and treatment of cervical cancer at the same time.

POINT-OF-CARE TESTING DURING COVID-19

Point-of-care tests are diagnostic tests performed at or near the place where a specimen is collected, and they provide results within minutes rather than hours. These may be molecular, antigen, or antibody tests.

Rapid point-of-care tests provide results within minutes (depending on the test) and are used to diagnose current or detect past SARS-CoV-2 infections in various settings, such as:

- Physician offices
- Urgent care facilities
- Pharmacies
- School health clinics
- Long-term care facilities and nursing homes
- Temporary locations, such as drive-through sites managed by local organizations

REGULATORY REQUIREMENTS FOR POINT-OF-CARE AND RAPID TESTING

There are four different types of Clinical Laboratory Improvement Amendments (CLIA) certificates, any one of which is appropriate for point-of-care testing. A CLIA Certificate of Waiver is appropriate for SARS-CoV-2 point-of-care testing and can be obtained as follows:

1. Complete an application (Form CMS-116), available on the Centers for Medicare & Medicaid Services (CMS) CLIA website or from a local state agency.
2. Send the completed application to the address of the local state agency for the state where testing will be performed.

3. Pay the CLIA Certificate of Waiver fee, following instructions provided by the state agency.

Laboratories or point-of-care testing sites that have applied for a CLIA Certificate of Waiver to perform SARS-CoV-2 point-of-care testing can begin testing and reporting SARS-CoV-2 results as soon as they have submitted their application to the state agency, as long as they meet any additional state licensure requirements that apply. A noncertified point-of-care testing site will be treated as operating under a Certificate of Waiver while their application is being processed. The point-of-care testing site must keep its certificate information current. The state agency should be notified of any changes to the laboratory or testing site ownership, name, address, or director within 30 days.

During the COVID-19 public-health emergency, the CMS allows a laboratory or testing site to use its existing Certificate of Waiver to operate a temporary COVID-19 testing site in an off-site location, such as a nursing home or drive-through location. A temporary COVID-19 testing site can only perform CLIA-waived or the FDA-authorized point-of-care tests for SARS-CoV-2 and must be under the direction of the existing laboratory or testing site director.

TESTS THAT CAN BE USED FOR POINT-OF-CARE AND RAPID SARS-CoV-2 TESTING

Refer to the U.S. Food and Drug Administration (FDA) website for a list of the SARS-CoV-2 point-of-care and rapid tests that have received Emergency Use Authorization (EUA) (www.fda.gov/medical-devices/coronavirus-disease-2019-covid-19-emergency-use-authorizations-medical-devices/in-vitro-diagnostics-euas). Tests that have been authorized for use in a point-of-care setting will have a W, for Waived, in the Authorized Settings column of the FDA table. The laboratory or testing site must use a test authorized for point-of-care use by the FDA and must follow the manufacturer's instructions for each test. The instructions for use provide specific information on how to perform the test, which specimens can be used, and the people who may be tested. All of

233

the FDA-authorized tests for current SARS-CoV-2 infection are for use on symptomatic people. However, the CMS has indicated that CLIA will temporarily allow CLIA-certified laboratories and other testing sites to use SARS-CoV-2 point-of-care and rapid antigen tests on asymptomatic people for the duration of the COVID-19 public-health emergency.

REPORTING REQUIREMENTS FOR POINT-OF-CARE AND RAPID TESTING

A CLIA-certified laboratory or testing site must report all COVID-19 diagnostic and screening test results for current or past infections to the person who was tested or that person's health-care provider. Depending on the test manufacturer's instructions for use, which can be found on the FDA's EUA website, the laboratory or testing site may be required to report a negative test result as a "presumptive negative."

A CLIA-certified laboratory or testing site must also report all COVID-19 test results to their respective state, local, tribal, or territorial health department in accordance with the Coronavirus Aid, Relief, and Economic Security (CARES) Act; refer to the CMS interim final rule for regulatory reporting requirements. In addition, laboratories and testing sites can find out more about How to Report COVID-19 Laboratory Data.

The CMS-certified long-term care (LTC) facilities can submit point-of-care SARS-CoV-2 testing data, including antigen testing data, to the CDC's National Healthcare Safety Network (NHSN). This CDC- and CMS-preferred pathway to submit data to the CDC's NHSN applies only to CMS-certified long-term care facilities. Test data submitted to NHSN will be reported to appropriate state and local health departments using standard electronic laboratory messages. Other types of LTC facilities can also report testing data in NHSN for self-tracking or to fulfill state or local reporting requirements, if any. While NHSN is the CDC- and CMS-preferred pathway, Medicare and Medicaid-certified LTC facilities can submit data through the other mechanisms described in the Current Methods of Submission section of HHS Laboratory Reporting Guidance to meet the reporting requirements.

SPECIMEN COLLECTION AND HANDLING OF POINT-OF-CARE AND RAPID TESTS

Each point-of-care test has been authorized for use with certain specimen types and should only be used with those specimen types. Proper specimen collection and handling are critical for all COVID-19 testing, including those tests performed in point-of-care settings. A specimen that is not collected or handled correctly can lead to inaccurate or unreliable test results.

For personnel collecting specimens or working within six feet of patients suspected to be infected with SARS-CoV-2, maintain proper infection control and use recommended personal protective equipment (PPE), which could include an N95 or higher-level respirator (or face mask if a respirator is not available), eye protection, gloves, and a lab coat or gown.

For personnel handling specimens but not directly involved in the collection (e.g., self-collection) and not working within six feet of the patient, follow standard precautions. It is recommended that personnel wear well-fitting cloth masks, facemasks, or respirators at all times while at the point-of-care site where the testing is being performed.

Disinfect surfaces within six feet of the specimen collection and handling area before, during, and after testing and at these times:
- Before testing begins each day
- Between each specimen collection
- At least hourly during testing
- When visibly soiled
- In the event of a specimen spill or splash
- At the end of every testing day

The CDC Recommends the Following Practices When Performing Point-of-Care Tests
BEFORE THE TEST
- Perform a risk assessment to identify what could go wrong, such as breathing in infectious material or touching contaminated objects and surfaces. Then
  - Implement appropriate control measures to prevent these potentially negative outcomes from happening.

235

- Find more information on Risk Assessment Best Practices and Risk Assessment templates.
- Learn more about the CDC's guidelines for safe handling and processing of COVID-19 samples.
- Use a new pair of gloves each time a specimen is collected from a different person. If specimens are tested in batches, also change gloves before putting a new specimen into a testing device. Doing so will help to avoid cross-contamination.
- Do not reuse used test devices, reagent tubes, solutions, swabs, lancets, or fingerstick collection devices.
- Store reagents, specimens, kit contents, and test devices according to the manufacturer's instructions found in the package insert.
- Discard tests and test components that have exceeded the expiration date or show signs of damage or discoloration (such as reagents showing any signs of alteration).
- Do not open reagents, test devices, and cassettes until the test process is about to occur. Refer to the manufacturer's instructions to see how long a reagent, test device, or cassette can be used after opening.
- Label each specimen with appropriate information to definitively connect that specimen to the correct person being tested.
- When transferring specimens from a collection area to a testing area, follow the instructions for the point-of-care test used.

DURING THE TEST

- Follow all of the manufacturer's instructions for performing the test in the exact order specified.
- Perform regular quality control and instrument calibration, as applicable, according to the manufacturer's instructions. If quality control or calibration fails, identify and correct issues before proceeding with patient testing.
- When processing multiple specimens successively in batches, ensure proper timing for each specimen and

each step of the testing process, as specified by the test manufacturer.

AFTER THE TEST

- Read and record results only within the amount of time specified in the manufacturer's instructions. Do not record results from tests that have not been read within the manufacturer's specified timeframe.
- Decontaminate the instrument after each use. Follow the manufacturer's recommendations for using an approved disinfectant, including proper dilution, contact time, and safe handling.
- Handle laboratory waste from testing suspected or confirmed COVID-19 patient specimens in the same manner as all other biohazardous waste in the laboratory. Currently, there is no evidence to suggest that laboratory waste needs additional packaging or disinfection procedures.

Chapter 19 | **Precision Medicine for Cancer Diagnostics**

WHAT IS BIOMARKER TESTING FOR CANCER TREATMENT?

Biomarker testing is a way to look for genes, proteins, and other substances (called "biomarkers" or "tumor markers") that can provide information about cancer. Each person's cancer has a unique pattern of biomarkers. Some biomarkers affect how certain cancer treatments work. Biomarker testing may help you and your doctor choose a cancer treatment for you.

There are also other kinds of biomarkers that can help doctors diagnose and monitor cancer during and after treatment.

Biomarker testing is for people who have cancer. People with solid tumors and people with blood cancer can get biomarker testing.

Biomarker testing for cancer treatment may also be called:
- Tumor testing
- Tumor genetic testing
- Genomic testing or genomic profiling
- Molecular testing or molecular profiling
- Somatic testing
- Tumor subtyping

A biomarker test may be called a "companion diagnostic test" if it is paired with a specific treatment.

This chapter includes text excerpted from "Biomarker Testing for Cancer Treatment," National Cancer Institute (NCI), March 24, 2021.

Biomarker testing is different from genetic testing that is used to find out if someone has inherited mutations that make them more likely to get cancer. Inherited mutations are those you are born with. They are passed on to you by your parents.

HOW ARE BIOMARKER TESTS USED TO SELECT CANCER TREATMENT?

Biomarker tests can help you and your doctor selects a cancer treatment for you. Some cancer treatments, including targeted therapies and immunotherapies, may only work for people whose cancers have certain biomarkers.

For example, people with cancer that has certain genetic changes in the epidermal growth factor receptor (EGFR) gene can get treatments that target those changes, called "EGFR inhibitor." In this case, biomarker testing can find out whether someone's cancer has an EGFR gene change that can be treated with an EGFR inhibitor.

Biomarker testing could also help you find a study of new cancer treatment (a clinical trial) that you may be able to join. Some studies enroll people based on the biomarkers in their cancer, instead of where in the body cancer started growing. These are sometimes called "basket trials."

For some other clinical trials, biomarker testing is part of the study. For example, studies, such as NCI-MATCH and NCI-COG Pediatric MATCH are using biomarker tests to match people to treatments based on the genetic changes in their cancers.

IS BIOMARKER TESTING PART OF PRECISION MEDICINE?

Yes, biomarker testing is an important part of precision medicine, also called "personalized medicine." Precision medicine is an approach to medical care in which disease prevention, diagnosis, and treatment are tailored to the genes, proteins, and other substances in your body.

For cancer treatment, precision medicine means using biomarker and other tests to select treatments that are most likely to help you, while at the same time sparing you from getting treatments that are not likely to help.

The idea of precision medicine is not new, but recent advances in science and technology have helped speed up the pace of this area of research. Scientists now understand that cancer cells can have many different changes in genes, proteins, and other substances that make the cells grow and spread. They have also learned that even two people with the same type of cancer may not have the same changes in their cancer. Some of these changes affect how certain cancer treatments work.

Even though researchers are making progress every day, the precision medicine approach to cancer treatment is not yet part of routine care for most patients. But, it is important to note that even the "standard" approach to cancer treatment (selecting treatments based on the type of cancer you have, its size, and whether it has spread) is effective and is personalized to each patient.

SHOULD YOU GET BIOMARKER TESTING TO SELECT CANCER TREATMENT?

Talk with your health-care provider to discuss whether biomarker testing for cancer treatment should be part of your care. Doctors usually suggest genomic biomarker testing (also called "genomic profiling") for people with cancer that has spread or come back after treatment (what is called "advanced cancer").

Biomarker testing is also done routinely to select treatment for people who are diagnosed with certain types of cancer – including nonsmall cell lung cancer, breast cancer, and colorectal cancer.

HOW IS BIOMARKER TESTING DONE?

If you and your health-care providers decide to make biomarker testing part of your care, they will take a sample of your cancer cells. If you have a solid tumor, they may take a sample during surgery. If you are not having surgery, you may need to have a biopsy of your tumor.

If you have blood cancer or are getting a biomarker test known as a "liquid biopsy," you will need to have a blood draw. You might get a liquid biopsy test if you cannot safely get a tumor biopsy, for example, because your tumor is hard to reach with a needle.

Your samples will be sent to a special lab where they will be tested for certain biomarkers. The lab will create a report that lists the biomarkers in your cancer cells and if there are any treatments that might work for you. Your health-care team will discuss the results with you to decide on a treatment.

For some biomarker tests that analyze genes, you will also need to give a sample of your healthy cells. This is usually done by collecting your blood, saliva, or a small piece of your skin. These tests compare your cancer cells with your healthy cells to find genetic changes (called "somatic mutations") that arose during your lifetime. Somatic mutations cause most cancers and cannot be passed on to family members.

ARE THERE DIFFERENT TYPES OF BIOMARKER TESTS?

Yes, there are many types of biomarker tests that can help select cancer treatment. Most biomarker tests used to select cancer treatment look for genetic markers. But, some look for proteins or other kinds of markers.

Some tests check for one certain biomarker. Others check for many biomarkers at the same time and may be called "multigene tests" or "panel tests." One example is the Oncotype DX test, which looks at the activity of 21 different genes to predict whether chemotherapy is likely to work for someone with breast cancer.

Some tests are for people with a certain type of cancer, such as melanoma. Other tests look for biomarkers that are found in many cancer types, and such tests can be used by people with different kinds of cancer.

Some tests, called "whole-exome sequencing," look at all the genes in your cancer. Others, called "whole-genome sequencing," look at all the DNA (both genes and outside of genes) in your cancer.

Still, other biomarker tests look at the number of genetic changes in your cancer (known as "tumor mutational burden"). This information can help figure out if a type of immunotherapy known as "immune checkpoint inhibitors" may work for you.

Biomarker tests, known as "liquid biopsies" look in blood or other fluids for biomarkers from cancer cells. There are two liquid biopsy tests approved by the U.S. Food and Drug Administration (FDA), called "Guardant360 CDx" and "FoundationOne Liquid CDx."

WHAT DO THE RESULTS OF A BIOMARKER TEST MEAN?

The results of a biomarker test could show that your cancer has a certain biomarker that is targeted by a known therapy. That means that the therapy may work to treat your cancer.

The results could also show that your cancer has a biomarker that may prevent a certain therapy from working. This information could spare you from getting a treatment that will not help you.

In many cases, biomarker testing may find changes in your cancer that will not help your doctor make treatment decisions. For example, genetic changes that are thought to be harmless (benign) or whose effects are not known (a variant of unknown significance) are not used to make treatment decisions.

Based on your test results, your health-care provider may recommend a treatment that has not been approved by the FDA as a treatment for the type of cancer that you have but is approved for the treatment of a different type of cancer. However, the therapy may still work for you because your cancer has the biomarker that the treatment targets.

Some biomarker tests can find genetic changes that you may have been born with (inherited) that increase your risk of cancer or other diseases. These genetic changes are also called "germline mutation." If such a change is found, you may need to get another genetic test to confirm whether you truly have an inherited mutation that increases cancer risk.

Finding out that you have an inherited mutation that increases cancer risk may affect you and your family. For that reason, your health-care provider may recommend that you speak with a genetic health-care provider (such as a genetic counselor, clinical geneticist, or certified genetic nurse) to help you understand what the test results mean for you and your family.

WILL BIOMARKER TESTING HELP FOR CANCER TREATMENT?

Biomarker tests do not help everyone who gets them. There could be several different reasons why they may not help you.

One reason is that the test might not find a biomarker in your cancer that matches with available therapy.

Even if your cancer has a biomarker that matches an available treatment, the therapy may not work for you. Sometimes other features of your cancer or your body affect how well a treatment works, such as how the medicine is broken down in your body.

Another reason the treatment might not work is that not all of your cancer cells have the same biomarkers. That means that a biomarker test may find a treatment that will kill some, but not all, of your cancer cells. Cancer cells that are not killed by the treatment could keep growing, preventing the treatment from working or causing cancer to come back.

One other reason biomarker tests might not help is because the biomarkers in your cancer can change over time. But, a test only captures a "snapshot" of the changes at one point in time. So, the results of a biomarker test done in the past may not reflect the biomarkers in your cancer now. Your health-care provider may want to test your cancer again if it comes back after treatment.

HOW MUCH DOES BIOMARKER TESTING FOR CANCER TREATMENT COST?

The cost of biomarker testing varies widely depending on the type of test you get, the type of cancer you have, and your insurance plan.

For people with advanced cancer, some biomarker tests are covered by Medicare and Medicaid. Private insurance providers often cover the cost of a biomarker test if there is enough proof that the test is required to guide treatment decisions. Tests without enough proof to support their value may be considered experimental and are likely not covered by insurance.

Many clinical trials involve biomarker testing. If you join one of these clinical trials, the cost of biomarker testing might be covered. The study coordinator can give you more information about related costs.

Chapter 20 | Cinematic Rendering and Digital Twin Technology

CINEMATIC RENDERING

Various methods for postprocessing medical imaging data from computed tomography (CT) and magnetic resonance imaging (MRI) scans have been used in the field of medicine since the 1980s. As they are only viewed in one plane, traditional axial slices produce images that can be at times hard to interpret.

The quality of images achieved by any animation software, such as programs used in the entertainment industry, especially to create animated films, inspired people across the globe to create a new technology, known as "cinematic rendering."

Cinematic rendering is a modern three-dimensional reconstruction technology that can generate accurate images from conventional CT scan and is now licensed for clinical use. The technology relies on light trajectory methods and global lighting models to replicate images from all around the world. In various viewpoints, three-dimensional reconstructions may reveal structure descriptions and diseases of complicated anatomy.

Three-dimensional (3-D) photographs can be mixed with additional data to feed into cinematic rendering techniques to better explain the intricate functioning of organs like the heart. This allows doctors to see how organs function in real time, and will help them schedule operations, describe surgical procedures to patients, and identify diseases more accurately. Such procedures ensure that technology will assist in getting the correct decision for patients on time, resulting in faster care and improved public health.

Potential Advantages of Cinematic Rendering in Healthcare Sector
PATIENT EDUCATION

The high image quality given by 3-D technology can help patients and healthcare providers communicate more effectively as 3-D photographs are much superior to conventional flat and cross-sectional images in shades of grey. They help doctors and surgeons visualize medical symptoms and opt for various options to treat patients.

Three-dimensional photographs are often one-of-a-kind, personalized, and accurate replicas of real organs and diseases. When compared to conventional medical images, three-dimensional images can help patients better understand their condition and stick to treatment plans.

UNDERSTANDING ANATOMY

Medical imaging is becoming a more effective instrument of anatomy instruction. Digital anatomy can be improved even further with three-dimensional technology, which provides benefit by offering more accurate, patient-based representations of normal and altered anatomy consistent with a variety of diseases. Students may use a 3-D technology workstation to understand the anatomy of various organs and diseases at any time.

PLANNING A SURGICAL PROCEDURE

Surgical technique has been transformed by three-dimensional picture and model-based planning. Surgical preparation involves the theoretical integration of many images and is completely dependent on the surgeon's skill. In a single image, three-dimensional technology creates an accurate depiction of the structures. Picture recognition also allows for the depiction of anatomical images from various angles. In comparison to conventional (cross-sectional or flat) images, more realistic images can accurately represent what physicians see during surgery and procedures.

DIGITAL TWIN TECHNOLOGY

A digital twin technology is a computer program that takes real-world data of a physical object or system as input and generates predictions or projections of how those inputs will influence that physical object or system as output. In short, it is a virtual replica of physical devices used to run simulations before actual devices are built and deployed.

Stakeholders can review healthcare management plans, capabilities, staffing, and treatment models to decide what steps to take and prepare for potential problems by building a digital twin of a hospital. Bed shortages, nurse scheduling, and operating rooms will all benefit from a digital twin. This knowledge would aid in the optimization of patient treatment, medical expense, and workforce efficiency. Digital twin technology can virtualize a hospital setting and create a risk-free environment to test the effects of improvements. This is critical in healthcare as it allows for well-informed rational assessments in a deeply dynamic and responsive setting.

The technology can also be used to construct customized medicine by modeling an individual's genetic structure, physiological traits, and lifestyle. Doctors may use digital twin technology to model organs for a variety of reasons, including detecting undiagnosed diseases, experimenting with therapies, and optimizing surgery readiness.

A few healthcare industries and service providers that deal with digital twin technology are as follows:

Virtonomy

From design to preclinical assessment to postmarket monitoring, Virtonomy assists medical device producers during the product life cycle. Manufacturers can better understand the target anatomy, find the best match of the unit to treat most patients, find the correct in-vivo form, and improve health outcomes by using digital twins.

This medical equipment manufacturer functions to reduce the time-to-market delivery of medical technology development, accelerates medical research, and lowers the prices of healthcare products. Their automated clinical trial approach is built on a large database of patients with a wide range of physiological, demographic, and pathological characteristics.

Babylon Health

Beyond the use of digital twin technology, Babylon also assists people in obtaining trustworthy medical advice, scheduling appointments with trained physicians, electronically sending prescriptions to pharmacies, and providing direct links to doctor's notes and their video recordings.

By integrating artificial intelligence (AI) and health practitioners, Babylon Health strives to provide safe and reliable healthcare. The "Healthcheck" app created by Babylon helps users to consider their current health status and how they can be improved in the future. The AI-powered app builds a digital twin after users complete a questionnaire about their diet and family background, allowing them to gain insights into their own health and risk factors for future illnesses, as well as realistic tips for remaining healthy.

References

1. "Cinematic Rendering for Three-Dimensional Reconstructions of the Chest Wall: a New Reality," Scielo, February 7, 2020.
2. Fellner, Franz, A. "Introducing Cinematic Rendering: A Novel Technique for Post-Processing Medical Imaging Data," Research Gate, April 7, 2021.
3. Shaw, Keith; Fruhlinger, Josh. "What Is a Digital Twin and Why Is It Important to IoT?" Network World, January 31, 2019.
4. Garcia, Diego Arias; Roseman, Julianne. "How Digital Twin Technology is Disrupting Healthcare," Plug and Play, February 17, 2021.
5. Shah, Siddharth. "Top 4 Technologies in Medical Imaging," Imaging Technology News (ITN), October 16, 2019.

Chapter 21 | Food Allergy Lab Fits on Your Keychain

Food allergies and other types of food hypersensitivities affect millions of Americans and their families. Food allergies occur when the body's immune system reacts to certain proteins in food. Food allergic reactions vary in severity from mild symptoms involving hives and lip swelling to severe, life-threatening symptoms, often called "anaphylaxis," that may involve fatal respiratory problems and shock. While promising prevention and therapeutic strategies are being developed, food allergies currently cannot be cured. Early recognition and learning how to manage food allergies, including which foods to avoid, are important measures to prevent serious health consequences.

INDIVIDUALS WITH ALLERGIES CAN TEST THEIR MEAL AT THE RESTAURANT TABLE

More than 50 million Americans have food allergies and often just trace amounts of allergens can trigger life-threatening reactions. The National Institute of Biomedical Imaging and Bioengineering (NIBIB)-funded researchers at Harvard Medical School had developed a $40 device that fits on a key chain and can accurately test for allergens, such as gluten or nuts, in a restaurant meal in less than 10 minutes.

Food allergies are extremely common. Those fortunate enough not to be affected are likely to have a friend or family member who

This chapter contains text excerpted from the following sources: Text in this chapter begins with excerpts from "Food Allergies," U.S. Food and Drug Administration (FDA), May 5, 2021; Text under the heading "Individuals with Allergies Can Test Their Meal at the Restaurant Table" is excerpted from "Food Allergy Lab Fits on Your Keychain," National Institute of Biomedical Imaging and Bioengineering (NIBIB), October 25, 2017. Reviewed June 2021.

struggles to avoid dangerous reactions to food allergens every day. In the United States, federal regulations require packaged foods to disclose the presence of some of the most common allergens, such as gluten, nuts, and milk products, which is helpful, but not always accurate.

When it comes to eating out, people with allergies have had to rely on their knowledge of what ingredients contain the allergens they must avoid, and on the efforts of the restaurant to provide dishes that eliminate allergens; and they must work to avoid cross-contamination between different ingredients in the kitchen. All in all, this approach generally leaves those with allergies with little choice but to completely avoid any foods that have the chance of containing an allergen, either in the natural ingredients or because of contact with other foods containing allergens during preparation in a restaurant kitchen.

Recognizing this widespread public-health problem, researchers at Harvard Medical School in Boston have developed a system called "integrated exogenous antigen testing" (iEAT). The purpose of the iEAT system is to give those who suffer from food allergies a rapid, accurate device that allows them to personally test foods in less than 10 minutes.

Development of the iEAT system was led by cosenior team leaders Ralph Weissleder, M.D., Ph.D., the Thrall Professor of Radiology, Professor of Systems Biology at Harvard, and Director of the Center for Systems Biology (CSB) at Massachusetts General Hospital (MGH); and Hakho Lee, Ph.D., Associate Professor in Radiology at Harvard, Hostetter MGH Research Scholar, and Director of the Biomedical Engineering Program at the CSB, MGH.

"This invention is a fortuitous combination of the interests and expertise of Drs. Weissleder and Lee in developing tools for early disease detection, magnetic sensors, and point-of-care diagnostics," said Shumin Wang, Ph.D., director of the NIBIB program in Biomagnetic and Bioelectric Devices. "They have taken technologies they developed for other medical problems, such as early cancer detection from blood samples, and applied them to solving the daily, potentially life-threatening difficulties of people with food allergies – a highly significant public-health problem that incurs 25 billion dollars in annual costs in the United States alone."

The device consists of three components. A small plastic test tube is used to dissolve a small sample of the food being tested and to add the magnetic beads that capture the food allergen of interest, such as gluten. A bit of that solution is then dropped onto electrode strips on a small module that is then inserted into the electronic keychain reader. The keychain reader has a small display that indicates whether the allergen is present, and if so, in what concentration. Testing showed that measurements of the concentration of the allergen are extremely accurate.

A high level of accuracy is very important. For example, even though federal standards say that a food is considered gluten free if it has a concentration of less than 20 mg per kg of gluten, everyone's sensitivity is different, and many people would have a reaction at much lower gluten concentrations. Extensive testing of iEAT revealed that the system could detect levels of gluten that were 200 times lower than the federal standard.

"High accuracy built into a compact system were the key goals of the project," says Weissleder. "Users can be confident that even if they are sensitive to very low levels, iEAT will be able to give them exact concentrations. Armed with accurate concentration levels they will not have to completely avoid potentially problematic foods, but will know whether an allergen is at a dangerous level for them or a concentration that is safe for them to eat."

Beyond obtaining the information they need in about 10 minutes using iEAT, a novel addition to the system was the development of a cell phone app, which offers the possibility of addressing food allergies at the community level. Using the app, users can compile and store the data they collect as they test different foods for various allergens at different restaurants and even in packaged foods. The app is set up to share this information online with both time and location stamps indicating when, where, and in what food or dish an allergen reading was taken. With the app, people will eventually have a personal record of levels that trigger a reaction. Others with the app will be able to find restaurants with foods they like to eat that consistently have no or low levels that are below the individual's triggering concentration.

"Although we believed iEAT could address a significant public-health problem, we were surprised at the amount of interest the device has generated. We are receiving calls from people asking if we can adapt iEAT to test for other substances, such as MSG or even pesticides," said Hakho Lee, cosenior leader of the project. "The good news is that we definitely can adapt the device to test for just about any allergen or substance."

Towards that end, the research team has granted a license to a local start-up company to make iEAT commercially available. The company plans to merge the three components into a single module to make it even easier and more convenient to use. Production on a larger scale is also expected to reduce the price of the unit considerably.

In addition to contributing to food safety at the individual and community levels in the United States, the inventors point out that the device would be very valuable for travelers in countries where there are no specific requirements for food labels. Another use of the system would be to trace the source of food contamination with bacteria, such as *E. Coli* or *Salmonella* to a specific food-processing site by testing DNA in the samples to potentially identify and contain an outbreak more quickly.

Chapter 22 | Wireless Patient Monitoring

WHY WIRELESS PATIENT MONITORING IS NEEDED?

Paramedics and other emergency medical services (EMS) providers often operate in confined spaces and/or mobile environments. They are required to manage multiple tasks, including the monitoring of a patient's vital signs. Currently, emergency medical responders must attach numerous wires and instruments to a patient to monitor vital signs. While the information received from these instruments is displayed on one screen, the entanglement of wires and the process of connecting and disconnecting the patient can be overwhelming and take up precious time and space in confined ambulatory transports (i.e., the back of an ambulance or an aircraft). EMS personnel need a hands-free, wireless technology that monitors all required patient vital signs from one location, and the ViSi Mobile® device meets this need by providing continuous noninvasive blood pressure (cNIBP) monitoring.

HOW WIRELESS PATIENT MONITORING WORKS?

In late 2012, the U.S. Department of Homeland Security Science and Technology Directorate (DHS S&T) partnered with Sotera Wireless, Inc. to develop a ViSi Mobile® device that can monitor vital signs without connecting wired sensors from the patient to other equipment. The device monitors blood pressure, 12-lead electrocardiograms, temperature, and respiration. The system works with existing devices, including traditional sensor patches

This chapter includes text excerpted from "Wireless Patient Monitoring," U.S. Department of Homeland Security (DHS), June 15, 2016. Reviewed June 2021.

attached to a patient that transmit data wirelessly back to a central monitor. The system is capable of operating in confined and "on the go" spaces (e.g., when a distressed patient is moved from the scene of an incident into an ambulance) and uses a single monitor that is lightweight and easier to transport than existing models on the market.

THE VALUE OF WIRELESS PATIENT MONITORING

This technology provides paramedics, clinicians, and other medical personnel with a hands-free, wireless device to monitor a patient's vital signs, creating a safer environment for both EMS personnel and patients. No longer will first responders have to worry about entangled wires and a heavy monitor to transport with the patient. If patients require movement downstairs or through tight door-ways, this wireless monitoring device poses fewer snag hazards and saves valuable time and space when connecting a patient to the ViSi sensors. Reducing snag hazards with just one device and a lightweight monitor will allow paramedics to respond to emergency incidents and perform daily operations more seamlessly and effectively. The technology also allows end-to-end, real-time connectivity between the emergency medical technician in the field and the emergency room. Data can be forwarded through a remote system from the ambulance to the hospital to give doctors, nurses, and other staff better situational awareness prior to the patient's arrival.

RAPID PROTOTYPE DEVELOPMENT TO TRANSITION

In keeping with its mission of providing first responders with solutions to fill critical technology gaps, DHS S&T's R-Tech program worked with Sotera Wireless to address the technology requirements identified by EMS subject matter experts with backgrounds in patient transport and vital sign monitoring. The continuous surveillance monitoring capabilities developed were tested during an operational field assessment (OFA) with EMS participants in San Diego, California in December 2013. Technological and operational feedback from this OFA has supported transitioning this device to the emergency medical response community. Since transitioning the product to the commercial market, Sotera Wireless has targeted the device for use in a hospital-based setting. The U.S. Food and Drug Administration (FDA) has approved the ViSi Mobile® device for continuous noninvasive blood pressure (cNIBP) monitoring.

Chapter 23 | Applications of Digital Technology in COVID-19 Pandemic

The coronavirus disease 2019 (COVID-19) is a highly transmissible and infectious disease caused by the severe acute respiratory syndrome coronavirus 2, commonly known as "SARS-CoV-2." It has caused a pandemic with a case fatality rate of 1 percent. With many cases and deaths recorded due to the virus, there are rising concerns about its effect on global economies, societies, and healthcare systems. The strategies used in restricting and controlling the outbreak have been similar to those employed during the plague that affected fourteenth-century Europe and include detection, containment, interruption of community transmission, isolation, and restricting public movement. Managing a pandemic also requires surveillance, case identification, and effective public awareness. Digital technology has played a significant part in bolstering the effectiveness of these containment measures.

Digital-health technologies such as artificial intelligence (AI), telehealth, and big data analytics help healthcare systems restructure their resources and services at the population level to avoid transmission through health services and ensure surveillance, reduced risk, and containment. Tackling the coronavirus disease (COVID-19) rests on two critical strategies: rapid tracing and notifying infected individuals. The immediate solution that several countries have adopted has been the introduction of mobile software applications. These apps have been used to alert at-risk individuals. They provide other advantages such as mass reach, speed in contact tracing, and maintaining specificity. Digital technology can be viewed as a method to complement the delivery of global-health services. Utilizing digital technology to help combat the COVID-19 outbreak involves using Bluetooth and application programming interfaces (APIs) supported by tech giants, such as Google and Apple. In 2019, 67 percent of the global population subscribed to a mobile device, and 65 percent were smartphones.

About 204 billion applications were downloaded in 2019, and 3.8 billion people worldwide were on social media. While communicating via Bluetooth on iOS and Android devices, a unique code is assigned for all the contacts in the vicinity of a person's device. If a positive result is detected, the app downloads the assigned codes to help public-health authorities. This is one of the measures to break the chain of transmission. Prevention and management of COVID-19 have become easier by the use of technologies such as machine learning and the Internet of Healthcare Things (IoHT).

At present, digital technology for COVID-19 management includes extensive drug and vaccine recovery efforts, simplification of clinical workload, precision treatments for those diagnosed with COVID-19, prediction, and analytics about future outbreaks, and methods for effective management. The efficiency of digital technology in the fight against COVID-19 depends significantly on its interconnecting ability. Many digital approaches use a combination of technologies that rely on telecommunication and the Internet. Various interconnected digital technologies are in use to help tackle COVID-19 at present, such as:

- SMS and instant messages for public awareness
- Machine learning and natural language processing for web-based epidemic intelligence
- Cybersecurity technologies and applications
- Smartphone apps such as contact tracing apps, chatbots, telemedicine, symptom reporting apps, and mobility pattern analysis
- Computer-aided sensors such as accelerometers, GPS sensors, and pressure sensors for drones
- Visualization tools to help update current caseload, recovery, and death toll statistics

- Digital diagnostics and genomics
- Wearable devices and sensors
- Social media and online searches for syndromic surveillance
- Data dashboards and interactive geospatial maps

South Korea used digital technology with coordinated government efforts that included surveillance, contact tracing, extensive testing, and strict quarantines, which helped reduce their caseload, having incurred only 0.5 COVID-19 deaths per 100,000 people compared to a death rate equal to ten times this value per capita in the United States.

A data dashboard called "UpCode" uses data from the Ministry of Health (MOH), Singapore to show infection trends among populations and recovery times of affected individuals. Germany developed a smartwatch application that collects sleep-pattern data, pulse rates to identify viral illness patterns. This data is presented in an interactive map online that healthcare authorities can utilize to identify hotspots. Germany showed a low mortality rate compared to other countries due to extensive testing and digital-health tools.

Countries worldwide used a combination of digital-technology resources to ensure efficient management of the COVID-19 pandemic. Some countries such as Germany and New Zealand successfully contained virus transmission through strict and immediate quarantines, travel restrictions, testing, tracking, isolation, and clinical management integrated with digital-technology services.

When using digital technology to tackle pandemics, it must involve six aspects of pandemic preparedness and response, which include:

- Contact tracing
- Quarantine and self-isolation
- Screening for infections
- Clinical management
- Planning and tracking
- Medical supplies

Screening for infections used technologies such as artificial intelligence, mobile applications, thermal cameras, online toolkits, and digital thermometers that were deployed by Singapore, Taiwan, and Iceland.

Tracking the spread of the virus in real-time involved data dashboards, migration maps, and machine-learning models, which were all employed by Singapore, Taiwan, and Sweden.

Germany, Singapore, and South Korea primarily used wearable technology, mobile applications, and global positioning systems (GPS) for contact tracing.

Quarantine and self-isolation are a significant step in managing outbreaks and breaking the chain of transmission. It requires the use of cameras, digital recorders, GPS systems, and artificial intelligence. These were the primary digital-technology services used by Iceland, South Korea, Australia, and Taiwan.

Clinical management includes diagnosing infected individuals, monitoring their status, providing a prognosis, providing necessary medical aid, and enabling telemedicine services and virtual healthcare. Canada, Australia, Ireland, and the United States used artificial intelligence for diagnosis, machine learning, and telehealth platforms to help contain the spread of COVID-19.

Countries with integrated digital technology in their pandemic response strategies could enhance surveillance, testing, planning, tracing, quarantine, and clinical management and have seen lower disease burdens, more tremendous success in containing and managing the spread of the highly infectious disease COVID-19.

The speed and accuracy with which COVID vaccines were developed is highly commendable and can be attributed to technological advances in technology, design, and manufacturing over the past 10 years or so which helped characterize the virus right down to its genetic detail. There are three major digital technologies that helped make COVID vaccines a reality. They are:

- **Digitalization.** When developing a potent vaccine, one can expect rows upon rows of data from trials which then needs to be contextualized and analyzed, and preserved. This involves data transfer through faster digitalization and better data management. Product lifecycle management systems are integrated with software such as Emerson's DeltaV Distributed

Control System (DCS) and the Syncade Manufacturing Execution System (MES) to help digitally alter, share and use data, recipes, and procedures involved in vaccine development. Integration and cloud computing provide faster data transfers and increase the speed at which the viable product, in this case, vaccines, enters the market. Operators and processing equipment for manufacture of vaccines need to be flexible which can be achieved by the use of scheduling software and process control systems. These approaches help increase production volume of vaccines and improve resource availability. Production delays are avoided through modular automation software and instrumentation.

- Single-use technology (SUT) has helped advance manufacturing speeds in the pharmaceutical industry. In SUT, a presterilized bag is fixed into a support structure with ports for instrumentation. Processing occurs in the bag thereby eliminating the need for sterilization or cleaning post the process.

- **Instrument to application.** For SUT applications, a pH sensor is installed in the reactor bag through a port to stay in contact with the medium. This sensor is connected to a transmitter that converts its analog signals to pH units. The transmitter integrates the medium's pH readings into the DCS and MES systems using digital fieldbus communication. Data transfer from instrumentation helps batch reporting and data analysis.

- Vaccine delivery and shipping are monitored by technology such as GPS beacons, a temperature monitor, and a scannable barcode that alerts manufacturers on deviations in routes, and temperature ranges. Modern technology and digital tools have made it possible to combat the spread of COVID-19 with the rapid and efficient development of viable and safe vaccines.

References

1. Whitelaw, Sera, et al. "Applications of Digital Technology in COVID-19 Pandemic Planning and Response," *The Lancet Digital Health,* June 29, 2020.
2. Budd, Jobie, et al. "Digital Technologies in the Public-Health Response to COVID-19," *Nature Medicine,* August 7, 2020.
3. Owusu, Priscilla N. "Digital Technology Applications for Contact Tracing: The New Promise for COVID-19 and Beyond?" Global Health Research and Policy, BioMed Central, August 3, 2020.
4. Newmarker, Chris. "These Technologies Are Speeding COVID-19 Vaccines to Market," Pharmaceutical Processing World, April 8, 2021.

Part 4 | **Role of Technology in Treatment**

Chapter 24 | Medical Treatment Technology

Chapter Contents

Section 24.1 | Genomic Medicine

This section contains text excerpted from the following sources: Text in this section begins with excerpts from "Division of Genomic Medicine," National Human Genome Research Institute (NHGRI), April 5, 2021; Text beginning with the heading "Genomic Medicine: Population-Wide Implementation Research" is excerpted from "Genomic Medicine Year in Review 2020: Population-Wide Implementation Research Has Arrived," Centers for Disease Control and Prevention (CDC), May 11, 2021; Text beginning with the heading "Genomic Medicine: Implementation and Outcomes" is excerpted from "Genomic Medicine is Here: We Need More Data on Implementation and Outcomes," Centers for Disease Control and Prevention (CDC), May 11, 2021.

Genomic medicine is an emerging medical discipline that involves using genomic information about an individual as part of their clinical care (e.g., for diagnostic or therapeutic decision-making) and the health outcomes and policy implications of that clinical use. Already, genomic medicine is making an impact in the fields of oncology, pharmacology, rare and undiagnosed diseases, and infectious disease.

The nation's investment in the Human Genome Project (HGP) was grounded in the expectation that knowledge generated as a result of that extraordinary research effort would be used to advance our understanding of biology and disease and to improve health. In the years since the HGP's completion there has been much excitement about the potential for so-called "personalized medicine" to reach the clinic. A 2011 report from the National Academy of Sciences (NAS) has called for the adoption of "precision medicine," where genomics, epigenomics, environmental exposure, and other data would be used to more accurately guide individual diagnosis. Genomic medicine, as defined above, can be considered a subset of precision medicine.

The translation of new discoveries to use in patient care takes many years. Genomic medicine is beginning to fuel new approaches in certain medical specialties. Oncology, in particular, is at the leading edge of incorporating genomics, as diagnostics for genetic and genomic markers are increasingly included in cancer screening, and to guide tailored treatment strategies.

DIVISION OF GENOMIC MEDICINE
The division plans direct and facilitates multidisciplinary research to identify genetic contributions to human health and to advance

approaches for the use of genomic data to improve diagnosis, treatment, and prevention of disease; through research grants, research training grants, and contracts. The division also:

- Determines program priorities in genomic medicine and related areas and recommends funding levels
- Assesses needs for research and research training in genomic medicine and related areas
- Prepares reports and analyses to assist Institute staff and advisory groups in carrying out their responsibilities
- Collaborates with the other National Human Genome Research Institute (NHGRI) extramural research divisions to establish a balance of resources, personnel, and research and training budgets to achieve NHGRI goals
- Provides expert advice to the director of NHGRI on various aspects of genomic medicine
- Collaborates with the other NHGRI divisions, other National Institutes of Health Institutes and Centers (ICs), and other agencies and entities, national and internationally and maintains an awareness of research efforts in relevant program areas

GENOMIC MEDICINE: POPULATION-WIDE IMPLEMENTATION RESEARCH

Advances in genomic medicine continue at a steady pace. In a December 2019 paper, The Genomic Medicine Working Group of the National Advisory Council for Human Genome Research of the NHGRI identified 10 papers with the most significant advances in the field. In their 2019 end of the year blog, they featured 5 of these papers based on their potential for near-term impact on clinical practice and public health.

The NHGRI Working Group has again selected its ten most significant advances among the 45 recognized accomplishments published during the year and chose the four applications that were evaluated in population-wide implementation studies.

POPULATION-BASED WHOLE-GENOME SEQUENCING

Whole-genome sequencing (WGS) is being used increasingly to identify genetic causes of rare diseases. Nevertheless, WGS has so far been used mostly in specialized centers rather than on a nationwide scale. The working group chose a study conducted in 57 National Health Service hospitals in the United Kingdom as well as 26 hospitals in other countries. WGS results were reviewed for over 13,000 patients, three quarters of whom had either a rare disease or other unusual phenotypes. Genetic diagnoses were made in 16 percent of patients, leading to specific treatment decisions in some. The paper not only shows the diagnostic utility of genome sequencing but also how it can be deployed in multiple populations.

POPULATION-BASED GENOMIC SCREENING TO IDENTIFY AND INTERVENE ON GENETIC CONDITIONS

The working group chose two 2020 studies on population screening for three genetic conditions that have designated as tier 1 applications (hereditary breast and ovarian cancer, Lynch syndrome, and familial hypercholesterolemia). The first study uses electronic health records (EHRs) among individuals in whom a pathogenic/likely pathogenic variant in a tier 1 gene was discovered through Geisinger's health MyCode Community Health Initiative.

The second study describes the use of DNA-based screening in over 26,000 Healthy Nevada Project (HNP) volunteers to find identifiable monogenic risk for these three conditions. Both studies showed that 1 percent of unselected populations have pathogenic/likely pathogenic variants associated with the three genetic conditions and that most participants are unaware of their increased risk. The studies establish proof of concept for the use of DNA-based screening in the general population.

ROLE OF EXOME SEQUENCING IN NEWBORN SCREENING

Newborn screening (NBS) is a well-established public-health program that tests all babies at birth for rare, treatable conditions that require immediate intervention. Tandem mass spectrometry (MS/MS) is the main screening method for inborn errors of metabolism

(IEMs). The working group chose a study that evaluated whole-exome sequencing (WES) as an adjunct method to MS/MS in NBS in California. Residual dried blood spots and data were obtained for IEM cases from 4.5 million infants. WES was found to have a sensitivity of 88 percent and specificity of 98.4 percent, as compared with 99 percent and 99.8 percent, respectively for MS/MS. Although WES alone is generally not sensitive or specific enough to be a primary screen, it can be useful as a secondary test for infants with abnormal MS/MS screening results. WES can reduce false-positive results and facilitate timely and more specific diagnoses. The study is the largest population-based sequencing effort, allowing evaluation of WES as a tool for NBS.

POPULATION-WIDE NONINVASIVE PRENATAL TESTING

Noninvasive prenatal testing (NIPT) is an emerging genomic application that uses circulating fetal cells in maternal blood to conduct whole-genome sequencing. The test is increasingly used in the clinical management of high-risk pregnancies, but its yield as a prenatal test in all pregnant women is unknown. In this population study, NIPT was performed in over 73,000 pregnancies in the Netherlands. 343 fetuses with trisomies were detected, and another 207 had other abnormalities. Comparing NIPT with invasive diagnostic testing (e.g., amniocentesis), the positive predictive value was greater than 95 percent for trisomies 21 and 18 but much lower for other abnormalities. These results illustrate how NIPT may be useful in population-wide pregnancy screening for trisomies 21 and 18.

FUTURE OF PUBLIC-HEALTH GENOMIC IMPACT

Diagnosis of rare diseases, newborn screening, noninvasive prenatal testing and adult genetic screening are four promising areas for public-health genomics in 2020. The highlighted papers are pilot or proof of concept population-based implementation studies. More data on implementation, benefits, harms and costs are needed before evidence-based guidelines can drive public-health implementation.

GENOMIC MEDICINE: IMPLEMENTATION AND OUTCOMES

The use of genomic tests in clinical research and practice continues to accelerate in the United States and around the world. For almost a decade, the Genetic Testing Registry (GTR) at the National Institutes of Health has continued to track the growth and development of genomic tests. As of October 28, 2020, the GTR lists 76,835 tests offered by 582 laboratories on 16,494 disease conditions involving 18,696 human genes. The Public Health Genomics and Precision Health Knowledge Base (PHGKB) also tracks the growth of genomic tests, associated guidelines, levels of evidence, as well as implementation studies and programs. PHGKB currently lists over 1,000 existing guidelines and recommendations about the use of genomic tests.

Despite this growth in capability and application, implementation and outcome data remain too scarce. Two recent commentaries reviewed implementation issues, initiatives, and challenges in the global implementation of genomic medicine and are worthy of a brief discussion.

In the first paper, Phillips and coauthors reviewed the status of implementation and reimbursement of next-generation sequencing (NGS) in routine clinical practice. They examined the use, payment, and gaps in data on implementation of NGS globally using three common examples of NGS: (1) noninvasive prenatal testing (NIPT), which examines fetal DNA circulating in the mother's blood for genetic abnormalities, (2) whole-exome sequencing (WES)/whole-genome sequencing (WGS) for the diagnosis of genetic disorders, and (3) tumor sequencing (TS), which is increasingly used for targeted cancer treatment and prognosis. They found that NIPT is available and widely used in 90 + countries. In the United States, based on commercial insurance 2019 data, about half a million NIPT tests, 5,600 WGS/WES tests, and 70,300 TS tests were reimbursed. NGS is increasingly used in Canada, Europe, the Middle East, and Asia, and to a lesser extent in Central/South America and Africa. In the U.S., almost all insured individuals have NIPT coverage, mostly for high-risk pregnancies (e.g., advanced maternal age, family history). More than half of insured persons have WES/WGS and TS coverage, with lesser coverage among Medicaid enrollees. In addition, there is no central source of information on implementation across countries and clinical applications. Much of the available information comes from U.S. peer-reviewed publications that provide data on selected tests and health-care systems.

In the second paper, Belcher and coauthors review global approaches to the implementation of genomic medicine. Between 2017 and 2020, the Global Genomic Medicine Collaborative identified 65 initiatives worldwide. These initiatives are cataloged here. Each entry provides information on goals and policy issues, details of populations, diseases, and testing methods. Most initiatives focus on research to understand the contribution of genetics to disease and the technical improvements in sequencing capacity, information management, workforce development, and public education and awareness. Most of the initiatives (71 percent) are in high-income countries. Although there are currently no initiatives in low-income countries, there are multinational initiatives, such as the Human Heredity and Health in Africa consortium and the GenomeAsia 100K consortium that include countries with low- to upper middle-income. Less than a third of the initiatives include policy and/or implementation road maps for integrating genomic medicine into routine health services.

These papers, just two of the rapidly growing publications on genomic medicine implementation included in PHGKB, illustrate the progress and challenges in the implementation of the young field of genomic medicine.

DATA VERSUS GENOMIC MEDICINE IMPLEMENTATION

Among the many challenges to genomic medicine implementation, one critical issue is the ability to generate, enable access to, and assess data on implementation and clinical outcomes. Without population-level data, it is not possible to develop an understanding of the benefits and harms associated with genomic medicine in the real world. In addition to randomized clinical trials, available population-level data sources should be expanded, as well as collaboration across countries and multiple stakeholders, such as industry, payers, and government. Data are also needed on the full range of clinical applications of genomic tests. It is essential to assess the clinical utility (health benefits versus harms), especially among underserved populations. While many studies have assessed the clinical utility of genomic tests, not all tests with demonstrated clinical utility are fully implemented to achieve a population health benefit. At the same time, many tests without known clinical utility are still be implemented.

THE ROLE OF IMPLEMENTATION SCIENCE

The field of implementation science (IS) is intended to support the integration of findings from scientific evidence into routine care. IS promotes an ongoing cycle of discovery-implementation in learning health-care systems. Until recently, IS had minor contributions to the field of genomics, as evidenced by the number and proportion of IS genomic publications, as well as research funding. More recent NIH initiatives have focused on creating networks and research infrastructures for the use of IS in the implementation of genomic applications with the highest level of evidence, such as hereditary cancers and familial hypercholesterolemia. The crucial importance of IS to fulfill the promise of genomics was also highlighted in the recent National Human Genome Research Institute 2020 strategic vision for the next decade.

Ultimately, implementation science initiatives in genomic medicine will require the engagement of diverse stakeholders including scientists, bioinformaticians, clinicians, health-care providers, policy analysts, industry, academia, patients, community members, and government. The implementation of genomic medicine is complex and multifaceted. Its current and future success in saving lives and improving health should not leave anyone behind.

Section 24.2 | **Precision Medicine**

This section includes text excerpted from "Precision Medicine," U.S. Food and Drug Administration (FDA), September 27, 2018.

Most medical treatments are designed for the "average patient" as a one-size-fits-all approach, which may be successful for some patients but not for others. Precision medicine, sometimes known as "personalized medicine" is an innovative approach to tailoring disease prevention and treatment that takes into account differences in people's genes, environments, and lifestyles. The goal of precision medicine is to target the right treatments to the right patients at the right time.

Advances in precision medicine have already led to powerful new discoveries and the U.S. Food and Drug Administration (FDA)-approved treatments that are tailored to specific characteristics of individuals, such as a person's genetic makeup, or the genetic profile of an individual's tumor. Patients with a variety of cancers routinely undergo molecular testing as part of patient care, enabling physicians to select treatments that improve chances of survival and reduce exposure to adverse effects.

NEXT-GENERATION SEQUENCING TESTS

Precision care will only be as good as the tests that guide diagnosis and treatment. Next-generation sequencing (NGS) tests are capable of rapidly identifying or sequencing large sections of a person's genome and are important advances in the clinical applications of precision medicine.

Patients, physicians, and researchers can use these tests to find genetic variants that help them diagnose, treat, and understand more about human diseases.

THE FDA's ROLE IN ADVANCING PRECISION MEDICINE

The FDA is working to ensure the accuracy of NGS tests, so that patients and clinicians can receive accurate and clinically meaningful test results.

The vast amount of information generated through NGS poses novel regulatory issues for the FDA. While current regulatory approaches are appropriate for conventional diagnostics that detect a single disease or condition (such as blood glucose or cholesterol levels), these new sequencing techniques contain the equivalent of millions of tests in one. Because of this, the FDA has worked with stakeholders in industry, laboratories, academia, and patient and professional societies to develop a flexible regulatory approach to accommodate this rapidly evolving technology that leverages consensus standards, crowd-sourced data, and state-of-the-art open-source computing technology to support NGS test development. This approach will enable innovation in testing and research and will speed access to accurate, reliable genetic tests.

STREAMLINING THE FDA's REGULATORY OVERSIGHT OF NGS TESTS

In April 2018, the FDA issued two final guidances that recommend approaches to streamline the submission and review of data supporting the clinical and analytical validity of NGS-based tests. These recommendations are intended to provide an efficient and flexible regulatory oversight approach: as technology advances, standards can rapidly evolve and be used to set appropriate metrics for fast-growing fields, such as NGS. Similarly, as clinical evidence improves, new assertions could be supported. This adaptive approach would ultimately foster innovation among test developers and improve patients' access to these new technologies.

CLINICAL DATABASES GUIDANCE

The final guidance "Use of Public Human Genetic Variant Databases to Support Clinical Validity for Genetic and Genomic-Based In Vitro Diagnostics" (www.fda.gov/media/99200/download) allows developers to use data from FDA-recognized public databases of genetic variants to help support a test's clinical validity and outlines how database administrators can seek recognition for their databases if they meet certain quality recommendations. This

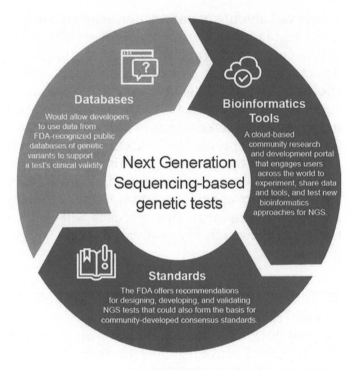

Figure 24.1. Next-Generation Genetic Tests

approach incentivizes data sharing and provides a more efficient path to market.

ANALYTICAL VALIDATION GUIDANCE

The final guidance "Considerations for Design, Development, and Analytical Validation of Next Generation Sequencing (NGS) – Based In Vitro Diagnostics (IVDs) Intended to Aid in the Diagnosis of Suspected Germline Diseases" (www.fda.gov/media/99208/download) offers recommendations for designing, developing and validating NGS tests. The guidance also encourages community engagement in developing NGS-related standards by standards developing organizations (SDOs) since standards can more rapidly evolve with changes in technology and knowledge and can therefore be used to set appropriate metrics, such as specific performance thresholds for fast-growing fields.

THE FDA's BIOINFORMATICS PLATFORM

The FDA created a cloud-based community research and development portal that engages users across the world to share data and tools to test, pilot, and validate existing and new bioinformatics approaches to NGS processing.

Section 24.3 | Drug Delivery Systems

This section includes text excerpted from "Drug Delivery Systems: Getting Drugs to Their Targets in a Controlled Manner," National Institute of Biomedical Imaging and Bioengineering (NIBIB), October 2016. Reviewed June 2021.

WHAT ARE DRUG DELIVERY SYSTEMS?

Drug delivery systems are engineered technologies for the targeted delivery and/or controlled release of therapeutic agents.

Drugs have long been used to improve health and extend lives. The practice of drug delivery has changed dramatically in the past few decades and even greater changes are anticipated in the near future. Biomedical engineers have contributed substantially to our understanding of the physiological barriers to efficient drug delivery, such as transport in the circulatory system and drug movement through cells and tissues; they have also contributed to the development of several new modes of drug delivery that have entered clinical practice.

Yet, with all of this progress, many drugs, even those discovered using the most advanced molecular biology strategies, have unacceptable side effects due to the drug interacting with parts of the body that are not the target of it. Side effects limit our ability to design optimal medications for many diseases such as cancer, neurodegenerative diseases, and infectious diseases. Drug delivery systems control the rate at which a drug is released and the location in the body where it is released. Some systems can control both.

HOW ARE DRUG DELIVERY SYSTEMS USED IN CURRENT MEDICAL PRACTICE?

Clinicians historically have attempted to direct their interventions to areas of the body at risk or affected by a disease. Depending on the medication, the way it is delivered, and how our bodies respond, side effects sometimes occur. These side effects can vary greatly from person to person in type and severity. For example, an oral drug for seasonal allergies may cause unwanted drowsiness or an upset stomach.

Administering drugs locally rather than systemically (affecting the whole body) is a common way to decrease side effects and drug toxicity while maximizing a treatment's impact. A topical (used on the skin) antibacterial ointment for a localized infection or a cortisone injection of a painful joint can avoid some of the systemic side effects of these medications.

There are other ways to achieve targeted drug delivery, but some medications can only be given systemically.

WHAT TECHNOLOGIES ARE NIBIB-FUNDED RESEARCHERS DEVELOPING FOR DRUG DELIVERY?

Current research on drug delivery systems can be described in four broad categories: routes of delivery, delivery vehicles, cargo, and targeting strategies.

Routes of Delivery

Medications can be taken in a variety of ways, such as by swallowing, inhalation, absorption through the skin, or intravenous injection. Each method has advantages and disadvantages, and not all methods can be used for every medication. Improving current delivery methods or designing new ones can enhance the use of existing medications.

Microneedle arrays are one example of a new method to deliver medications through the skin. In these arrays, dozens of microscopic needles, each far thinner than a strand of hair, can be fabricated to contain a medicine. The needles are so small that, although they penetrate the skin, they do not reach nerves in the skin, thus delivering medications painlessly. These patches are easy to use and do not require refrigeration or special disposal methods, so they could be used by patients themselves at home. This technology could be especially helpful in low-resource communities that may not have many health-care providers or adequate storage facilities for traditional, refrigerated medicines.

Delivery Vehicles

Biotechnology advances are leading to improved medications that can target diseases more effectively and precisely. Researchers have begun to reformulate drugs so they may be more safely used in specific conditions. The more targeted a drug is, the lower its chance of triggering drug resistance, a cautionary concern surrounding the use of broad-spectrum antibiotics.

Nanotechnology is opening up new avenues for drug delivery vehicles. The NIBIB-funded researchers have reported promising results in developing a treatment for glioblastoma, a devastating brain cancer. In rat models of the disease, they have shown that tumors can be penetrated and shrunken when injected with nanoparticles. The nanoparticles target the tumor by delivering an altered gene, or suicide gene, that is programmed for cell death. The nanoparticle method replaces a type of gene therapy using viruses, which can have unpredictable outcomes.

Other NIBIB-funded researchers are developing a system of drug delivery using a type of bacteria that has a two-part navigation system – magnetic and oxygen sensing. They have tested the delivery system in mice, achieving remarkable success in delivering drugs to tumors. The bacteria seek out oxygen-poor zones, which are a feature of tumors. Using a computer-programmed magnetic field to direct the bacteria to tumors, the researchers found that the bacteria were drawn deep into the oxygen-starved tumors, away from healthy cells. This process could open the door for directing drug-laden bacteria to tumors deep in the body.

Cargo

Perhaps the most obvious route to improving disease treatment would be to focus on the medications themselves. In addition to drugs and novel vaccines, researchers are also exploring the use of genes, proteins, and stem cells as treatments.

NIBIB-funded researchers are pursuing ways to improve the immune response against cancer and infection using nanovaccines that have unique structures and incorporate inorganic materials. In one study, they injected mice with a vaccine formulated with silica rods that assemble like a stack of match sticks. The scaffold of rods is capable of recruiting, housing, and manipulating immune cells to generate a powerful immune response. Researchers found that the nanovaccine could delay tumor growth in mice with lymphoma, cancer affecting the infection-fighting cells of the immune system.

In another study, researchers prolonged survival for mice with melanoma by treating them with a nanovaccine that combines a bacterial DNA – programmed to trigger an immune response – and a nano-sized inorganic substance that helps the nanovaccine remain longer in the tumor environment. Once inside, the nanovaccine instructs the immune cells to recognize cancer cells as foreign and attack them.

Targeting Strategies

Working backward is sometimes an effective way to solve a problem. In drug delivery research, this means starting with a delivery method. The target may be whole organs (heart, lung, brain), tissue types (muscle, nerve), disease-specific structures (tumor cells), or structures inside of cells. Using this reverse engineering approach, NIBIB-funded researchers developed a plant virus nanoparticle that can target and attach itself to prostate cancer cells. When labeled with fluorescent dyes, the viral nanoparticles can show researchers whether cancer cells have spread into the bone at earlier stages of the disease than with traditional bone scans.

Made from modified viruses, viral nanoparticles take advantage of the natural ways that viruses have developed to slip past immune defenses and enter cells. This means they do not need to be modified as much as other types of nanoparticles to behave in desired ways, and their actions within the human body are well understood. Plant-based viral nanoparticles are also biodegradable, harmless to polychromatic scanning electron microscopy of a 3D vaccine consisting of microsized, porous silica rods. Further research aims to develop viral nanoparticles that can deliver chemotherapy drugs directly to tumors. Such an advance would reduce the severe side effects usually associated with cancer treatment.

WHAT ARE SOME IMPORTANT AREAS FOR FUTURE RESEARCH IN DRUG DELIVERY SYSTEMS?

As scientists study how diseases develop and progress, they are also learning more about the different ways our bodies respond to illness and the influence of specific environmental or genetic cues. Coupled with advances in technology, this increased understanding suggests new approaches for drug delivery research. Key areas for future research include:

Crossing the Blood-Brain Barrier

The blood-brain barrier (BBB) works constantly to allow essential substances from the bloodstream into the central nervous system and keep out harmful substances. Delivering drugs into the brain is critical to the successful treatment of certain diseases such as brain tumors, Alzheimer disease (AD), and Parkinson disease (PD), but better methods are needed to cross or bypass the BBB. One method currently under study uses advanced ultrasound techniques that disrupt the BBB briefly and safely so medications can target brain tumors directly, with no surgery required.

Enhancing Targeted Intracellular Delivery

Just as the immune system defends the body against disease, each cell also has internal processes to recognize and get rid of potentially harmful substances and foreign objects. These foreign agents may include drugs enclosed in targeted delivery vehicles. So as researchers work to develop reliable methods of delivering treatments to targeted cells, further engineering is still needed to ensure the treatments reach the correct structures inside cells. Ideally, future healthcare will incorporate smart delivery systems that can bypass cellular defenses, transport drugs to targeted intracellular sites, and release the drugs in response to specific molecular signals.

Combining Diagnosis and Treatment

The full potential of drug delivery systems extends beyond treatment. By using advanced imaging technologies with targeted delivery, doctors may someday be able to diagnose and treat diseases in one step, a new strategy called "theranostics."

Section 24.4 | Artificial Pancreas Device System

This section contains text excerpted from the following sources: Text beginning with the heading "What Is the Pancreas?" is excerpted from "What Is the Pancreas? What Is an Artificial Pancreas Device System?" U.S. Food and Drug Administration (FDA), August 30, 2018; Text under the heading "The FDA's Efforts to Advance Artificial Pancreas Device Systems" is excerpted from "The Artificial Pancreas Device System," U.S. Food and Drug Administration (FDA), August 30, 2018.

WHAT IS THE PANCREAS?

The pancreas is an organ in the body that secretes several hormones, including insulin and glucagon, as well as digestive enzymes that help break down food. Insulin helps cells in the body take up glucose (sugar) from the blood to use for energy, which lowers blood glucose levels. Glucagon causes the liver to release stored glucose, which raises blood glucose levels.

Type 1 diabetes occurs when the pancreas produces little or none of the insulin needed to regulate blood glucose. Type 2 diabetes occurs when the pancreas does not produce enough insulin or the body becomes resistant to the insulin that is present. Patients with type 1 diabetes and some patients with type 2 diabetes inject insulin, and occasionally glucagon, to regulate their blood glucose, which is critical to lower their risk of long-term complications, such as blindness, kidney failure, and cardiovascular disease.

When managing diabetes, many patients must vigilantly test blood glucose with a glucose meter, calculate insulin doses, and administer necessary insulin doses with a needle or insulin infusion pump to lower blood glucose. Glucagon may be injected in an emergency to treat severe low blood glucose. Some patients benefit from additional monitoring with a continuous glucose monitoring system.

WHAT IS AN ARTIFICIAL PANCREAS DEVICE SYSTEM?

The artificial pancreas device system is a system of devices that closely mimics the glucose regulating function of a healthy pancreas.

Most artificial pancreas device systems consist of three types of devices already familiar to many people with diabetes: a continuous glucose monitoring system (CGM) and an insulin infusion pump. A blood glucose device (glucose meter) is used to calibrate the CGM.

A computer-controlled algorithm connects the CGM and insulin infusion pump to allow continuous communication between the two devices. Sometimes an artificial pancreas device system is referred to as a "closed-loop system," an "automated insulin delivery system," or an "autonomous system for glycemic control."

An artificial pancreas device system will not only monitors glucose levels in the body but also automatically adjusts the delivery of insulin to reduce high blood glucose levels (hyperglycemia) and minimize the incidence of low blood glucose (hypoglycemia) with little or no input from the patient.

The U.S. Food and Drug Administration (FDA) is collaborating with diabetes patient groups, diabetes care providers, medical device manufactures, researchers, and academic investigators to foster innovation by clarifying agency expectations for clinical studies and product approvals.

The FDA's guidance, The Content of Investigational Device Exemption (IDE) and Premarket Approval (PMA) Applications for artificial pancreas device systems (www.fda.gov/media/80644/download), addresses requirements for clinical studies and premarket approval applications for an artificial pancreas device system and provided a flexible regulatory approach to support the rapid, safe and effective development of artificial pancreas device systems.

COMPONENTS OF AN ARTIFICIAL PANCREAS DEVICE SYSTEM

1. **Continuous glucose monitor (CGM).** A CGM provides a steady stream of information that reflects the patient's blood glucose levels. A sensor placed under the patient's skin (subcutaneously) measures the glucose in the fluid around the cells (interstitial fluid) which is associated with blood glucose levels. A small transmitter sends information to a receiver. A CGM continuously displays both an estimate of blood glucose levels and their direction and rate of change of these estimates.

2. **Blood glucose device (BGD).** Currently, to get the most accurate estimates of blood glucose possible from a CGM,

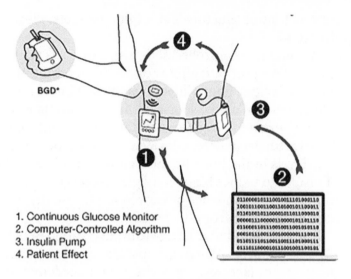

1. Continuous Glucose Monitor
2. Computer-Controlled Algorithm
3. Insulin Pump
4. Patient Effect

Figure 24.2. The Artificial Pancreas Device System

the patient needs to periodically calibrate the CGM using a blood glucose measurement from a BGD; therefore, the BGD still plays a critical role in the proper management of patients with an APDS. However, over time, it is anticipated that improved CGM performance may do away with the need for periodic blood glucose checks with a BGD.

3. **Control algorithm.** A control algorithm is a software embedded in an external processor (controller) that receives information from the CGM and performs a series of mathematical calculations. Based on these calculations, the controller sends dosing instructions to the infusion pump. The control algorithm can be run on any number of devices including an insulin pump, computer, or cellular phone. The FDA does not require the control algorithm to reside on the insulin pump.

4. **Insulin pump.** Based on the instructions sent by the controller, an infusion pump adjusts the insulin delivery to the tissue under the skin.

5. **The patient.** The patient is an important part of the Artificial Pancreas Delivery System. The concentration

of glucose circulating in the patient's blood is constantly changing. It is affected by the patient's diet, activity level, and how his or her body metabolizes insulin and other substances.

THE FDA's EFFORTS TO ADVANCE ARTIFICIAL PANCREAS DEVICE SYSTEMS

The FDA supports and fosters medical device innovation as it upholds its mission of ensuring that medical devices are safe and effective. The FDA is helping advance the development of an artificial pancreas device system, an innovative device that automatically monitors blood glucose and provides appropriate insulin doses in people with diabetes who use insulin.

The FDA has been working together with diabetes patient groups, diabetes care providers, medical device manufacturers, and researchers to advance the development of an artificial pancreas. The FDA's efforts include prioritizing the review of research protocol studies, providing clear guidelines to the industry, setting performance and safety standards, fostering discussions between government and private researchers, sponsoring public forums, and finding ways to shorten study and review time.

There have been tremendous strides made in the research and development of an Artificial Pancreas Device System. On September 28, 2016, the FDA approved the first hybrid closed loop system, Medtronic's MiniMed 670G System, intended to automatically monitor blood sugar and adjust basal insulin doses in people with type 1 diabetes. There are also many research projects underway looking at the feasibility of these device systems in hospital settings.

Chapter 25 | Surgical Treatment Technology

Chapter Contents

Section 25.1 | **Computer-Assisted Surgical Systems**

This section includes text excerpted from "Computer-Assisted Surgical Systems," U.S. Food and Drug Administration (FDA), March 13, 2019.

WHAT ARE COMPUTER-ASSISTED SURGICAL SYSTEMS?

Different types of computer-assisted surgical systems can be used for preoperative planning, surgical navigation and to assist in performing surgical procedures. Robotically-assisted surgical (RAS) devices are one type of computer-assisted surgical system. Sometimes referred to as "robotic surgery," RAS devices enable the surgeon to use computer and software technology to control and move surgical instruments through one or more tiny incisions in the patient's body (minimally invasive) for a variety of surgical procedures.

The benefits of a RAS device may include its ability to facilitate minimally invasive surgery and assist with complex tasks in confined areas of the body. The device is not actually a robot because it cannot perform surgery without direct human control.

RAS devices generally have several components, which may include:

- A console, where the surgeon sits during surgery. The console is the control center of the device and allows the surgeon to view the surgical field through a 3D endoscope and control the movement of the surgical instruments.
- The bedside cart that includes three or four hinged mechanical arms, a camera (endoscope), and surgical instruments that the surgeon controls during surgical procedures.
- A separate cart that contains supporting hardware and software components, such as an electrosurgical unit (ESU), suction/irrigation pumps, and light source for the endoscope.

Most surgeons use multiple surgical instruments and accessories with the RAS device, such as scalpels, forceps, graspers, dissectors, cautery, scissors, retractors, and suction irrigators.

COMMON USES OF ROBOTICALLY-ASSISTED SURGICAL DEVICES

The FDA has cleared RAS devices for use by trained physicians in an operating room environment for laparoscopic surgical procedures in general surgery cardiac, colorectal, gynecologic, head and neck, thoracic and urologic surgical procedures. Some common procedures that may involve RAS devices are gallbladder removal, hysterectomy and prostatectomy (removal of the prostate).

RECOMMENDATIONS FOR PATIENTS AND HEALTH-CARE PROVIDERS ABOUT ROBOTICALLY-ASSISTED SURGERY
Health-Care Providers

Robotically-assisted surgery is an important treatment option that is safe and effective when used appropriately and with proper training. The FDA does not regulate the practice of medicine and therefore does not supervise or provide accreditation for physician training nor does it oversee training and education related to legally marketed medical devices. Instead, training development and implementation are the responsibility of the manufacturer, physicians, and health-care facilities. In some cases, professional societies and specialty board certification organizations may also develop and support training for their specialty physicians. Specialty boards also maintain the certification status of their specialty physicians.

Physicians, hospitals, and facilities that use RAS devices should ensure that proper training is completed and that surgeons have appropriate credentials to perform surgical procedures with these devices. Device users should ensure they maintain their credentialing. Hospitals and facilities should also ensure that other surgical staff that uses these devices complete proper training.

Users of the device should realize that there are several different models of robotically-assisted surgical devices. Each model may operate differently and may not have the same functions. Users should know the differences between the models and make sure to get appropriate training on each model.

If you suspect a problem or complications associated with the use of RAS devices, the FDA encourages you to file a voluntary report through MedWatch, the FDA Safety Information

290

and Adverse Event Reporting program. Health-care personnel employed by facilities that are subject to the FDA's user facility reporting requirements should follow the reporting procedures established by their facilities. Prompt reporting of adverse events can help the FDA identify and better understand the risks associated with medical devices.

Patients

Robotically-assisted surgery is an important treatment option but may not be appropriate in all situations. Talk to your physician about the risks and benefits of robotically-assisted surgeries, as well as the risks and benefits of other treatment options.

Patients who are considering treatment with robotically-assisted surgeries should discuss the options for these devices with their health-care provider, and feel free to inquire about their surgeon's training and experience with these devices.

FREQUENTLY ASKED QUESTIONS ON RASD
Why Did the FDA Issue the February 28, 2019, Safety Communication?

The FDA has become aware of the increasing use of Robotically-Assisted Surgical Devices (RASD) for the prevention of cancer and treatment of patients with cancer. It is important for health-care providers and patients to understand that the FDA has not granted marketing authorization to any RASD system specifically for the prevention or treatment of cancer.

Are RASD Permitted to Be Used in Patients Who Have Cancer?

RASD has been evaluated by the FDA and cleared for use in certain types of surgical procedures commonly performed in patients with cancer, such as hysterectomy, prostatectomy, and colectomy. These clearances are based on short-term (30 days) patient follow-up. The safety and effectiveness of RASD, for the prevention and treatment of cancer, based on cancer-related outcomes, such as overall survival, recurrence, and disease-free survival have not been established.

What Is Known about Using RASD to Perform Mastectomy Procedures for the Prevention and Treatment of Breast Cancer?

There is little evidence on the safety and effectiveness of the use of RASD in patients undergoing mastectomy for the prevention or treatment of breast cancer, and the FDA has not granted any RASD system marketing authorization for mastectomy. For patients undergoing mastectomy, the surgical approach used with RASD differs from conventional surgical approaches. The impact of these differences on the prevention of cancer, overall survival, recurrence, and disease-free survival has not been established.

What Is Known about Using RASD for the Treatment of Cervical Cancer?

Researchers are aware of limited reports that conclude that min-imally invasive surgery (which included laparoscopic surgery or surgery using RASD) was associated with a lower rate of long-term survival compared with open abdominal surgery. Other reports have demonstrated no significant difference in long-term survival when these types of surgical procedures are compared. Clinicians and patients should be aware of this information when making treatment decisions.

Section 25.2 | Surgical Robots for Tumor Treatment

This section contains text excerpted from the following sources: Text in this section begins with excerpts from "Robotic & Minimally Invasive Surgery," National Cancer Institute (NCI), July 24, 2017. Reviewed June 2021; Text beginning with the heading "Caution When Using Robotically-Assisted Surgical Devices" is excerpted from "Caution When Using Robotically-Assisted Surgical Devices in Women's Health including Mastectomy and Other Cancer-Related Surgeries: FDA Safety Communication," U.S. Food and Drug Administration (FDA), February 27, 2019.

The National Institutes of Health's (NIH) Foregut Team offers robotic-assisted surgery for a variety of tumor types of the chest and abdomen. The robotic surgery platform is designed to over-come the limitations of both open and traditional laparoscopic surgery by giving surgeons magnified stereoscopic vision and the ability to work within confined spaces. In addition, robotic-assisted procedures are associated with a reduced need for oral pain medications and a shorter length of hospitalization. The surgeons of the NIH Foregut Teamwork with patients to select a surgical treatment and determine whether robotic surgery is right for them.

Robotic surgery for foregut cancers at NIH was initiated by Dr. R. Taylor Ripley in collaboration with anesthesiologists, thoracic nursing team leaders, and a surgical technologist in June 2015. The thoracic robotics program was introduced first to treat tumors of the esophagus, lung, mediastinum, chest wall, and diaphragm. Soon after, the robotic surgery program was expanded by Dr. Jeremy L. Davis to treat abdominal tumors including the stomach, pancreas, liver, colon, and rectum.

Both Dr. Ripley and Dr. Davis received advanced training in robotic surgery at Memorial Sloan Kettering Cancer Center. As part of the multi-disciplinary NIH Foregut Team, robotic surgery is a complex surgical treatment option offered in the setting of innovative clinical cancer research.

CAUTION WHEN USING ROBOTICALLY-ASSISTED SURGICAL DEVICES

Since robotically-assisted surgical devices became available in the U.S., robotically-assisted surgical procedures were widely adopted because they may allow for quicker recovery and could improve surgical precision. However, the U.S. Food and Drug Administration (FDA) is concerned that health-care providers and patients may not be aware that the safety and effectiveness of these devices have not been established for use in mastectomy procedures or the prevention or treatment of cancer. Patients and health-care providers should also be aware that the FDA encourages health-care providers who use robotically-assisted surgical devices to have specialized training and practice in their use.

RECOMMENDATIONS FOR PATIENTS

Before you have robotically-assisted surgery to prevent or treat cancer:

- Be aware that that the safety and effectiveness of using robotically-assisted surgical devices in mastectomy procedures or in the prevention or treatment of cancer have not been established.
- Discuss the benefits, risks, and alternatives of all available treatment options with your health-care provider to make the most informed treatment decisions.
- Before choosing your surgeon, it is recommended to asking the following questions:
  - Ask your surgeon about her or his training, experience, and patient outcomes with robotically-assisted surgical device procedures.
  - Ask how many robotically-assisted surgical procedures like yours she or he has performed.
  - Ask your surgeon about possible complications and how often they happen.

If you had treatment with a robotically-assisted surgical device for any cancerous condition and experienced a complication, it is encouraged you file a report through MedWatch, the FDA Safety Information and Adverse Event Reporting program.

Section 25.3 | Robotic Angiography Gantry

"Robotic Angiography Gantry," © 2021 Omnigraphics. Reviewed June 2021.

A gantry is a type of robotic device known as a "Cartesian" or "linear" robot. A gantry robot comprises a device called a "manipulator" placed upon an overhead system. This overhead system permits a free range of movement across a horizontal plane. A gantry robot utilizes the x,y,z coordinate system. This type of robotics finds applications in pick and place operations, large-scale movement, and welding purposes. Gantry robots are generally used for scanning, electronics assembly, automatic inspection, automation of industry processes, and digital printing.

In recent times, the mechanics of a gantry robot have been integrated into the medical field for ergonomic reasons. Robotics in medicine has been highly beneficial as it reduces the error margin and employment costs while increasing precision in delivering medical services. There are different types of robots used in healthcare delivery systems, such as:

- **Care robots.** They are still gaining traction as a substitute for caregivers. It is also useful in helping nurses manage their workload with precision.
- **Surgical robots.** The most common use of robots in medicine is in the field of surgery. Robot-assisted surgeries are gaining popularity due to their precision and reduced error rate.
- Exoskeletons aid in rehabilitation postsurgery
- Hospital robots are used to deliver medications, transport laboratory samples, and disinfection

An angiography is a procedure used to visualize blockages and the flow of blood in the heart and other organs such as the kidneys or the brain. It is administered with a special dye through catheterization and imaging with x-rays. The procedure takes 30 to 60 minutes, and the x-ray images help the doctor insert the catheter. The catheter is directed into the organ through an artery, and the dye is injected. X-rays help monitor the flow of the dye within the organ and highlight any blockages if present. The x-ray images obtained from the procedure are called "angiograms."

Robotic angiography gantries are a part of the image-guided therapy approach in medicine. The robotic angiographic gantry is more manageable for patients to access as it is not fixed to the floor or ceiling. This is highly beneficial during open surgeries as well. Some robotic gantries are laser-guided for better positioning and advanced imaging. These properties of the gantry are advancements of technologies found on C-arm systems with fixed bases. The C-arm gantry used in healthcare is capable of rotational angiography with the help of x-ray imaging with x-ray image intensifiers or flat panel detectors.

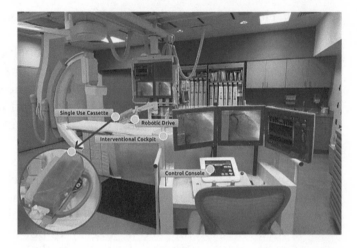

Figure 25.1. Robotic Angiography Gantry *(Source: Securities and Exchange Commission (SEC).)*

BENEFITS OF ROBOTIC ANGIOGRAPHY

Robotic angiography gantries have a variety of benefits such as:

- Increased precision
- Higher patient outcomes
- More than three axes of movement along any desirable length
- Ease of programming
- Ease of access for patients
- Fewer limitations from floor space constraints
- Better image resolutions
- Reduced radiation dose for the patient
- Higher mobility

The latest robotic angiography gantries are increasingly mobile and are provided with wheels that can move the device to any part of the room. These gantries offer the combined features of fixed systems and the mobility of C-arm systems. They can be positioned over a surface for observation and then kept aside to use the room space for other purposes. Robotic gantries are ergonomically efficient and are the future of medical imaging where convenience is the primary goal.

References

1. "GE Introduces Robotic Angiography Gantry That Addresses Ergonomic Issues," Diagnostic and Interventional Cardiology (DAIC), December 1, 2020.
2. "What Are Gantry Robots?" Robot Worx, November 14, 2012.
3. "What Are the Main Types of Robots Used in Healthcare?" Medical Device Network, January 2, 2020.
4. Fornell, Dave. "Advances in Angiographic Imaging Systems," Imaging Technology News (ITN), January 30, 2015.
5. "Amendment No. 1 to Form S-1 Registration Statement," U.S. Securities and Exchange Commission (SEC), May 26, 2015.

Section 25.4 | Technologies Enhance Tumor Surgery

This section includes text excerpted from "Technologies Enhance Tumor Surgery," *NIH News in Health*, National Institutes of Health (NIH), February 2016. Reviewed June 2021.

For surgeons, removing a tumor is a balancing act. Cut out too much and you risk removing healthy tissues that have important functions. Remove too little and you may leave behind cancer cells that could grow back into a tumor over time.

The NIH-funded researchers are developing new technologies to help surgeons determine exactly where tumors end and healthy tissue begins. Their ultimate goal is to make surgery for cancer patients safer and more effective.

"Currently, surgeons view MRI and CT scans taken prior to an operation to establish where a tumor is located and to plan a surgical approach that will minimize damage to healthy tissues," says Dr. Steven Krosnick, an NIH expert in image-guided surgery. "But, once the operation has begun, surgeons generally rely only on their eyes and sense of touch to distinguish tumor from healthy tissue."

Surgeons go through many years of training to understand the subtle cues that can distinguish tumors from normal surroundings. Sometimes the tumor is a slightly different color than healthy tissue, or it feels different. It might also bleed more readily or could contain calcium deposits. Even with these cues, however, surgeons do not always get it right.

"In a lot of cases, we leave tumor behind that could be safely removed if only we were able to better visualize it," says Dr. Daniel Orringer, a neurosurgeon at the University of Michigan.

In today's operating rooms, pathologists can often help surgeons determine if all of a tumor has been taken out. A pathologist may view the edges of the tissue under a microscope and look for cancer cells. If they are found, the surgeon will remove more tissue from the patient and send these again to the pathologist for review. This process can occur repeatedly while the patient remains on the operating table and continue until no cancer cells are detected.

"Each time a pathologist analyzes tissue during an operation, it can take up to 30 minutes because the tissue has to be frozen, thinly sliced, and stained so it can be viewed under the microscope," Krosnick says. "If multiple rounds of tissue are taken, it can greatly increase the length of the surgery."

In the days following an operation, the pathologist conducts a more thorough review of the tissue. If cancer cells are found at the margins, the patient may undergo a second surgery to remove the cancer that was left behind.

Orringer is part of a research team that's testing a new technology that could help surgeons tell the difference between a tumor and healthy brain tissue during surgery. The team developed a special microscope with NIH support that shoots a pair of low-energy lasers at the tissue. That causes the chemical bonds in the tissue's molecules to vibrate. The vibrations are then analyzed by a computer and used to create detailed images of the tissue.

From a molecular point of view, the components of a tumor differ from those in healthy tissue. This specialized microscope can reveal differences between the tissues that cannot be seen with the naked eye.

"Our technology enables us to get a microscopic view of human tissues without taking them out of the body," Orringer says. "We can see cells, blood vessels, the connections between brain cells… all of the microscopic components that make up the brain."

Orringer and colleagues developed a computer program that can quickly analyze the images and assess whether or not cancer cells are present. This type of analysis could help surgeons decide whether all of a tumor has been cut out. To date, Orringer has used the specialized microscope to help remove cancer tissue in nearly 100 patients with brain tumors.

Other researchers are taking different approaches. For example, Dr. Quyen Nguyen – a head and neck surgeon at the University of California, San Diego – has developed a fluorescent molecule that's currently being tested in clinical trials. The patient receives an injection of the molecules before surgery. When exposed to certain types of light, these molecules cause cancer cells to glow, making them easier to spot and remove. The surgeon then uses a near-infrared camera to visualize the glowing tumor cells while operating.

Nguyen is also developing a fluorescent molecule to light up nerves. Accidental nerve injury during surgery can leave patients with loss of movement or feeling. In some cases, sexual function may be impaired.

"Nerves are really, really small, and they are often buried in soft tissue or encased within the bone. When we have to do cancer surgery, they can be encased in cancer itself," Nguyen says. The fluorescent molecule could help surgeons detect hard-to-spot nerves, so they can be protected. The nerve-tagging molecule is now being tested in animal studies.

Other NIH-funded researchers are focusing on ways to speed up cancer surgeries. Dr. Milind Rajadhyaksha, a researcher at Memorial Sloan Kettering Cancer Center, has developed a microscope technique to reduce the amount of time it takes to perform a common surgery for removing nonmelanoma skin cancers.

Each year about two million people in the U.S. undergo Mohs surgery, in which a doctor successively removes suspicious areas until the surrounding skin tissue is free of cancer. The procedure can take several hours because each time more tissue is removed, it has to be prepared and reviewed under a microscope to determine if cancer cells remain. This step can take up to 30 minutes.

The technique developed by Rajadhyaksha shortens the time for assessing removed tissue to less than five minutes, which greatly reduces the overall length of the procedure. Tissue is mounted in a specialized microscope that uses a focused laser line to do multiple scans of the tissue. The resulting image "strips" are then combined, such as a mosaic, into a complete microscopic image of the tissue.

About 1,000 specialized skin surgeries have already been performed guided by this technique. Rajadhyaksha is currently developing an approach that would allow doctors to use the technology directly on a patient's skin before any tissue has been removed. This would allow doctors to identify the edges of tumors before the start of surgery and reduce the need for several presurgical "margin-mapping" biopsies.

Section 25.5 | Smart Operating Rooms of the Future

This section includes text excerpted from "NIH-Supported Technologies of the Future," MedlinePlus, National Institutes of Health (NIH), July 14, 2017. Reviewed June 2021.

NIH-SUPPORTED TECHNOLOGIES OF THE FUTURE

The National Institute of Biomedical Imaging and Bioengineering's (NIBIB) Surgery of the Future app lets users see different medical technologies that are coming down the pipeline. Read about a few of these breakthrough technologies below.

Silk Screws

Silk has been used to stitch up wounds for centuries. Now, researchers have created silk screws and plates to repair fractured bones. Unlike metal, silk can safely break down in the body. This means that patients who receive temporary silk devices to hold their bones in place would not need a second surgery to remove them. Developer: David Kaplan, Tufts University.

Biopsy Guidance

The Clear Guide ONE is a device that helps target tumors for biopsy. The tool attaches to an ultrasound probe, which produces images of the inside of the body. It helps the physician see the path the needle would take if inserted at that spot. Developer: Clear Guide Medical.

High-Intensity Focused Ultrasound

High-intensity focused ultrasound lets surgeons operate deep within the body without making a cut. In a procedure that uses this technology, multiple beams of ultrasound focus on a target in the body. At the focal point, the energy from the ultrasound beam causes the temperature of the tissue to rise and then destroy it. It does this while leaving surrounding tissue unharmed. Developer: Kullervo Hynynen, Sunnybrook Research Institute.

Flexible Endoscope with Fluorescent Capabilities

Researchers have developed a flexible endoscope that can help spot precancerous growths in the colon. The endoscope has a single optical fiber that uses laser light and shows images of fluorescent molecules, which stick to the precancerous growths. Developers: Eric Seibel, University of Washington, and Thomas D. Wang, University of Michigan.

Minimally Invasive Neurosurgical Intracranial Robot

Researchers are creating robots to use inside an MRI (magnetic resonance imaging) machine so surgeons can more easily see tumors. One researcher is developing a worm-like robot that could be directed inside the brain while a patient has an MRI scan. Developer: Jaydev Desai, Georgia Institute of Technology.

Fluorescent Tumor Paint

Researchers created fluorescent molecules that cause cancer cells to glow. The molecules can be injected before surgery and are just taken up by cancer cells. Surgeons can see the glowing cancer tissue or tumors using a special camera. Researchers are also developing molecules to light up nerves, which can get wrapped up in tumors. Developer: Quyen Nguyen, University of California, San Diego.

Self-Stitching Surgical Robot

This robot can stitch soft tissues all by itself. It has 3D and special light cameras to keep track of tissue position. Developers: Axel Krieger and Peter Kim, Children's National Health System.

Tremor-Reducing Instrument

This hand-held tool reduces a surgeon's shaking when operating on small structures, such as the eye. It estimates the tremor of the surgeon and then adjusts to provide smooth control. Developer: Cameron Riviere, Carnegie Mellon University.

Biodegradable Stent

Each year, approximately half a million Americans receive a stent to hold open an artery in their heart that has been unclogged during a procedure called "angioplasty." A stent is a small wire-mesh tube. It is usually made of stainless steel or another metal. NIBIB-funded researchers have invented a new material that makes a stent dissolve over time. This new solution could eliminate some of the disadvantages of metal stents. Developer: Joachim Kohn, Rutgers University.

Chapter 26 | Technology and the Future of Mental-Health Treatment

Technology has opened a new frontier in mental-health support and data collection. Mobile devices such as cell phones, smartphones, and tablets are giving the public, doctors, and researchers new ways to access help, monitor progress, and increase understanding of mental well-being.

Mobile mental-health support can be very simple but effective. For example, anyone with the ability to send a text message can contact a crisis center. New technology can also be packaged into an extremely sophisticated app for smartphones or tablets. Such apps might use the device's built-in sensors to collect information on a user's typical behavior patterns. If the app detects a change in behavior, it may provide a signal that help is needed before a crisis occurs. Some apps are stand-alone programs that promise to improve memory or thinking skills. Others help the user connect to a peer counselor or to a health-care professional.

Excitement about the huge range of opportunities has led to a burst of app development. There are thousands of mental-health apps available in iTunes and Android app stores, and the number is growing every year. However, this new technology frontier includes a lot of uncertainty. There is very little industry regulation and very little information on app effectiveness, which can lead consumers to wonder which apps they should trust.

This chapter includes text excerpted from "Technology and the Future of Mental Health Treatment," National Institute of Mental Health (NIMH), September 2019.

Before focusing on the state of the science and where it may lead, it is important to look at the advantages and disadvantages of expanding mental-health treatment and research into a mobile world.

THE PROS AND CONS OF MENTAL-HEALTH APPS

Experts believe that technology has a lot of potential for clients and clinicians alike. A few of the advantages of mobile care include:

- **Convenience.** Treatment can take place anytime and anywhere (e.g., at home in the middle of the night or on a bus on the way to work) and may be ideal for those who have trouble with in-person appointments.
- **Anonymity.** Clients can seek treatment options without involving other people.
- **An introduction to care.** Technology may be a good first step for those who have avoided mental-healthcare in the past.
- **Lower cost.** Some apps are free or cost less than traditional care.
- **Service to more people.** Technology can help mental-health providers offer treatment to people in remote areas or to many people in times of sudden need (e.g., following a natural disaster or terror attack).
- **Interest.** Some technologies might be more appealing than traditional treatment methods, which may encourage clients to continue therapy.
- **24-hour service.** Technology can provide round-the-clock monitoring or intervention support.
- **Consistency.** Technology can offer the same treatment program to all users.
- **Support.** Technology can complement traditional therapy by extending an in-person session, reinforcing new skills, and providing support and monitoring.
- **Objective data collection.** Technology can quantitatively collect information such as location, movement, phone use, and other information.

This new era of mental-health technology offers great opportunities but also raises a number of concerns. Tackling potential problems will be an important part of making sure new apps provide benefits without causing harm. That is why the mental-health community and software developers are focusing on:

- **Effectiveness.** The biggest concern with technological interventions is obtaining scientific evidence that they work and that they work as well as traditional methods.
- **For whom and for what.** Another concern is understanding if apps work for all people and for all mental-health conditions.
- **Privacy.** Apps deal with very sensitive personal information so app makers need to be able to guarantee privacy for app users.
- **Guidance.** There are no industry-wide standards to help consumers know if an app or other mobile technology is proven effective.
- **Regulation.** The question of who will or should regulate mental-health technology and the data it generates needs to be answered.
- **Overselling.** There is some concern that if an app or program promises more than it delivers, consumers may turn away from other, more effective therapies.

CURRENT TRENDS IN APP DEVELOPMENT

Creative research and engineering teams are combining their skills to address a wide range of mental-health concerns. Some popular areas of app development include:

Self-Management Apps

"Self-management" means that the user puts information into the app so that the app can provide feedback. For example, the user might set up medication reminders, or use the app to develop tools for managing stress, anxiety, or sleep problems. Some software can use additional equipment to track heart rate, breathing patterns, blood pressure, etc., and may help the user track progress and receive feedback.

Apps for Improving Thinking Skills

Apps that help the user with cognitive remediation (improved thinking skills) are promising. These apps are often targeted toward people with serious mental illnesses.

Skill-Training Apps

Skill-training apps may feel more like games than other mental-health apps as they help users learn new coping or thinking skills. The user might watch an educational video about anxiety management or the importance of social support. Next, the user might pick some new strategies to try and then use the app to track how often those new skills are practiced.

Illness Management, Supported Care

This type of app technology adds additional support by allowing the user to interact with another human being. The app may help the user connect with peer support or may send information to a trained health-care provider who can offer guidance and therapy options. Researchers are working to learn how much human interaction people need for app-based treatments to be effective.

Passive Symptom Tracking

A lot of effort is going into developing apps that can collect data using the sensors built into smartphones. These sensors can record movement patterns, social interactions (such as the number of texts and phone calls), behavior at different times of the day, vocal tone and speed, and more. In the future, apps may be able to analyze these data to determine the user's real time state of mind. Such apps may be able to recognize changes in behavior patterns that signal a mood episode such as mania, depression, or psychosis before it occurs. An app may not replace a mental-health professional, but it may be able to alert caregivers when a client needs additional attention. The goal is to create apps that support a range of users, including those with serious mental illnesses.

Data Collection

Data collection apps can gather data without any help from the user. Receiving information from a large number of individuals at the same time can increase researchers' understanding of mental health and help them develop better interventions.

RESEARCH VIA SMARTPHONE?

Dr. Patricia Areán's pioneering BRIGHTEN study showed that research via smartphone app is already a reality. The BRIGHTEN study was remarkable because it used technology to both deliver treatment interventions and also to actually conduct the research trial. In other words, the research team used technology to recruit, screen, enroll, treat, and assess participants. BRIGHTEN was especially exciting because the study showed that technology can be an efficient way to pilot test promising new treatments and that those treatments need to be engaging.

A NEW PARTNERSHIP: CLINICIANS AND ENGINEERS

Researchers have found that interventions are most effective when people like them, are engaged and want to continue using them. Behavioral health apps will need to combine the engineers' skills for making an app easy to use and entertaining with the clinician's skills for providing effective treatment options.

Researchers and software engineers are developing and testing apps that do everything from managing medications to teaching coping skills to predicting when someone may need more emotional help. Intervention apps may help someone give up smoking, manage symptoms, or overcome anxiety, depression, posttraumatic stress disorder (PTSD), or insomnia. While the apps are becoming more appealing and user-friendly, there still is not a lot of information on their effectiveness.

EVALUATING APPS

There are no review boards, checklists, or widely accepted rules for choosing a mental-health app. Most apps do not have peer-reviewed research to support their claims, and it is unlikely that every mental-health app will go through a randomized, controlled research trial to test effectiveness. One reason is that testing is a slow process and technology evolves quickly. By the time an app has been put through rigorous scientific testing, the original technology may be outdated.

Currently, there are no national standards for evaluating the effectiveness of the hundreds of mental-health apps that are available. Consumers should be cautious about trusting a program. However, there are a few suggestions for finding an app that may work for you:

- **Ask a trusted health-care provider for a recommendation.** Some larger providers may offer several apps and collect data on their use.
- Check to see if the app offers recommendations for what to do if symptoms get worse or if there is a psychiatric emergency.
- Decide if you want an app that is completely automated or an app that offers opportunities for contact with a trained person.
- **Search for information on the app developer.** Can you find helpful information about his or her credentials and experience?
- **Beware of misleading logos.** The National Institute of Mental Health (NIMH) has not developed and does not endorse any apps. However, some app developers have unlawfully used the NIMH logo to market their products.
- **Search the PubMed database offered by the U.S. National Library of Medicine (NLM).** This resource contains articles on a wide range of research topics, including mental-health app development.
- If there is no information about a particular app, check to see if it is based on a treatment that has been tested. For example, research has shown that Internet-based cognitive-behavioral therapy (CBT) is as effective as conventional CBT for disorders that respond well to

CBT, such as depression, anxiety, social phobia, and panic disorder.

- **Try it.** If you are interested in an app, test it for a few days and decide if it is easy to use, holds your attention, and if you want to continue using it. An app is only effective if keeps users engaged for weeks or months.

Chapter 27 | **Enabling New Cancer Technologies**

INTEGRATION AND VALIDATION OF EMERGING TECHNOLOGIES TO ACCELERATE CANCER RESEARCH

These exploratory and developmental projects are advancing the development and validation of new enabling technologies and tools for basic and clinical cancer research. The focus of these projects includes: enhancing experimental and analytical capabilities to understand the complexities of cancer, developing new technologies to advance cancer diagnosis, designing predictive models of cancer progression and responses to treatment, and generating new approaches to improve cancer-related data quality. Investigators in this program are also performing technology validation to ensure that new approaches could be readily adopted by the cancer research community.

These projects are being funded to overcome persistent challenges in cancer research and have the potential to lead to new capabilities in cancer research areas.

PATIENT-DERIVED XENOGRAFTS DEVELOPMENT NETWORK

Patient-derived xenografts (PDX) models describe an experimental method where tissue from a cancer patient's tumor is implanted in a mouse. These models are emerging as an important approach for translational cancer research. For example, scientists can perform PDX trials where they test drug treatments in mice to understand a tumor's response to therapy and potential biomarkers of an effective treatment. These PDX trials can help researchers determine

This chapter includes text excerpted from "Develop New Enabling Cancer Technologies," National Cancer Institute (NCI), October 22, 2018.

the most promising cancer drugs or drug combinations to test in specific populations of cancer patients.

However, PDX models are often developed in isolated programs, leading to a lack of standardization in these systems, as well as issues validating and replicating the results. Also, isolated collections of PDX models are often too small to reflect the diversity of patient tumors found in large-scale clinical trials.

PDXNet is addressing research challenges related to PDX models. PDX Development and Trial Centers (PDTCs) are developing PDX models on a large scale, advancing standardization procedures for these experimental systems, and designing model validation methods to advance the translation of PDX findings to clinical cancer treatments. The PDTCs are determining the best PDX trial approaches for the experimental testing of cancer drugs in molecularly defined tumors.

Minority (M)-PDTCs are developing racially and ethnically diverse PDX models that can be used to test cancer treatments. These centers aim to advance the understanding of disparities observed in the outcomes of cancer treatments among racially and ethnically diverse populations.

Interactions and collaborations across PDXNet, as well as data sharing with the broader community, are supported by the PDXNet Data Commons and Coordinating Center (PDCCC).

The National Cancer Institute (NCI) also supports interdisciplinary collaborative projects between PDXNet and researchers outside the network to accelerate drug testing in PDX model collections.

Along with investigators developing PDX models, the Patient-Derived Models Repository at the Frederick National Laboratory for Cancer Research plays an important role in PDXNet. This repository is developing PDX models from tissue samples across the country, stored in a PDX bank that can be shared with investigators in the PDTCs and the cancer research community.

ACTIVITIES TO PROMOTE TECHNOLOGY RESEARCH COLLABORATIONS FOR CANCER RESEARCH

There are two unique NCI programs related to APTRC that focus on supporting technology development for advancing cancer research.

The Innovative Molecular Analysis Technologies (IMAT) program supports innovative, data-generating platforms and methods while the Informatics Technologies for Cancer Research (ITCR) program supports data processing and visualization technologies.

The NCI is accelerating the development of new enabling cancer technologies by leveraging expertise in IMAT and ITCR through multidisciplinary collaborations between investigators in these programs. These collaborative projects bring together complementary technology platforms and approach to enhance their capabilities for studies of cancer.

NOVEL TECHNOLOGIES TO FACILITATE RESEARCH USING NEXT GENERATION PATIENT-DERIVED CANCER MODELS

Research projects in this program are developing technology tools to accelerate and enhance studies across the spectrum of cancer research using advanced human-derived next-generation cancer models, including 3D organoids and conditionally reprogrammed cells. These projects are specifically advancing cancer models developed as part of the Human Cancer Models Initiative (HCMI). The technology tools being examined by investigators of the program include new laboratory methods and reagents for screening studies and computational approaches for data analysis from experiments using next-generation cancer models. The goal of these research projects is to enhance the adoption, sharing, and use of next-generation cancer models to advance cancer research progress.

SMALL BUSINESS INNOVATION RESEARCH AND SMALL BUSINESS TECHNOLOGY TRANSFER RESEARCH GRANTS AND CONTRACTS FOR ENABLING TECHNOLOGIES

The NCI supports grants and contracts with small businesses developing new enabling technologies for cancer research. The range of projects supported through these investments spans the breadth of Cancer Moonshot, with some of the currently active projects focusing on the development of experimental models to study cancer disparities and the design of new cancer detection technologies, for example.

EVALUATION OF PROSTATE SPECIFIC MEMBRANE ANTIGEN-BASED PET IMAGING OF HIGH-RISK PROSTATE CANCER

At this time, there are limited ways to stratify high-risk prostate cancer patients. To address this issue, researchers with NCI's Center for Cancer Research are investigating the clinical use of positron emission tomography (PET) imaging on patients with high-risk prostate cancer. The PET offers the opportunity to develop an approach to image Prostate-Specific Membrane Antigen (PSMA), a protein that is expressed in prostate cancer tissue and associated with cancer aggressiveness. By comparing the PSMA PET scans with complication-free survival outcomes, the researchers hope to understand if PSMA imaging could be used to identify subsets of prostate cancer patients and guide treatment decisions.

NCI PROGRAM FOR NATURAL PRODUCTS DISCOVERY

The NCI Program for Natural Product Discovery (NPNPD) is advancing natural product research and the discovery of new molecules in nature that impact biological processes of cancer. The NCI Natural Products Repository of the NPNPD has over 230,000 extracts of plants, microbes, algae, and marine species, which are being used for the generation of more than a million research-ready, partially purified natural product samples. The NPNPD collection of natural product extracts and partially purified samples is being sent to research centers performing drug screens around the world. Once researchers identify an extract with potential anti-cancer activity, the NPNPD uses automated techniques to quickly identify and isolate the active compound for more detailed studies.

Chapter 28 | **Role of Technology in the Treatment for Osteopenia**

Osteopenia is a common skeletal condition characterized by below-normal bone mineral density (BMD) and accelerated loss of bone mass that leads to osteoporosis. If BMD loss is not mitigated, patients become osteoporotic and are at increased risk of bone fractures, particularly of the hips and spine. Such fractures reduce independent living, shorten life, and increase morbidity. Clinical guidelines for treating osteopenia include both dietary modifications and high-impact exercise. While a healthy diet and high-impact exercise can be effective in maintaining BMD, compliance is low. The alternative is prescribed medications (e.g., bisphosphonates), which effectively inhibit the decline in BMD and can even increase BMD. However, rare but serious adverse events with prolonged administration of bisphosphonates limit their use to patients with osteoporotic levels of BMD, when the antifracture benefits of medications considerably outweigh their potential for harm.

Bone Health Technologies has developed OsteoBoost™, a wearable vibration device designed to provide controlled, safe, and therapeutic mechanical stimulation localized to the hips and spine in order to mitigate bone mass loss and fracture risk.

This chapter includes text excerpted from "NIA Small Business Showcase: Bone Health Technologies," National Institute on Aging (NIA), National Institutes of Health (NIH), August 8, 2020.

Osteopenia affects about 43 million Americans. There is a need for an effective, nondrug intervention to prevent early progression of bone loss prior to patients reaching an osteoporotic state.

Although whole-body vibration treatment has been shown to be effective at mitigating bone loss, it is inconvenient because it requires the user to stand still on a vibrating platform for 20 to 30 minutes per day. In contrast, OsteoBoost™ is a wearable belt that allows the user to do normal activities while getting the daily vibration treatment. OsteoBoost™ also targets therapeutic vibration to the hips and lower spine, two of the most common anatomic regions for osteoporotic fractures. In addition, the OsteoBoost™ advantages are offered in a low-cost solution.

INTELLECTUAL PROPERTY

Bone Health Technologies has intellectual property (IP) covering the method of delivering vibration through a body-worn device placed over the sacrococcygeal region. This area is critical to target the two key skeletal areas affected by osteoporotic fractures: the hips and spine. The company also has IP on the use of accelerometers and pressure sensors to ensure proper fit of the belt and application of the correct magnitude of vibration. Lastly, the company has filed a series of patents protecting the broad methods and the enabling features of their commercial design and future embodiments.

PRODUCT DEVELOPMENT AND REGULATORY STRATEGY

Bone Health Technologies is developing two versions of the OsteoBoost™ device. Accordingly, the company has a two-pronged approach to both product development and regulatory approval. They have already developed their first device, called "OsteoBoost™," which is available over the counter as a Class I medical device (following the regulatory pathway for whole-body vibration devices). Bone Health Technologies has registered with FDA for marketing of OsteoBoost™.

The second device, called "OsteoBoost™ Pro," will be a Class II medical device with indications for use focused on treating osteopenia. OsteoBoost™ Pro has additional features that enable treatment parameters to be automatically optimized for each patient with each treatment session. The data from the ongoing pivotal clinical trial will support a de novo FDA submission for clearance of OsteoBoost™ Pro.

COMMERCIALIZATION STRATEGY

Bone Health Technologies is developing two versions of the OsteoBoost™ device for commercial release. To enable the company to bring the technology to the market quickly, they have developed their first device, called "OsteoBoost™," which is already available over the counter. OsteoBoost™ can be purchased through the company's website, www.osteoboost.com. The second device, called "OsteoBoost™ Pro," will be a Class II medical device. The data from the ongoing pivotal clinical trial will support a de novo, the U.S. Food and Drug Administration (FDA) submission for clearance of OsteoBoost™ Pro as a treatment for osteopenia. The commercial launch of OsteoBoost™ Pro is expected in early 2022.

Chapter 29 | **Nutrigenomics**

The importance of diet and nutrition in the etiology of a number of metabolic and autoimmune diseases, affecting mortality and morbidity is well recognized. However, the exact nature of how diet impacts health and disease is not clearly understood. Several studies involving children of famine cohorts clearly demonstrate that nutrition is not only important at every stage in the life of an individual but also plays a critical role in the health and disease from in-utero to old age, thus providing a broad window of opportunity for nutrition in disease prevention. In addition, nutrients and dietary components alter gene expression, modulate protein and metabolite levels in target tissues, modify cellular and metabolic pathways, affect epigenetic phenomena, and modify response to drugs. These nutrient-host interactions thus influence an individual's predisposition to disease and potential therapeutic response. However, the exact nature of these interactions and underlying causal mechanisms are poorly understood.

Current nutritional research methodologies often fail to explore nutrient-host interactions beyond associations. For this reason, there exists a critical need for novel approaches and methodologies employed in nutrition research that allow for the characterization of nutrient host interactions and how they play a critical role in health and disease.

In the genomic era, the high throughput omic technologies are emerging as reliable technical platforms for generating high dimensional biological data, for studying the impact of environmental exposures such as diet, on multiple biological pathways affecting human health and disease in ways that complement conventional

This chapter includes text excerpted from "Nutrigenetics and Nutrigenomics Approaches for Nutrition Research," National Institutes of Health (NIH), November 1, 2017. Reviewed June 2021.

scientific approaches. In recent years, there is a lot of enthusiasm for the application of these methodologies to nutrition research. Specifically, the field of nutrigenetics explores the impact of genetic variants on nutrient metabolism whereas nutrigenomics explores the gene expression, function, and regulation in response to nutrient intake and collectively comprises the approaches namely transcriptomics, proteomics, epigenomics, and metabolomics that enable analysis of multiple mRNA species, proteins and metabolites, respectively. Such approaches can be targeted to a defined set of analytes, or untargeted allowing the analysis of global molecular species. The molecular signatures from these approaches can provide valuable insights into pathophysiological processes and yield potentially clinically relevant markers of diseases.

While the field is still in its initial stages, the application of these omic approaches to well-designed animal and human nutritional intervention studies and disease models holds great promise for understanding the impact of nutrients and dietary constituents on host metabolism and allow for identification of unique metabolic signatures critical for patho-physiological processes, in response to multiple, cumulative nutrient exposures. When applied to various transgenic and disease models and target tissues, these approaches have the ability to yield mechanistic information on the role of nutrients in the etiology and provide temporal changes associated with the disease process. The initial literature in this area already indicates a great promise on how omic approaches can be successfully applied to nutrition research to unravel nutrient-gene interactions both at the basic and population level.

Collaboration between investigators with demonstrated expertise in nutrition research and omics techniques is highly encouraged.

Examples of the application of nutrigenetics and nutrigenomics approaches to nutrition research include but are not limited to:

- Impact of genetic polymorphisms on nutrient absorption, transport, and metabolism
- Impact of nutrients and dietary components on gene expression that affects nutrient absorption, transport,

and metabolism in target tissues and relevant bio-
specimens in health
- Mechanisms by which specific nutrients/dietary
  components modulate intestinal physiology
  (transporters), barrier function, inflammation, and/or
  microbiome composition
- Mechanisms by which nutrient sensing in the gut is
  transduced to extra-intestinal organs and tissues
- Studies that explore the interaction/competition
  between various nutrients for their absorption,
  transport, metabolism, and elimination
- Studies that explore the interaction/competition
  between various nutrients and drugs for their
  absorption, transport, metabolism, and elimination
- Impact of nutrient excess and deficiency in health and
  diseases
- Mechanism of action of prebiotics and resistant
  starches on intestinal function and host metabolism
- Mechanism of action of probiotics and secreted
  probiotic factors on intestinal function and host
  metabolism

RESEARCHES ON NUTRIGENETICS
The National Cancer Institute
The National Cancer Institute (NCI) has multiple interests in nutrigenetic and nutrigenomic-based mechanistic studies including
vitamins, minerals and other nutritive agents present in food that
reduce the risk of cancer. Genetic variations present in individuals
may alter their susceptibility to cancer. Specific interests include
strategies to facilitate precision medicine using nutrition-focused
interventions to reduce cancer risks in various populations including those mediated by host-microbiome interactions.

National Center for Complementary and Integrative Health
The National Center for Complementary and Integrative
Health (NCCIH) is particularly interested in nutrigenetic and

321

nutigenomic-based mechanistic studies of interaction and competition between nutrient-nutrient, nutrient-drug, dietary supplements, and probiotics/prebiotics on host-microbial metabolism, immunologic/inflammatory signaling, neuro-hormonal pathways, and target tissues [including bioavailability, absorption, transport, metabolism, and excretion studies] that impact the basic fundamentals that will eventually lead to a better understanding of the gut-brain function in health promotion and disease prevention. The NCCIH is also interested in the impact of [selected] nutrients, dietary supplements, the ketogenic diet, and probiotic/prebiotic modulation of specific conditions including pain. In addition, the NCCIH is interested in studying mechanisms for how botanical products, fish oil, and other dietary supplements, and prebiotics in helping to identify their relationship to pain and inflammation.

Chapter 30 | Nanotechnology

Chapter Contents

Section 30.1 | What Is Nanotechnology?

This section includes text excerpted from "Nanotechnology," National Institute for Occupational Safety and Health (NIOSH), Centers for Disease Control and Prevention (CDC), March 27, 2020.

Nanotechnology involves the manipulation of nanometer length matter (one-billionth of a meter) to produce new materials, structures, and devices. The U.S. National Nanotechnology Initiative (NNI) defines technology as nanotechnology only if it involves all of the following:

- Research and technology development involves structures with at least one dimension in the 1–100 nanometer range.
- Creating and using structures, devices, and systems that have new properties and functions because of their nanometer-scale dimensions
- Ability to control or manipulate on the atomic scale

Nanostructured materials do not represent a new phenomenon. For example, the red and yellow hues in stained glass are the result of the presence of nanometer-sized gold and silver particles. However, the ability to probe, manipulate, understand and engineer matter at atomic scales has only recently become a possibility. In a 1959 lecture titled "There is plenty of room at the bottom," the Nobel laureate Professor Richard P. Feynman introduced the idea of a new and exciting field of research based on manipulating matter at the atomic level. At the time, Professor Feynman's predictions were based on theoretical speculation.

However, developments, such as the invention of the scanning tunneling microscope in 1981 have since made nanoscale science a reality. Nanotechnology is now a rapidly growing field of research and development that is cutting across many traditional boundaries.

WORKER RISKS

Workers within nanotechnology-related industries have the potential to be exposed to uniquely engineered materials with novel sizes, shapes, and physical and chemical properties. Occupational health risks associated with manufacturing and using nanomaterials are not yet clearly understood. Minimal information is currently available on dominant exposure routes, potential exposure levels, and material toxicity of nanomaterials.

CURRENT RESEARCH

Studies have indicated that low solubility nanoparticles are more toxic than larger particles on a mass-for-mass basis. There are strong indications that particle surface area and surface chemistry are responsible for observed responses in cell cultures and animals. Studies suggest that some nanoparticles can move from the respiratory system to other organs. Research is continuing to understand how these unique properties may lead to specific health effects.

FREQUENTLY ASKED QUESTIONS IN NANOTECHNOLOGY
What Kind of Nanomaterials (Nanoparticles) Are in Production in the United States?

An increasing number of products and materials are becoming commercially available. These include nanoscale powders, solutions, suspensions as well as composite materials and devices containing nanomaterials. Nanoscale titanium dioxide is currently used in cosmetics, sunblock creams, and self-cleaning windows. Nanomaterials are increasingly being used in optoelectronic, electronic, magnetic, medical imaging, drug delivery, cosmetic, catalytic, and other applications. Nano-coatings and nano-composites are being used in a wide range of consumer products from bicycles to automobiles.

How Many Workers Are Potentially Exposed to Nanoparticles?

By one estimate, there are 400,000 workers worldwide in the field of nanotechnology, with an estimated 150,000 of those in the United States. The National Science Foundation has estimated that approximately six million workers will be employed in nanotechnology industries worldwide by 2020.

How Many Workers May Be Exposed to Nanoparticles?

Nanomaterials that can be inhaled, ingested, or can penetrate skin indicate a potential for exposure and present the possibility of potential health effects. Processes that lead to airborne nanometer-diameter particles, respirable nanostructured particles (typically smaller than four micrometers), and respirable droplets of nanomaterial suspensions, solutions, and slurries are of particular concern for potential inhalation exposures.

What Effects Do Nanoparticles Have on Worker's Health?

Results from experimental animal studies with engineered nanomaterials have provided evidence that some nanoparticle exposures can result in serious health effects involving pulmonary and cardiovascular systems and possibly other organ systems. The National Institute for Occupational Safety and Health (NIOSH) researchers have conducted or participated in the following research activities that have determined that:

- Asbestos and carbon nanotubes (CNTs) affect similar molecular signaling pathways in cultured lung cells, with asbestos exhibiting greater potency.
- Nano or ultrafine titanium dioxide (TiO_2) causes pulmonary inflammation and neuro-immune responses.
- Ultrafine TiO_2 or carbon black causes more inflammation than fine TiO_2 or carbon black on a mass-dose basis.
- Dispersion of ultrafine carbon black nanoparticles in the lungs of rats following intratracheal instillation results in an inflammatory response that is greater than agglomerated ultrafine carbon black.
- Pulmonary exposure to single-walled carbon nanotubes (SWCNTs) and multi-walled carbon nanotubes (MWCNTs) in mice causes acute and chronic systemic responses associated with adverse cardiovascular effects.
- SWCNTs, MWCNTs, and carbon nanofibers (CNFs) have equal or greater potency in causing adverse health

effects in laboratory animals, including pulmonary inflammation and fibrosis, in comparison with other inhaled particles (ultrafine TiO_2, carbon black, crystalline silica, and asbestos).

- CNTs are genotoxic and can transform lung epithelial cells after long-term, low-dose in vitro exposure.
- Preliminary research has indicated that mice exposed to both MWCNTs and methylcholanthrene (a known cancer initiator) are significantly more likely to develop tumors than those exposed to just MWCNT alone.

How Should Workplace Exposures to Nanomaterials Be Measured?

An exposure assessment should review the process and material flow plans for the facility and identify tasks and workers that may be exposed to nanomaterials. Staff interviews and a preliminary walk-through of the facility should be performed to ensure that all activities and potential exposure pathways are identified prior to sampling. Information collected should include the potential magnitude, duration, and frequency of exposure during different job tasks, or at specific processes, and the amounts of materials being used. Current work practices and existing engineering controls should be evaluated.

Exposure assessment and control verification approaches can be performed with traditional industrial hygiene sampling methods that include the use of samplers placed at static locations (area sampling), samples collected in the breathing zone of the employee (personal sampling), and measurements with real time direct reading instrumentation. An integrated sampling strategy should include the use of both direct reading instrumentation and filter-based samples. Direct-reading instrumentation can be used to datalog particle concentrations. Filter-based samples can be used to identify the nanomaterial of interest with electron microscopy and elemental analysis.

Should Workplace Exposures to Nanomaterials Be Controlled, and If So, How?

Identifying appropriate control methods depends on knowing the characteristics of the nanomaterial, how exposures to nanomaterials can occur in the workplace, what are the potential effects of workplace exposure to a given material, and how can exposures to nanomaterials be measured accurately and reliably.

What Are the Potential Applications of Nanotechnology in Occupational Safety and Health?

Nanotechnology holds great promise for society, and occupational safety and health are no exception. Engineered nanomaterials may support the development of the following: high-performance filter media, respirators, coatings in nonsoiling/dust-repellant/self-cleaning clothes, fillers for noise absorption materials, fire retardants, protective screens for prevention of roof falls, and curtains for ventilation control in mines, catalysts for emissions reduction, and clean-up of pollutants and hazardous substances.

Nanotechnology-based sensors and communication devices may help empower workers during work-based emergencies so that they can take preventative steps to reduce their exposure to the risk of injury. The smallness of their size coupled with wireless technology may facilitate the development of wearable sensors and systems for real time occupational safety and health management. Nanotechnology-based fuel cells, lab-on-chip analyzers, and optoelectronic devices all have the potential to be useful in the safe, healthy, and efficient design of work itself.

HEALTH-CARE BENEFITS OF NANOTECHNOLOGY

Nanotechnology is already broadening the medical tools, knowledge, and therapies currently available to clinicians. Nanomedicine, the application of nanotechnology in medicine, draws on the natural scale of biological phenomena to produce precise solutions for disease prevention, diagnosis, and treatment. Below are some examples of recent advances in this area:

- Commercial applications have adapted gold nanoparticles as probes for the detection of targeted sequences of nucleic acids, and gold nanoparticles are also being clinically investigated as potential treatments for cancer and other diseases.

- Better imaging and diagnostic tools enabled by nanotechnology are paving the way for earlier diagnosis, more individualized treatment options, and better therapeutic success rates.
- Nanotechnology is being studied for both the diagnosis and treatment of atherosclerosis, or the buildup of plaque in arteries. In one technique, researchers created a nanoparticle that mimics the body's "good" cholesterol, known as "high-density lipoprotein" (HDL), which helps to shrink plaque.
- The design and engineering of advanced solid-state nanopore materials could allow for the development of novel gene sequencing technologies that enable single-molecule detection at low cost and high speed with minimal sample preparation and instrumentation.
- Nanotechnology researchers are working on a number of different therapeutics where a nanoparticle can encapsulate or otherwise help to deliver medication directly to cancer cells and minimize the risk of damage to healthy tissue. This has the potential to change the way doctors treat cancer and dramatically reduce the toxic effects of chemotherapy.
- Research in the use of nanotechnology for regenerative medicine spans several application areas, including bone and neural tissue engineering. For instance, novel materials can be engineered to mimic the crystal mineral structure of human bone or used as a restorative resin for dental applications. Researchers are looking for ways to grow complex tissues with the goal of one day growing human organs for transplant. Researchers are also studying ways to use graphene nanoribbons to help repair spinal cord injuries; preliminary research shows that neurons grow well on the conductive graphene surface.
- Nanomedicine researchers are looking at ways that nanotechnology can improve vaccines, including vaccine delivery without the use of needles. Researchers also are working to create a universal vaccine scaffold

for the annual flu vaccine that would cover more strains and require fewer resources to develop each year.

Section 30.2 | **Nanomedicine**

This section includes text excerpted from "Nanomedicine," National Institutes of Health (NIH), September 1, 2016. Reviewed June 2021.

Nanomedicine, an offshoot of nanotechnology, refers to highly specific medical intervention at the molecular scale for curing disease or repairing damaged tissues, such as bone, muscle, or nerve. A nanometer is one-billionth of a meter, too small to be seen with a conventional lab microscope. It is at this size scale – about 100 nanometers or less – that biological molecules and structures operate in living cells.

The National Institutes of Health (NIH) vision for Nanomedicine is built upon the strengths of the NIH-funded researchers in probing and understanding the biological, biochemical, and biophysical mechanisms of living tissues. Since the cellular machinery operates at the nanoscale, the primary goal of the program – characterizing the molecular components inside cells at a level of precision that leads to reengineering intracellular complexes – is a monumental challenge.

The teams selected to carry out this initiative consist of researchers with deep knowledge of biology and physiology, physics, chemistry, math and computation, engineering, and clinical medicine. The choice and design of experimental approaches are directed by the need to solve clinical problems (e.g., treatment of sickle cell disease, blindness, cancer, and Huntington disease). These are very challenging problems, and great breakthroughs are needed to achieve the goals within the projected 10-year timeframe. The initiative was selected for the NIH Roadmap (now common fund) precisely because of the challenging, high-risk goals, and the NIH team is working closely with the funded investigators to use the funds and the intellectual resources of the network of investigators to meet those challenges.

TEN-YEAR PROGRAM DESIGN – HIGH RISK, HIGH REWARD

The Centers were funded with the expectation that the first half of the initiative would be more heavily focused on basic science with increased emphasis on the application of this knowledge in the second five years. This was a novel, experimental approach to translational medicine that began by funding basic scientists interested in gaining a deep understanding of an intracellular nanoscale system and necessitated collaboration with clinicians from the outset in order to properly position work at the centers so that during the second half of the initiative, studies would be applied directly to medical applications. The program began with eight Nanomedicine Development Centers (NDCs), and four centers remain in the second half of the program.

CLINICAL CONSULTING BOARDS

The program has established the Clinical Consulting Boards (CCBs) for each of the continuing centers. These boards consist of at least three disease-specific clinician-scientists who are experts in the target disease(s). The intent is for the CCBs to provide advice and insight into the needs and barriers regarding resource and personnel allocations as well as scientific advice as needed to help the centers reach their translational goals. Each CCB reports directly to the NIH project team.

TRANSLATIONAL PATH

In 2011, the PIs of the NDCs worked with their CCBs to precisely define their translational goals and the translational research path needed to reach those goals by the end of the initiative in 2015. To facilitate this, the NIH project team asked them to develop critical decision points along their path. These critical decision points differ from distinct milestones because they may be adjusted based on successes, challenges, barriers, and progress. Similarly, the timing of these decision points may be revised as the centers progress. Research progress and critical decision points are revisited several times a year by the CCB and the NIH team, and when a decision point is reached, the next steps are re-examined for relevance, feasibility, and timing.

TRANSITION PLAN

Throughout the program, various projects have been spun off of work at all the centers and most have received funding from other sources. This was by design as work at each center has been shifting from basic science to translational studies. Centers will not be supported by the common fund after 10 years. It is expected that work at the centers will be more appropriately funded by other sources. Preclinical targets will likely be developed, and the work at each center will be focused on a specific disease so the work will need to transition out of the experimental space of the common fund.

Section 30.3 | Nanotechnology at NIOSH

This section contains text excerpted from the following sources: Text in this section begins with excerpts from "Nanotechnology at NIOSH," National Institute for Occupational Safety and Health (NIOSH), Centers for Disease Control and Prevention (CDC), March 29, 2018; Text under the heading "The NIOSH's Research on Nanotechnology: FAQs" is excerpted from "Nanotechnology – Frequently Asked Questions," National Institute for Occupational Safety and Health (NIOSH), Centers for Disease Control and Prevention (CDC), March 29, 2018; Text beginning with the heading "Nanotechnology Research Center" is excerpted from "Nanotechnology Research Center," National Institute for Occupational Safety and Health (NIOSH), Centers for Disease Control and Prevention (CDC), January 16, 2019.

The National Institute for Occupational Safety and Health (NIOSH) is the leading federal agency conducting research and providing guidance on the occupational safety and health implications and applications of nanotechnology. Given the rapid growth and global reach of nanotechnology, the NIOSH established the Nanotechnology Research Center (NTRC) in 2004 to identify critical issues, create a strategic plan for investigating these issues, coordinate the NIOSH research effort, develop research partnerships, and disseminate information gained.

The NTRC is comprised of nanotechnology-related activities and projects consisting of and supported by a diverse group of scientists from various NIOSH divisions and laboratories.

TEN CRITICAL TOPIC AREAS
Toxicity and Internal Dose
- Investigating and determining the physical and chemical properties (e.g., size, shape, solubility) that influence the potential toxicity of nanoparticles
- Evaluating short and long-term effects that nanomaterials may have in organ systems and tissues (e.g., lungs)
- Determining biological mechanisms for potential toxic effects
- Creating and integrating models to assist in assessing possible hazards
- Determining if a measure other than mass is more appropriate for determining toxicity

Risk Assessment
- Determining the likelihood that current exposure-response data (human or animal) could be used in identifying and assessing potential occupational hazards
- Developing a framework for evaluating potential hazards and predicting potential occupational risk of exposure to nanomaterials

Epidemiology and Surveillance
- Evaluating existing epidemiological workplace studies where nanomaterials are used
- Identifying knowledge gaps where epidemiological studies could advance understanding of nanomaterials and evaluating the likelihood of conducting new studies
- Integrating nanotechnology health and safety issues into existing hazard surveillance methods and determining whether additional screening methods are needed
- Using existing systems to share data and information about nanotechnology

Engineering Controls and PPE

- Evaluating the effectiveness of engineering controls in reducing occupational exposures to nanoaerosols and developing new controls where needed
- Evaluating and improving current personal protective equipment
- Developing recommendations to prevent or limit occupational exposures (e.g., respirator fit testing)
- Evaluating suitability of control banding techniques where additional information is needed, and evaluating the effectiveness of alternative materials

Measurement Methods

- Evaluating methods of measuring the mass of respirable particles in the air and determining if this measurement can be used to measure nanomaterials
- Developing and field-testing practical methods to accurately measure airborne nanomaterials in the workplace
- Developing testing and evaluation systems to compare and validate sampling instruments

Exposure Assessment

- Determining key factors that influence the production, dispersion, accumulation, and reentry of nanomaterials into the workplace
- Assessing possible exposure when nanomaterials are inhaled or settle on the skin
- Determining how possible exposures differ by work process
- Determining what happens to nanomaterials once they enter the body

Fire and Explosion Safety

- Identifying physical and chemical properties that contribute to dustiness, combustibility, flammability, and conductivity of nanomaterials.

- Recommending alternative work practices to eliminate or reduce workplace exposures to nanoparticles.

Recommendations and Guidance

- Using the best available science to make interim recommendations for workplace safety and health practices during the production and use of nanomaterials.
- Evaluating and updating occupational exposure limits for mass-based airborne particles to ensure good continuing precautionary practices.
- Providing guidance and publications to help provide information on the best available science for nanomaterials.

Global Collaborations

- Establishing partnerships and collaborations to allow for identification and sharing of research needs, approaches, and results
- Developing and disseminating training and educational materials to workers and health and safety professionals

Applications

- Identifying uses of nanotechnology for application in occupational safety and health
- Evaluating and disseminating effective applications to workers and occupational safety and health professionals

THE NIOSH's RESEARCH ON NANOTECHNOLOGY: FAQs
Where Can You Find More Information about NIOSH's Research Pertaining to Nanotechnology?

More information on NIOSH's nanotechnology research program can be found on the NIOSH Nanotechnology topic page (www. cdc.gov/niosh/topics/nanotech/). This is designed to be a robust source of information on the NIOSH's research program, with new information added as it becomes available. Additional information can be found on the National Nanotechnology Initiative (NNI) website.

Why Is NIOSH Conducting Research on Nanotechnology?

The NIOSH is performing research to help answer questions that are critical for supporting the responsible development of nano-technology in the United States and the competitive global market. These questions include:

- Are workers exposed to nanomaterials in the manufacture and use of nanomaterials, and if so what are the characteristics and levels of exposures?
- Are there potential adverse health effects of working with nanomaterials?
- What work practices, personal protective equipment, and engineering controls are available, and how effective are they for controlling exposures to nanomaterials?
- NIOSH is addressing these questions through a program of multi-disciplinary research, communication, and partnerships with other agencies, organizations, and stakeholders.

What Knowledge or Expertise Does NIOSH Bring to This Research?

The NIOSH's research role stems from its mission as the federal institute that conducts research and makes recommendations in occupational safety and health. For more than 30 years, the NIOSH has led research to define and address occupational health concerns related to emerging technologies and workplace practices. To its research on nanotechnology and occupational health, the NIOSH brings:

- Experience in defining the characteristics and properties of ultrafine particles (such as welding fume and diesel particulate), which have some features in common with engineered nanomaterials
- Capability of conducting laboratory studies to determine advanced health effects laboratory studies

- Historic leadership in industrial hygiene policies and practices
- Close research partnerships with diverse stakeholders in industry, labor, the government, and academia

How Does NIOSH Relate to Other Government Efforts Associated with Research and Development in Technology?

The NIOSH is working in partnership with other government agencies primarily through participation in the U.S. National Nanotechnology Initiative, a federal research and development program established to coordinate the multiagency efforts in nanoscale science, engineering, and technology. This initiative is managed within the framework of the National Science and Technology Council (NSTC). The NIOSH is a member of the NTSC's Nanoscale Science, Engineering, and Technology Subcommittee (NSET). Within that subcommittee, NIOSH cochairs, with the U.S. Food and Drug Administration, the interagency Nanotechnology, Environmental and Health Implications (NEHI) Working Group.

NANOTECHNOLOGY RESEARCH CENTER

The NIOSH, through its Nanotechnology Research Center (NTRC), leads the federal government in research focused on providing guidance on the occupational safety and health implications and applications of advanced manufacturing, including nanomaterial manufacturing.

PROGRAM DESCRIPTION

The Nanotechnology Research Center (NTRC) conducts research to better understand the effects of advanced materials, including engineered nanomaterials, on human health and methods to control or eliminate exposures. Nanomaterials are extremely small particles (with at least one dimension between 1 and 100 nanometers) purposefully designed to have certain new or unique characteristics, such as strength or elasticity, needed to make advanced materials and products.

NIOSH is the leading federal agency conducting research and providing guidance on the occupational safety and health implications and applications of advanced materials and nanotechnology. Given the rapid growth and global reach of nanotechnology, NIOSH established the NTRC in 2004 to identify critical issues, create a strategic plan for investigating these issues, coordinate the NIOSH research effort, develop research partnerships, and disseminate information gained. The NTRC is comprised of nanotechnology- and advanced manufacturing-related activities and projects consisting of and supported by a diverse group of scientists from various NIOSH divisions and laboratories.

The NTRC works with partners in industry, labor, trade associations, professional organizations, other federal agencies, and academia. The NTRC focuses on these areas:

- Increasing understanding of hazards and related health risks to workers who make and use advanced materials, such as nanomaterials.
- Preventing occupational exposures to advanced materials, such as nanomaterials through understanding control technologies and protective technologies.

Much research is still needed to understand the impact of advanced manufacturing and nanotechnology on health and to determine appropriate exposure monitoring and control strategies. As hazards and risks associated with advanced materials and engineered nanomaterials continue to be explored and characterized, knowledge from that research will serve as a foundation for an anticipatory and proactive approach to the introduction and use of materials in advanced manufacturing. At this time, the limited evidence available suggests caution when potential exposures to free – unbound nanoparticles may occur.

BURDEN, NEED, AND IMPACT
Burden
Nanotechnology is the understanding and control of matter at dimensions between approximately 1 and 100 nanometers, where

unique phenomena enable novel applications. The President's 2019 Budget requests $1.4 billion for the National Nanotechnology Initiative, with a cumulative total of nearly $27 billion in nanotechnology research since 2001. However, less than 3 percent of the cumulative federal budget has been directed to study the Environmental, Health, and Safety (EHS) potential of engineered nanomaterials. The U.S. recognized that the historical investment was not sufficient to address EHS knowledge gaps, and the amount projected for FY 2019 EHS research is approximately 5 percent of the total NNI investment.

Air pollution (consisting of incidental nanoparticles) epidemiology has demonstrated that ultrafine particles can affect the lung, cardiovascular, and other organ systems; and are responsible for excess respiratory and cardiovascular mortality. Recent air pollution and animal studies have shown various ultrafine and nanoscale particles are linked to adverse neurological changes. Welding fumes, which contain several types of nanoparticles, are known to cause toxicological and carcinogenic effects. Development and commercialization of nanotechnology-based products and applications are occurring at a rapid rate, making it imperative that more information on the potential health hazards from exposure to engineered nanomaterials (ENMs) be generated. The number of workers exposed to EMNs is not known, but market reports indicate that large and growing quantities of ENMs are being used in commerce, and workers are involved throughout their manufacture, formulation, and use to create nanomaterial products.

While It is too early to identify the exact burden of ENMs to workers, it is reasonable to assume that health effects from exposure to ENMs could be similar to ultrafine air pollution or other dust and fumes that cause pulmonary and cardiovascular effects. Some ENMs appear to be 10–100 times more reactive or potent than their bulk counterparts, so one would expect a commensurate increase in burden for a given exposure. Based on these developing trends, burden in terms of morbidity and mortality has the potential to be large, significant, and costly. Failure to develop the technology responsibly, including worker protection, may ultimately place a burden on capital, entrepreneurial investment, and ultimate benefit to society.

Need

Nanotechnology is continuing to emerge, as commercial application of the technology is only about 20 years old. Consequently, there are many unanswered questions about the risk management continuum of hazard, exposure, risk, and control. Although hazard is the driver of these actions, the wide use of ENMs in commerce means workers potentially have exposure to them. Employers, workers, and other decision-makers are asking for information on all steps of risk management, from hazard identification to control approaches. Consequently, we must address all the steps in the hazard continuum.

Impact

The NIOSH is internationally recognized for its impact on health and safety issues related to advanced manufacturing and nanotechnology. Since its inception, the NTRC has published 12 guidance documents including Approaches to Safe Nanotechnology, Laboratory guidance, Engineering Control guidance and Small Business guidance, developed two recommended occupational exposure limits for ENMs, conducted over 100 field site visits, published over 1600 peer reviewed journal articles and actively participates in voluntary consensus standards development through organizations, such as the International Standards Organization, ASTM, and Organization for Economic Co-Operation and Development.

PROGRAM GOALS

A key leadership role for the NTRC is the development of goals and these have been identified in previous strategic plans.

The five overarching strategic goals of the NTRC are:
- **Strategic Goal 1.** Increase understanding of new hazards and related health risks to nanomaterial workers.
- **Strategic Goal 2.** Build upon initial data and information to further increase understanding of the initial hazard findings of engineered nanomaterials.

- **Strategic Goal 3.** Build upon initial guidance materials to further inform nanomaterial workers, employers, health professionals, regulatory agencies, and decision-makers about hazards, risks, and risk management approaches.
- **Strategic Goal 4.** Support epidemiologic studies for nanomaterial workers, including medical, cross-sectional, prospective cohort, and exposure studies.
- **Strategic Goal 5.** Assess and promote national and international adherence with risk management guidance.

NTRC Priority Goals

Based on the burden, need, and impact, the following goals are the top three priorities for the NTRC:

- **Priority 1 – Strategic Goal 1.** Increase understanding of new nanomaterials and related health risks to nanomaterial workers.
- This research will contribute to the body of knowledge about the adverse health effects in animals exposed to various ENMs. The findings will have a direct impact on risk assessment of potential outcomes for exposed workers; contribute to epidemiologic research; and provide background that can be used to create guidance on control technologies and medical surveillance.
- **Priority 2 – Strategic Goal 3.** Build upon initial guidance materials to inform nanomaterial workers, employers, health professionals, regulatory agencies, and decision-makers about hazards, risks, and risk management approaches.
- Various target audiences, such as nanotechnology workers and employers, occupational safety and health professionals, policy-makers, decision-makers, and/or the scientific community in research, manufacturing, construction, mining, oil, and gas, and healthcare will begin or continue to apply NIOSH guidance to responsibly develop, handle, and commercialize ENMs.

Through strategic planning, research, partnering with stakeholders, and making information widely available, the NTRC will continue supporting the responsible development of nanotechnology by translating research into effective risk management guidance and practices across the lifecycle of ENM-enabled products.

- **Priority 3 – Activity/Output Goal 3.1.3.** Use a nanomaterial hazard banding classification scheme to group ENMs.
- This research will investigate the evidence for developing predictive algorithms of structure-activity relationships and comparative toxicity for use in quantitative risk assessment. Findings from this research will provide the scientific basis for developing occupational exposure limits for individual nanomaterials or groups of nanomaterials.

These priorities have been integrated into the NIOSH Strategic Plan in research goals to better understand the potential respiratory health effects of exposure to nanomaterials and other advanced materials in the Construction and Manufacturing sectors, as a well as a goal to research the potential link of nanomaterial exposure to cancer and cardiovascular disease among manufacturing workers.

Section 30.4 | Nanotechnology in Cancer

This section includes text excerpted from "Cancer and Nanotechnology," National Cancer Institute (NCI), August 8, 2017. Reviewed June 2021.

Currently, scientists are limited in their ability to turn promising molecular discoveries into cancer patient benefits. Nanotechnology – the science and engineering of controlling matter, at the molecular scale, to create devices with novel chemical, physical, and/or biological properties that can provide technical control and tools to enable the development of new diagnostics, therapeutics, and preventions that keep pace with today's explosion in knowledge.

Nanotechnology has the potential to radically change how we diagnose and treat cancer. Although scientists and engineers have only recently (ca. the 1980s) developed the ability to industrialize technologies at this scale, there has been good progress in translating nano-based cancer therapies and diagnostics into the clinic and many more are in development.

Nanotechnology is the application of materials, functionalized structures, devices, or systems at the atomic, molecular, or macromolecular scales. At these length scales, approximately the 1–100 nanometer range as defined by the U.S. National Nanotechnology Initiative (NNI), unique and specific physical properties of matter exist, which can be readily manipulated for a desired application or effect. Furthermore, the nanoscale structures can be used as individual entities or integrated into larger material components, systems, and architectures.

BENEFITS OF NANOTECHNOLOGY FOR CANCER

Nanoscale devices are one hundred to ten thousand times smaller than human cells. They are similar in size to large biological molecules ("biomolecules") such as enzymes and receptors. As an example, hemoglobin, the molecule that carries oxygen in red blood cells, is approximately 5 nanometers in diameter. Nanoscale devices smaller than 50 nanometers can easily enter most cells, while those smaller than 20 nanometers can move out of blood vessels as they circulate through the body. Because of their small size, nanoscale devices can readily interact with biomolecules on both the surface and inside cells. By gaining access to so many areas of the body, they have the potential to detect disease and deliver treatment in ways unimagined before now.

Biological processes, including ones necessary for life and those that lead to cancer, occur at the nanoscale. Thus, in fact, we are composed of a multitude of biological nano-machines. Nanotechnology provides researchers with the opportunity to study and manipulate macromolecules in real time and during the earliest stages of cancer progression. Nanotechnology can provide rapid and sensitive detection of cancer-related molecules, enabling scientists to detect molecular changes even when they occur only in a small percentage of cells. Nanotechnology also has the potential to generate entirely novel and highly effective therapeutic agents.

Ultimately and uniquely, the use of nanoscale materials for cancer comes down to its ability to be readily functionalized and easily tuned; its ability to deliver and/or act as the therapeutic, diagnostic, or both; and its ability to passively accumulate at the tumor site, to be actively targeted to cancer cells, and to be delivered across traditional biological barriers in the body, such as dense stromal tissue of the pancreas or the blood-brain barrier that highly regulates delivery of biomolecules to/from, our central nervous system.

Passive Tumor Accumulation

An effective cancer drug delivery should achieve high accumulation in tumors and spare the surrounding healthy tissues. The passive localization of many drugs and drug carriers due to their extravasation through leaky vasculature (named the Enhanced Permeability and Retention [EPR] effect) works very well for tumors. As tumor mass grows rapidly, a network of blood vessels needs to expand quickly to accommodate tumor cells' need for oxygen and nutrient. This abnormal and poorly regulated vessel generation (i.e., angiogenesis) results in vessel walls with large pores (40 nm to 1 um); these leaky vessels allow relatively large nanoparticles to extravasate into tumor masses. As fast-growing tumor mass lacks a functioning lymphatic system, clearance of these nanoparticles is limited and further enhances the accumulation. Through the EPR effect, nanoparticles larger than 8 nm (between 8–100 nm) can passively target tumors by freely pass through large pores and achieve higher intratumoral accumulation. The majority of current nanomedicines for solid tumor treatment rely on EPR effect to ensure high drug accumulation thereby improve treatment efficacy. Without targeting cell types expressing targeting ligand of interest, this drug delivery system is called "passive targeting."

Before reaching to the proximity of tumor site for EPR effect to take place, passive targeting requires drug delivery system to be long-circulating to allow a sufficient level of drug to the target area. To design nano-drugs that can stay in blood longer, one can "mask" these nano-drugs by modifying the surface with water-soluble polymers, such as polyethylene glycol (PEG); PEG is often used to make water-insoluble nanoparticles to be water-soluble in many preclinical research laboratories. PEG-coated liposomal doxorubicin (Doxil) is used clinically for breast cancer leveraging passive tumor accumulation. As in vivo surveillance system for macromolecules (i.e., scavenger receptors of the reticuloendothelial system, RES) reportedly showed faster uptake of negatively charged nanoparticles, nano-drugs with a neutral or positive charge are expected to have a longer plasma half-life.

Utilizing EPR effect for passive tumor-targeting drug delivery is not without problems. Although EPR effect is a unique phenomenon in solid tumors, the central region of metastatic or larger tumor mass does not exhibit EPR effect, a result of an extreme hypoxic condition. For this reason, there are methods used in the clinics to artificially enhance EPR effect: slow infusion of angiotensin II to increase systolic blood pressure, topical application of NO-releasing agents to expand blood, and photodynamic therapy, or hyperthermia-mediated vascular permeabilization in solid tumors.

Passive accumulation through EPR effect is the most acceptable drug delivery system for solid tumor treatment. However, size or molecular weight of the nanoparticles is not the sole determinant of the EPR effect, other factors, such as surface charge, biocompatibility, and in vivo surveillance system for macromolecules should not be ignored in designing the nanomedicine for efficient passive tumor accumulation.

Active Tumor Targeting

EPR effect, which serves as nanoparticle "passive tumor targeting" scheme is responsible for accumulation of particles in the tumor region. However, EPR does not promote uptake of nanoparticles into cells; yet nanoparticle/drug cell internalization is required for some of the treatment modalities relying on drug activation within the cell nucleus or cytosol. Similarly, delivery of nucleic acids (DNA, siRNA, miRNA) in genetic therapies requires escape of these molecules from endosome so they can reach desired subcellular compartments. In addition, EPR is heterogenous and its strength vary among different tumors and/or patients. For these reasons, active targeting is considered an essential feature for next generation nanoparticle therapeutics. It will enable certain modalities of therapies not achievable with EPR and improve effectiveness of treatments which can be accomplished using EPR, but with less than satisfactory effect. Active targeting of nanoparticles to tumor cells, microenvironment or vasculature, as well as directed delivery to intracellular compartments, can be attained through nanoparticle surface modification with small molecules, antibodies, affibodies, peptides, or aptamers.

Passive targeting (EPR effect) is the process of nanoparticles extravasating from the circulation through the leaky vasculature to the tumor region. The drug molecules carried by nanoparticle are released in the extracellular matrix and diffuse throughout the tumor tissue. The particles carry surface ligands to facilitate active targeting of particles to receptors present on target cell or tissue. Active targeting is expected to enhance nanoparticle/drug accumulation in tumor and also promote their prospective cell uptake through receptor mediated endocytosis. The particles, which are engineered for vascular targeting, incorporate ligands that bind to endothelial cell-surface receptors. The vascular targeting is expected to provide synergistic strategy utilizing both targeting of vascular tissue and cells within the diseased tissue.

Most of the nanotechnology-based strategies which are approved for clinical use or are in advanced clinical trials rely on EPR effect. It is expected that next-generation nanotherapies will use targeting to enable and enhance intracellular uptake, intracellular trafficking, and penetration of physiological barriers which block drug access to some tumors.

Transport across Tissue Barriers

Nanoparticle or nano-drug delivery is hampered by tissue barriers before the drug can reach the tumor site. Tissue barriers for efficient transporting of nano-drugs to tumor sites include tumor stroma (e.g., biological barriers) and tumor endothelium barriers (e.g., functional barriers). Biological barriers are physical constructs or cell formation that restrict the movement of nanoparticles. Functional barriers can affect the transport of intact nanoparticles or nanomedicine into the tumor mass: elevated interstitial fluid pressure and acidic environment for examples. It is important to design nanoparticles and strategies to overcome these barriers to improve cancer treatment efficacy.

Tumor microenvironment (TME) is a dynamic system composed of abnormal vasculature, fibroblasts and immune cells, all embedded in an extracellular matrix (ECM). TME poses both biological and functional barriers to nano-drug delivery in cancer treatment. Increase cell density and abnormal vasculature elevate the interstitial fluid pressure within a tumor mass. Such pressure gradient is unfavorable for free diffusion of the nanoparticles and is often a limiting factor for the enhanced permeability and retention (EPR) effect. When tumor mass reaches 106 cells in number, metabolic strains ensue. Often, cells in the core of this proliferating cluster are distanced by 100–200 um from the source of nutrient: 200 um is a limiting distance for oxygen diffusion. As a result, cancer cells in the core live at pO2 levels below 2.5–10 mmHg and become hypoxic; anoxic metabolic pathway can kick in and generate lactic acid. Nanoparticles become unstable in an acidic environment and delivery of the drugs to target tumor cells will be unpredictable. ECM of the tumor provides nutrient for cancer cells and stromal cell. It is a collection of fibrous proteins and polysaccharides and expands rapidly in aggressive cancer as the result of stromal cell proliferation. The most notorious biological barrier to cancer treatment is pancreatic stroma in pancreatic ductal adenocarcinoma (PADC). Pancreatic cancer stroma has the characteristics of an abnormal and poorly functioning vasculature, altered extracellular matrix, infiltrating macrophages and proliferation of fibroblasts. Not only tumor-stroma interactions have been shown to promote pancreatic cancer cell invasion and metastasis, but TME and tumor stroma also create an unfavorable environment for drug delivery and other forms of cancer treatments.

Because EPR effect is a clinically relevant phenomenon for nano-carriers' tumor penetration, strategies have been developed to address the tumor endothelium barrier. Strategies to reduce interstitial fluid pressure to improve tumor penetration include ECM-targeting pharmacological interventions to normalize vasculature within TME; hypertonic solutions to shrink ECM cells; hyperthermia, radiofrequency (RF) or high-intensity focused ultrasound (HIFU) to enhance nano-drug transport and accumulation. These strategies can also alleviate hypoxic conditions in larger tumor mass. Although TME and tumor mass pose a harsh and acidic environment for nano-carrier stability, pH-responsive nano-carrier designs leveraging this unique feature are gaining interest in recent years. Many of the strategies described above are used to address the tumor stroma barrier.

Another formidable tissue barrier for drugs and nanoparticle delivery is the blood-brain barrier (BBB). The BBB is a physical barrier in the central nervous system to prevent harmful substances from entering the brain. It consists of endothelial cells which are sealed in a continuous tight junction around the capillaries. Outside the layer of the epithelial cell is covered by astrocytes that further contribute to the selectivity of substance passage. As BBB keeps harmful substances from the brain, it also restricts the delivery of therapeutics for brain diseases, such as brain tumors and other neurological diseases. There have been tremendous efforts in overcoming the BBB for drug delivery in general. The multivalent feature of nanoparticles makes nano-carriers appealing in designing the BBB-crossing delivering strategies. One promising nanoparticle design has transferrin receptor-targeting moiety to facilitate transportation of these nanoparticles across the BBB.

EARLIER DETECTION AND DIAGNOSIS

In the fight against cancer, half of the battle is won based on its early detection. Nanotechnology provides new molecular contrast agents and materials to enable earlier and more accurate initial diagnosis as well as in continual monitoring of cancer patient treatment.

Although not yet deployed clinically for cancer detection or diagnosis, nanoparticles are already on the market in numerous medical screens and tests, with the most widespread use of gold nanoparticles in home pregnancy tests. Nanoparticles are also at the heart of the Verigene® system from Nanosphere and the T2MR system from T2 Biosystems, currently used in hospitals for a variety of indications.

For cancer, nanodevices are being investigated for the capture of blood-borne biomarkers, including cancer-associated proteins circulating tumor cells, circulating tumor DNA, and tumor-shed exosomes. Nano-enabled sensors are capable of high sensitivity, specificity, and multiplexed measurements. Next-generation devices couple capture with genetic analysis to further elucidate a patient's cancer and potential treatments and disease course.

Already clinically established as contrast agents for anatomical structure, nanoparticles are being developed to act as molecular imaging agents, reporting on the presence of cancer-relevant genetic mutations or the functional characteristics of tumor cells. This information can be used to choose a treatment course or alter a therapeutic plan. Bioactivatable nanoparticles that change properties in response to factors or processes within the body act as dynamic reporters of in vivo states and can provide both spatial and temporal information on disease progression and therapeutic response.

Imaging In Vivo

Current imaging methods can only detect cancers once they have made a visible change to tissue, by which time, thousands of cells will have proliferated and perhaps metastasized. And even when visible, the nature of the tumor – malignant or benign – and the characteristics that might make it responsive to a particular treatment must be assessed through tissue biopsies. Furthermore, while some primary malignancies can be determined to be metastatic, tumor preseeding of metastatic sites and micro-metastases are extremely difficult to detect with modern imaging modalities, even if the tissue in which they commonly occur are known, a "priori." Finally, surgical resection of tumor tissue remains the standard of care for many tumor types and surgeons must weigh the consequences of removing often vital healthy tissue versus the cancerous mass which has grown nonuniformly within. Ultimately, removal of cancer cells at the single-cell level is not possible with current surgical techniques.

Nanotechnology-based imaging contrast agents being developed and translated today, offer the ability to specifically target and greatly enhance detection of tumor in vivo by way of conventional scanning devices, such as magnetic resonance imaging (MRI), positron emission tomography (PET), and computed tomography (CT). Moreover, current nanoscale imaging platforms are enabling novel imaging modalities not traditionally utilized for clinical cancer treatment and diagnosis, for example, photoacoustic tomography (PAT), Raman spectroscopic imaging, and multimodal imaging (i.e., contrast agents specific to several imaging modalities simultaneously). Nanotechnology enables all of these platforms by way of its ability to carry multiple components simultaneously (e.g., cancer cell-specific targeting agents or traditional imaging contrast agents) and nanoscale materials that are themselves the contrast agents of which enable greatly enhanced signal.

The NCI-funded research has produced many notable examples over the last several years. For example, researchers at Stanford University and Memorial Sloan Kettering Cancer Center developed multimodal nanoparticles capable of delineating the margins of brain tumors both preoperatively and intraoperatively. These MRI-PAT-Raman nanoparticles are able to be used both to track tumor growth and surgical staging, by way of MRI, but also in the same particle be used during surgical resection of brain tumor to give the surgeon 'eyes' down to the single cancer cell level, increasing the potential tumor-specific tissue removal.

For metastatic melanoma, researchers at MSKCC and Cornell University have developed silica-hybrid nanoparticles ('C-dots') that deliver both PET and optical imaging contrast in the same platform. These nanoparticles are actively targeted to cancer with cRGDY peptides that target this specific tumor type and have already made it successfully through initial clinical trials.

Another clinical cancer imaging problem being addressed by nanoscale solutions is prostate cancer. Researchers at Stanford University recently have been developing nanotechnologies that give both anatomical size and location of prostate cancer cells (nanobubbles for ultrasound imaging) and functional information to avoid overdiagnosis/treatment as well as to monitor progression (self-assembling nanoparticles for photoacoustic imaging). The nanoplatforms developed by this group are coupled directly to their recently approved handheld transrectal ultrasound and photoacoustic (TRUSPA) device. Ultimately offering a more effective, integrated, and less invasive technique to image and biopsy prostate cancers for diagnosis and prognostication prior to performing common interventions (surgical resection, radiotherapy, etc.).

Similarly, gold nanoparticles are being used to enhance light scattering for endoscopic techniques that can be used during colonoscopies. One really powerful potential that has always been envisioned for nanotechnology in cancer has been the potential to simultaneously image and deliver therapy in vivo and several groups have been pushing forward these 'theranostic' nanoscale platforms. One group at Emory University has been developing one of these for ovarian and pancreatic cancers, which are traditionally harder to deliver therapeutics to. Their platform for pancreatic cancer can break through the fibrotic stromal tissue of which these tumors are protected by the pancreas. After traversing through this barrier, they are composed of magnetic iron cores which allow MRI contrast for diagnosis and deliver small-molecule drugs directly to cancer cells to treat.

Finally, nanotechnology is enabling the visualization of molecular markers that identify specific stages and cancer cell death induced by therapy, allowing doctors to see cells and molecules undetectable through conventional imaging. A group at Stanford has developed the Target-Enabled in Situ Ligand Assembly (TESLA) nanoparticle system. This is based on nanoparticles that form directly in the body after IV injection of molecular precursors. The precursors contain specific sequences of atoms that can only form larger nanoparticles after being cleaved by enzymes produced by cancer cells during apoptosis (i.e., cell death) and carry various image contrast agents to monitor (PET, MRI, etc.) local tumor response to therapies. Being able to track cancer cell death in vivo and at the molecular level is extremely important for delivering effective dosing regimens and/or precisely administering novel therapies or combinations.

Sensing In Vitro

Nanotechnology-enabled in vitro diagnostic devices offer high sensitivity and selectivity, and the capability to perform simultaneous measurements of multiple targets. Well-established fabrication techniques (e.g., lithography) can be used to manufacture integrated, portable devices or point-of-care systems. A diagnostic device or biosensor contains a biological recognition element, which through biochemical reaction can detect the presence, activity, or concentration of a specific biological molecule in the solution. This reaction could be associated, for example, with: binding of antigen and antibody, hybridization of two single-stranded DNA fragments, or binding of capture ligand to the cell surface epitope. A transducer part of the detection device is used to convert the biochemical event into a quantifiable signal which can be measured. The transduction mechanisms can rely on light, magnetic, or electronic effects.

Several devices have been designed for the detection of various biological signatures from serum or tissue. The bio-barcode assay was designed as a sandwich immunoassay in the laboratory of Chad Mirkin at Northwestern University. It utilizes magnetic nanoparticles (MNPs) which are functionalized with monoclonal antibodies specific to the target protein of interest and then mixed with the sample to promote capture of target proteins. The MNP-protein hybrid structures are then combined with gold nanoparticle (Au-NP) probes which carry DNA barcodes. Target protein-specific DNA barcodes are released into solution and detected using the scanometric assay with sensitivities in femto-picomolar range.

James Heath's laboratory at Caltech designed sandwich immunoassay devices that rely on DNA-encoded antibody libraries (DEAL). The DEAL technique uses DNA-directed immobilization of antibodies in microfluidic channels allowing to convert a prepatterned single-stranded (ss) DNA barcode microarray into an antibody microarray. ssDNA oligomers attached onto the sensor surface are robust and can withstand elevated temperatures of channel fabrication. Subsequent flow-through of the DNA-antibody conjugates in channels transforms the DNA microarray into an antibody microarray and allows to perform multiplex surface-bound sandwich immunoassays. These devices allow for on-chip blood separation and measurement of large protein panels directly from blood.

The diagnostic magnetic resonance (DMR) sensor platform was designed in the laboratory of Ralph Weissleder at Massachusetts General Hospital. The DMR mechanism exploits changes in the transverse relaxation signal of water molecules in a magnetic field as a sensing mechanism for magnetic nanoparticle labeled analytes. Highly integrated systems including microfluidic processing circuits and nuclear magnetic resonance (NMR) detection heads with a high signal-to-noise ratio were built and are capable of detecting the presence of cells, vesicles, and proteins in clinical samples.

Shan Wang's laboratory at Stanford University designed Giant Magnetoresistive (GMR) biosensors for protein detection. These nanosensors operate by changing their electrical resistance in response to changes in the local magnetic field. They were adapted to detection of biological signatures in solution by implementing a traditional sandwich assay directly on GMR nanosensors. Antibodies are immobilized on the GMR sensor surface and are used as capture probes for the sample containing target proteins. A magnetic particle is used to label the biomolecule of interest in the sample and a GMR sensor is used for signal transduction. These sensors were used to measure protein levels in complex sample mixtures and also were employed to assess the kinetics of protein interactions.

The devices described above are capable of analyzing large panels of biological signatures at the same time providing for a high level of multiplexing. The data analysis can establish correlations among different biomarker levels and map correlations of network signaling and thus provide tools for patient stratification based on their response to different treatments and ultimately improve the therapeutic efficacy of the one selected. New advancements in microfluidic technologies opened opportunities to integrate sample preparation and sample processing with biosensors and to realize fully integrated devices that directly deliver full data for a medical diagnosis from a single sample.

Measuring Response to Therapy and the Liquid Biopsy

Measurement of an individual patient's response to therapeutics during the course of their disease is the basis for precise and prognostic medical care. Accurate and disease-relevant monitoring can allow for optimized treatment regimens (e.g., therapeutic course correction, drug combinations, and dose attenuation), preemptive clinical decision making (e.g., therapeutic responders versus nonresponders, and more), and patient stratification for clinical trials. Beyond the more traditional gold standards of in vivo imaging, tissue biopsy, and in vitro diagnostics available for this purpose, the "liquid biopsy" offers the ability to measure response to therapy by way of simple and serial blood draws. Traditional biopsies involve resection of small volumes of the tumor tissue directly, and thus, remain invasive procedures that cannot offer the sampling necessitated to track disease progression relative to the course of therapy or the dynamics of its evolving biology. Liquid biopsies rely on the fact that tumors shed material (e.g., cells, DNA, other cancer-specific biomolecules) into circulation, over time and in response to therapy. Although, the amount of materials shed by any given tumor and/or stage is typically at incredibly low concentrations relative to the rest of the blood's constituents (e.g., erythrocytes, leukocytes, thrombocytes, plasma, etc.). This requires specific and sensitive tools to detect, capture, and purify the circulating tumor material relative to the rest. Nanotechnology is enabling these tools to become reality.

Technological advances in the coupling of complex microfluidics and nanoscale materials have allowed the high-purity capture and downstream functional characterization of circulating tumor cells (CTCs), cell-free tumor DNA, microemboli, exosomes, proteins, neoantigens, and more. Examples include the capture and subsequent release of CTCs within microfluidic systems to maintain viable cells for downstream whole-genome sequencing, ex vivo expansion, RNA sequencing, and more. Of these examples, one type of device uses magnetic nanoparticles to enrich whole blood prior to magnetic separation within the microfluidic and the other device uses thermoresponsive nanopolymers that specifically capture CTCs as they flow through the microfluidic then release upon a change in temperature once blood processing is complete. In both cases, the detection sensitivities are very high (e.g., for enumeration greater than 95 percent) and capture purity is much higher than other nonnanomaterial based devices. Furthermore, the processing times are increasing every year as the technology evolves, currently averaging 10 mL blood per 30 minutes.

TREATMENT AND THERAPY

Cancer therapies are currently limited to surgery, radiation, and chemotherapy. All three methods risk damage to normal tissues or incomplete eradication of cancer. Nanotechnology offers the means to target chemotherapies directly and selectively to cancerous cells and neoplasms, guide in surgical resection of tumors, and enhance the therapeutic efficacy of radiation-based and other current treatment modalities. All of this can add up to a decreased risk to the patient and an increased probability of survival.

Research on nanotechnology cancer therapy extends beyond drug delivery into the creation of new therapeutics available only through the use of nanomaterial properties. Although small compared to cells, nanoparticles are large enough to encapsulate many small molecule compounds, which can be of multiple types. At the same time, the relatively large surface area of nanoparticles can be functionalized with ligands, including small molecules, DNA or RNA strands, peptides, aptamers, or antibodies. These ligands can be used for therapeutic effect or to direct nanoparticle fate in vivo. These properties enable combination drug delivery, multimodality treatment, and combined therapeutic and diagnostic, known as "theranostic," action. The physical properties of nanoparticles, such as energy absorption and reradiation, can also be used to disrupt diseased tissue, as in laser ablation and hyperthermia applications.

Integrated development of innovative nanoparticle packages and active pharmaceutical ingredients will also enable the exploration of a wider repertoire of active ingredients, no longer confined to those with acceptable pharmokinetic or biocompatibility behavior. In addition, immunogenic cargo and surface coatings are being investigated as both adjuvants to nanoparticle-mediated and traditional radio- and chemotherapy as well as stand-alone therapies.

Innovative strategies include the design of nanoparticles as artificial antigen-presenting cells and in vivo depots of immunostimulatory factors that exploit nanostructured architecture for sustained anti-tumor activity.

Delivering Chemotherapy

The traditional use of nanotechnology in cancer therapeutics has been to improve the pharmacokinetics and reduce the systemic toxicities of chemotherapies through the selective targeting and delivery of these anticancer drugs to tumor tissues. The advantage of nanosized carriers is that they can increase the delivered drug's overall therapeutic index through nanoformulations with chemo-therapeutics that are either encapsulated or conjugated to the sur-faces of nanoparticles. This capability is largely due to their tunable size and surface properties. Size is a major factor in the delivery of nanotechnology-based therapeutics to tumor tissues. Selective delivery of nanotherapeutic platforms depends primarily on the passive targeting of tumors through the enhanced permeability and retention (EPR) effect. This phenomenon relies on defects spe-cific to the tumor microenvironment, such as defects in lymphatic drainage, along with increased tumor vasculature permeability, to allow nanoparticles (lesser than 200 nm) to accumulate in the tumor microenvironment. Furthermore, the timing or site of drug release can be controlled by triggered events, such as ultrasound, pH, heat, or by material composition.

Several members of the Alliance are working towards developing nanomaterial-based delivery platforms that will reduce the toxicity of chemotherapeutics and increase their overall effectiveness. In the Centers for Cancer Nanotechnology Excellence, the Center for Multiple Myeloma Nanotherapy at Washington University is devel-oping a strategy for photodynamic therapy, which would bypass the toxicity that currently limits the effectiveness of chemotherapy for multiple myeloma patients. This strategy is designed for use in bone marrow, which is normally inaccessible to external radiation sources.

The Innovative Research in Cancer Nanotechnology awardees is focused on understanding the fundamental aspects of nanomaterial interactions with the biological system to improve on the development of cancer therapeutics and diagnostics. Several of these awardees are studying nanoparticle-based delivery and have proposed nanosystems that deliver chemotherapeutics by penetrating through physiological barriers for access to more restricted tumors via targeting and/or mechanical deformation of particles (Yang, Karathanasis, Kabanov). One of them is dedicated to using a synergistic approach for the delivery of paclitaxel and gemcitabine chemotherapeutics in mesoporous silica nanoconstructs (Nel).

Nano-Enabled Immunotherapy

Immunotherapy is a promising new front in cancer treatment encompassing a number of approaches, including checkpoint inhibition and cellular therapies. Although results for some patients have been spectacular, only a minority of patients being treated for just a subset of cancers experience durable responses to these therapies. Expanding the benefits of immunotherapy requires a greater understanding of tumor-host immune system interactions. New technologies for molecular and functional analysis of single cells are being used to interrogate tumor and immune cells and elucidate molecular indicators and functional immune responses to therapy. To this end, nano-enabled devices and materials are being leveraged to sort, image, and characterize T cells in the Alliance's NanoSystems Biology Cancer Center.

Nanotechnologies are also being investigated to deliver immunotherapy. This includes the use of nanoparticles for delivery of immunostimulatory or immunomodulatory molecules in combination with chemo- or radio-therapy or as adjuvants to other immunotherapies. Standalone nanoparticle vaccines are also being designed to raise sufficient T cell response to eradicate tumors, through co-delivery of antigen and adjuvant, the inclusion of multiple antigens to stimulate multiple dendritic cell targets, and continuous release of antigens for prolonged immune stimulation. Molecular blockers of immune-suppressive factors produced can also be coencapsulated in nanoparticle vaccines to alter the immune context of tumors and improve response, an approach being pursued in the Nano Approaches to Modulate Host Cell

Response for Cancer Therapy Center at UNC. Researchers in this Center are also investigating the use of nanoparticles to capture antigens from tumors following radiotherapy to create patient-specific treatments, similar in principle to a "dendritic cell-activating scaffold" currently in Phase I clinical trial.

Additional uses of nanotechnology for immunotherapy include immune depots placed in or near tumors for in situ vaccination and artificial antigen-presenting cells. These and other approaches will advance and be refined as our understanding of cancer immunotherapy deepens.

Delivering or Augmenting Radiotherapy

Roughly half of all cancer patients receive some form of radiation therapy over the course of their treatment. Radiation therapy uses high-energy radiation to shrink tumors and kill cancer cells. Radiation therapy kills cancer cells by damaging their DNA inducing cellular apoptosis. Radiation therapy can either damage DNA directly or create charged particles (atoms with an odd or unpaired number of electrons) within the cells that can in turn damage the DNA. Most types of radiation used for cancer treatment utilize x-rays, gamma rays, and charged particles. As such, they are inherently toxic to all cells, not just cancer cells, and are given in doses that are as efficacious as possible while not being too harmful to the body or fatal. Because of this tradeoff between efficacy and safety relative to tumor type, location, and stage, often the efficacy of treatment must remain at reduced levels in order to not be overtly toxic to surrounding tissue or organs near the tumor mass.

Nanotechnology-specific research has been focusing on radiotherapy as a treatment modality that could greatly benefit from nanoscale materials' properties and increased tumor accumulation. The primary mechanisms by which these nanoscale platforms rely on are either enhancement of the effect of the radiotherapy, augmentation of the therapy, and/or novel externally applied electromagnetic radiation modalities. More specifically, most of these nanotechnology platforms rely on the interaction between x-rays and nanoparticles due to the inherent atomic-level properties of the materials used. These include high-Z atomic number nanoparticles that enhance the Compton and photoelectric effects of conventional radiation therapy. In essence, increasing efficacy while maintaining the current radiotherapy dosage and its subsequent toxicity to the surrounding tissue. Other platforms utilize x-ray triggered drug-releasing nanoparticles that deliver the drug locally at the tumor site or to sensitize the cancer cells to radiotherapy in combination with the drug.

Another type of therapy that relies upon external electromagnetic radiation is photodynamic therapy (PDT). It is an effective anticancer procedure for a superficial tumor that relies on tumor localization of a photosensitizer followed by light activation to generate cytotoxic reactive oxygen species (ROS). Several nanomaterials platforms are being researched to this end. Often made of a lanthanide- or hafnium-doped high-Z core once injected these can be externally irradiated by x-rays allowing the nanoparticle core to emit the visible light photons locally at the tumor site. The emission of photons from the particles subsequently activates a nanoparticle-bound or local photosensitizer to generate singlet oxygen ($1O_2$) ROS for tumor destruction. Furthermore, these nanoparticles can be used as both PDT that generates ROS and for enhanced radiation therapy via the high-Z core. Although many of these platforms are initially being studied in vivo by intratumoral injection for superficial tumor sites, some are being tested for delivery via systemic injection to deep tissue tumors. The primary benefits to the patient would be local delivery of PDT to deep tissue tumor targets, an alternative therapy for cancer cells that have become radiotherapy resistant, and reduction in toxicity (e.g., light sensitivity) common to traditional PDT. Finally, other platforms utilize a form Cherenkov radiation to a similar end, of local photon emission to utilize as a trigger for local PDT. These can be utilized for deep-tissue targets as well.

Delivering Gene Therapy

The value of nanomaterial-based delivery has become apparent for new types of therapeutics, such as those using nucleic acids, which are highly unstable in systemic circulation and sensitive to degradation. These include DNA and RNA-based genetic therapeutics, such as small interfering RNAs (siRNAs), and microRNAs (miRNAs). Gene silencing therapeutics, siRNAs, have been reported to have significantly extended half-lives when delivered either encapsulated or conjugated to the surface of nanoparticles. These therapeutics are used in many cases to target 'undruggable' cancer proteins. Additionally, the increased stability of genetic therapies delivered by nanocarriers, and often combined with controlled release, has been shown to prolong their effects.

Members of the Alliance are exploring nanotechnology-based delivery of nucleic acids as effective treatment strategies for a variety of cancers. In particular, the nucleic acid-based nanoconstructs for the treatment of cancer center at Northwestern University are focused on the design and characterization of spherical nucleic acids for the delivery of RNA therapeutics to treat brain and prostate cancers. Project 1 of the Nano Approaches to Modulate Host Cell Response for Cancer Therapy Center at UNC-Chapel Hill targets vemurafenib resistant melanoma for direct suppression of drug resistance through the delivery of siRNA using their polymetformin nanoparticles. Among the Innovative Research in Cancer Nanotechnology awardees, the Ohio state project (Guo), is focused on the systematic characterization of in vitro and in vivo RNA nanoparticle behavior for optimized delivery of siRNA to tumor cells, as well as cancer immunotherapeutics.

CURRENT NANOTECHNOLOGY TREATMENTS

The use of nanotechnology for the diagnosis and treatment of cancer is largely still in the development phase. However, there are already several nanocarrier-based drugs on the market and many more nano-based therapeutics in clinical trials. The application of nanotechnology to medicine includes the use of precisely engineered materials to develop novel therapies and devices that may reduce toxicity as well as enhance the efficacy and delivery of treatments. As a result, the application of nanotechnology to cancer can lead to many advances in the prevention, detection, and treatment of cancer. The first nanotechnology-based cancer drugs have passed regulatory scrutiny and are already on the market including Doxil® and Abraxane®.

In recent years, the U.S. Food and Drug Administration (FDA) has approved numerous Investigational New Drug (IND) applications for nano-formulations, enabling clinical trials for breast, gynecological, solid tumor, lung, mesenchymal tissue, lymphoma, central nervous system, and genitourinary cancer treatments. The majority of these trials repurpose the previously approved technologies described above.

The NCI Alliance for Nanotechnology funds development of new technologies to bring the next generation of cancer treatments and diagnostics to the clinic.

SAFETY OF NANOTECHNOLOGY CANCER TREATMENT

Nanotechnology is a powerful tool for combating cancer and is being put to use in other applications that may reduce pollution, energy consumption, greenhouse gas emissions, and help prevent diseases. The NCI's Alliance for Nanotechnology in Cancer is working to ensure that nanotechnologies for cancer applications are developed responsibly.

There is nothing inherently dangerous about being nanosized. Our ability to manipulate objects at the nanoscale has developed relatively recently, but nanoparticles are as old as the earth. Many nanoparticles occur naturally (e.g., in volcanic ash and sea spray) and as by-products of human activities since the Stone Age (nanoparticles are in smoke and soot from fire). There are so many ambient incidental nanoparticles, in fact, that one of the challenges of nanoparticle exposure studies is that background incidental nanoparticles are often at order-of-magnitude higher levels than the engineered particles being evaluated.

As with any new technology, the safety of nanotechnology is continuously being tested. The small size, high reactivity, and unique tensile and magnetic properties of nanomaterials – the same properties that drive interest in their biomedical and industrial applications – have raised concerns about implications for the environment, health, and safety (EHS). There has been some as yet unresolved debate recently about the potential toxicity of a specific type of nanomaterial – carbon nanotubes (CNTs), which has been associated with tissue damage in animal studies. However, the majority of available data indicate that there is nothing uniquely toxic about nanoparticles as a class of materials.

In fact, most engineered nanoparticles are far less toxic than household cleaning products, insecticides used on family pets, and over-the-counter dandruff remedies. Certainly, the nanoparticles used as drug carriers for chemotherapeutics are much less toxic than the drugs they carry and are designed to carry drugs safely to tumors without harming organs and healthy tissue.

To insure that potential risks of nanotechnology are thoroughly evaluated, the NCI Alliance for Nanotechnology in Cancer makes the services of its Nanotechnology Characterization Laboratory (NCL) available to the nanotech and cancer research communities. The NCL, an intramural program of the Alliance, performs nanomaterial safety and toxicity testing in vitro (in the laboratory) and using animal models. The NCL tests are designed to characterize nanomaterials that enter the bloodstream, regardless of route. This testing is just one part of the NCL's cascade of tests to evaluate the physicochemical properties, biocompatibility, and efficacy of nanomaterials intended for cancer therapy and diagnosis. To date, the NCL has evaluated more than 125 different nanoparticles intended for medical applications.

The NCL works closely with the U.S. Food and Drug Administration (FDA) and National Institutes of Standards and Technology (NIST) to devise experiments that are relevant to nanomaterials, to validate these tests on a variety of nanomaterial types, and to disseminate its methods to the nanotech and cancer research communities. The NCL also facilitates the development of voluntary-consensus standards for reliably and proactively measuring and monitoring the environment, health, and safety ramifications of nanotech applications.

Whether actual or perceived, the potential health risks associated with the manufacture and use of nanomaterials must be carefully studied in order to advance our understanding of this field of science and to realize the significant benefits that nanotechnology has to offer society, such as for cancer research, diagnostics, and therapy.

Chapter 31 | **Robotics**

Chapter Contents

Section 31.1 | Robots for Better Health and Quality of Life

This section includes text excerpted from "NIH Funds Development of Robots to Improve Health, Quality of Life," National Institutes of Health (NIH), December 2, 2015. Reviewed June 2021.

As part of the National Robotics Initiative (NRI), the National Institutes of Health announced that it will fund the development of three innovative co-robots – robots that work cooperatively with people. Two of the robots will improve health and quality of life for individuals with disabilities, and the third will serve as a social companion for children that inspires curiosity and teaches the importance of hard work and determination. Funding for the NIH projects will total approximately $2.2 million over the next five years, subject to the availability of funds.

"When the general public thinks about the research that NIH supports, they do not usually imagine robots. But robots have a tremendous potential to contribute to the health and well-being of our society, whether they are helping an elderly person engage in physical activity or promoting the curiosity of a child," said Grace Peng, Ph.D., program director of Rehabilitation Engineering at the National Institute of Biomedical Imaging and Bioengineering, part of NIH. "These three highly innovative projects demonstrate the power of encouraging leaders in the field of robotics to focus their attention on solving issues that pertain to health."

The National Science Foundation, the National Aeronautics and Space Administration, the U.S. Department of Agriculture, and the U.S. Department of Defense also supported the development of new co-robots.

SMART-WALKER TO INCREASE MOBILITY FOR ELDERLY

As individuals age, their ability to walk without assistance diminishes, leading to a decrease in physical activity and quality of life. To stay in their homes, elderly with mobility issues often require costly home modifications such as replacing steps with ramps or installing wheelchair lifts. The goal of this project is to develop a four-legged robot that enhances mobility so that the elderly can remain physically active and enjoy a healthier life with reduced reliance on the assistance of caregivers or expensive home renovations.

The robot has two modes: smart power-assist walker and smart mule. In the smart power-assist walker mode, the user is situated within the robot and chooses the amount of powered assistance that is needed. In the smart mule mode, the robot walks alongside the user while carrying a load, for example groceries. The robot uses a 3-D computer vision-based sensing system to detect the user's motion and the environment. With its smart legs, the robot is able to easily overcome environmental obstacles in ways that powered wheelchairs cannot.

HAND-WORN DEVICE TO HELP PEOPLE WITH VISUAL IMPAIRMENT GRASP OBJECTS

This project proposed to create a hand-worn assistive device that uses computer vision to identify target objects in a user's environment, determine misalignment between the user's hand and the object, and then convey – via natural human-device interfaces – the hand motion needed to grasp the object. The device will contribute to the independent lives of the people with visual impairment in two major ways: It will enhance the individual's ability to travel independently by helping the user identify moveable obstacles and manipulate them so that they can pass, and it will assist in object grasping for nonnavigational purposes such as identifying and correctly maneuvering a specific door handle.

A SOCIAL-ROBOT COMPANION FOR KIDS

Curiosity, resilience to challenging environments, and a growth mindset – the belief that one's basic abilities can be improved through dedication and hard work – are important factors that influence a child's mental health, academic achievement, and general well-being. The goal of this project is to create an autonomous, long-term social robotic companion for children that will promote and assess curiosity and a growth mindset through various interactions. After developing the robot, the researchers plan to evaluate its influence by conducting a six-month longitudinal study in which children learn and play while interacting with the robot companion.

Section 31.2 | Robotic Cleaners

This section includes text excerpted from "A Human Support Robot for the Cleaning and Maintenance of Door Handles Using a Deep-Learning Framework," National Center for Biotechnology Information (NCBI), June 23, 2020.

Cleaning and disinfecting are very important steps in preventing the acquisition and spread of infectious diseases inside closed environments such as apartments, community centers, shopping malls, hospitals, etc. In particular, high-contact-point areas such as doors, lifts, handrails, etc., are major sources of contamination. The researchers revealed that the door handle and its connected areas are highly sensitive contact points that are prone to be contaminated, and a key medium for spreading the germs.

Therefore, the frequent cleaning or disinfection of doors handles is essential for preventing the acquisition and spread of infection. However, due to a shortage of human-power, the frequent cleaning of indoor areas has become a key challenge. In addition to that, involving human-power carries a high risk of infection while working for long time in such areas. Mobile robots can be used as a viable solution to the problems associated with conventional cleaning and disinfecting methods due to their proven ability to assist humans in diverse application areas such as hospitals, elderly homes, and industries.

Many robotic solutions have been designed and developed, targeting routine tasks in health-care facilities. The works demonstrate that service robots are used to deliver food and medicine. Ultraviolet (UV)-light-installed mobile robot was introduced by Danish-based company UVD Robot for efficiently disinfecting hospital rooms, which could slow the disease spread through viruses. These robots can disinfect anything much better than other techniques, using a mobile array of powerful short-wavelength ultraviolet-C (UVC) lights that emit enough energy to shred the DNA or RNA of any microorganisms exposed to them.

The researchers proposed an autonomous robot to performs bed baths in the pursuit of patient hygiene. In addition to this core functionality, the robot is equipped with a fall-detection system consisting of a video camera and a three-dimension (3-D) LiDAR to identify patients who have fallen to the ground. The robot can notify the medical staff for the assistance in an emergency condition of a person detected by the fall detection module and remote condition monitoring module. GeckoH13 has been developed as an automated solution for the cleaning of walls in health sectors. This robot can climb on walls with the aid of vacuum adhesion. The task is carried out by spraying different liquid mixers apart from steam. GeckoH13 is effective in sterilizing uniform wall surfaces to a great extent.

However, the cleaning of sensitive contact points such as door handles is highly challenging for service robots. To carry out this task, the service robot needs an optimal vision system to identify the target object and the surrounding environment, and generate a trajectory planning scheme corresponding to arm-manipulation function to safely perform the proper cleaning tasks. In the literature, various techniques have been developed for mobile robots to recognize a door and door handle, such as laser scanner technique, ultrasonic sensors, and image-processing schemes.

Laser scanning and ultrasonic sensors schemes have lot of limitations. They work mostly on a known model of a door and accuracy is not good. Image-processing-based schemes are widely studied for mobile robot object-recognition tasks. These are also widely studied for door and door-handle detection tasks. A door-frame detection model was proposed using Hough Transform to detect edges, and a fuzzy logic-based algorithm was used to find the relationship between them. However, the model was unable to differentiate doors from large objects typically indoors. In another work, a computer vision-based door-detection algorithm was reported for people who are blind conducting indoor activity. In another study, Huy-Hieu Pham used Kinect sensor-generated point cloud data and a 3D-image-processing scheme to detect a door and other indoor objects.

Deep learning (DL) is an emerging technique. It has been widely used for image classification and object detection. Generally, DL has different definition. In zhang et.al clearly described definition of DL. The authors stated that DL is a class of machine learning algorithms that learns the structure between inputs and outputs, besides learning the relationship between two or multiple variables but also the knowledge that manages the relationship as well as the insights that makes sense of the relation. DL-based object detection algorithms are widely used for various automation applications. To pick and place the objects, monitoring construction sites, recognized trash for cleaning robots, etc. These were also used for door and door-handle detection.

Another important aspect of the indoor cleaning environment is motion-planning and arm manipulation. Once the vision module can detect and localize the cleaning subject (doors, walls etc.), the information should be exploited by the robot platform such that it will move to the desired location and perform the cleaning task. The researchers proposed a motion-planning strategy for the opening of doors, using the concept of action primitives. In a similar line of work, a motion-planning and arm-manipulation technique was proposed for grasping books from any table, and returning them to a predetermined position.

However, the above-mentioned ML and DL studies were focused on door and door-handle detection for a mobile service robot in different applications that were not related to cleaning services. Moreover, very few studies have discussed integrating the vision module data for motion-planning and manipulation. Using a cleaning tool, the robot can spray the disinfecting liquids then clean the sprayed region with a cleaning brush to prevent infections. Furthermore, the indoor path-planning scheme was adopted for a robot to navigate indoors and clean multiple doors. The arm-manipulation function was added to control both the arm and cleaning tool to successfully accomplish the cleaning task.

OVERVIEW OF HUMAN SUPPORT ROBOT

The Human Support Robot (HSR) is a product from Toyota Ltd. Co. There is a wide range of sensors installed on the HSR platform.

Cleaning Module

The cleaning module comprises a disinfectant liquid spraying unit and a spindle-type cleaning brush; both units were attached to the HSR manipulator. The spraying unit is constructed with two spraying guns and a separate disinfection liquid tank. To spray the disinfectant, the disinfectant was drained by a small sucking unit from a tank and forwarded to an electric resistance boiler circuit to convert into steam. Then, the generated steam is sprayed onto the door handle through two spray-gun nozzles at different angles. After spraying the disinfectant liquid on the door handle, the cleaning brush is enabled for wiping the sprayed area. A horizontal and vertical zigzag cleaning pattern is adopted to spray the disinfectant and wipe function.

To wipe the entire sprayed region, the cleaning brush was rotated 360 degrees through a 12-volt DC motor. The function of the spraying unit and cleaning brush is controlled by an Arduino Mega micro-controller and HSR task-scheduler module. The task scheduler selects the module to be enabled to perform the disinfection task and the Arduino Mega micro-controller executes the task by generating the relay control signal for the spraying unit and PWM generation signals for enabling the DC motor. The tanks can be easily removed for maintenance and changing the cleaning substance, as required by the cleaning cycle.

Section 31.3 | Image-Guided Robotic Interventions

This section includes text excerpted from "Image-Guided Robotic Interventions Fact Sheet," National Institute of Biomedical Imaging and Bioengineering (NIBIB), December 2019.

WHAT ARE IMAGE-GUIDED ROBOTIC INTERVENTIONS?

Image-guided robotic interventions are medical procedures that integrate sophisticated robotic and imaging technologies, primarily to perform minimally invasive surgery. This integrated technology approach offers distinct advantages for both patients and physicians.

Imaging

In image-guided procedures, the surgeon is guided by images from various techniques, including magnetic resonance (MR) and ultrasound. Images can also be obtained using tiny cameras attached to probes that are small enough to fit into a minimal incision. The camera allows the surgery to be performed using a much smaller incision than in traditional surgery.

Robotics

The surgeon's hands and traditional surgical tools are too large for small incisions. Instead, thin, finger-like robotic tools are used to perform the surgery. As the surgeon watches the image on the screen, she uses a tele-manipulator to transmit and direct hand and finger movements to a robot, which can be controlled by hydraulic, electronic, or mechanical means.

Robotic tools can also be controlled by computer. One advantage of a computerized system is that a surgeon could potentially perform the surgery from anywhere in the world. This type of long-distance surgery is currently in the experimental phase. The experiments illustrate the life-saving potential for such surgeries when a delicate operation requires a specially trained surgeon who is in a distant location.

WHAT ARE THE ADVANTAGES OF MINIMALLY INVASIVE PROCEDURES?

Minimally invasive surgery can reduce the damage to surrounding healthy tissues, thus decreasing the need for pain medication and reducing patients' recovery time. For surgeons, image-guided interventions using robots also have the advantage of reducing fatigue during long operations, allowing the surgeon to perform the procedure while seated.

WHAT ARE SOME EXAMPLES OF IMAGE-GUIDED ROBOTIC INTERVENTIONS AND HOW ARE THEY USED?

Robotic Prostatectomy

Complete prostate removal is performed through a series of small incisions, compared with a single large incision of 4 to 5 inches in traditional surgery. The small incisions result in a shorter postoperative recovery, less scarring, and a faster return to normal activities.

Ablation Techniques for Early Cancers

Patients with early kidney cancer can be treated with minimally invasive procedures to destroy small tumors. Cryoablation uses cold energy to destroy the tumors. Doctors use computed tomography (CT) and ultrasound imaging to position a needle-like probe within each kidney tumor. Once in position, the tip of the probe is super-cooled to encase the tumor in a ball of ice. Alternate freeze/thaw cycles kill the tumor cells. Other minimally invasive methods of destroying early kidney cancers include heating the tumor cells, and surgical removal using a robotic device. Many patients can go home the same day and are able to perform regular activities in several days.

Orthopedics

Image-guided robotic procedures are improving the precision and outcome of a number of orthopedic procedures. For example, partial knee resurfacing surgeries aim to target only the damaged sections of the knee joint. Orthopedic surgeons are combining the use of a robotic surgical arm and fiber optic cameras in such procedures, which results in patients retaining more of their normal healthy tissue. Image-guided robotic procedures also improve total knee replacements, allowing precise alignment and positioning of knee implants. The result is more natural knee function, better range of motion, and improved balance for patients.

WHAT ARE NIBIB-FUNDED RESEARCHERS DEVELOPING IN THE AREA OF IMAGE-GUIDED ROBOTIC INTERVENTIONS?
Portable Robot Uses 3D Near-Infrared Imaging to Guide Needle Insertion into Veins

Drawing blood and inserting IV lines are the most commonly performed medical procedures in hospitals and clinics. However, for many patients it can be difficult to find veins and accurately insert the needle, resulting in patient injury. NIBIB-funded scientists are developing a portable, lightweight medical robot to help perform these procedures. The device uses 3D near-infrared imaging to identify an appropriate vein for the robot to insert the needle. The current goal is to integrate the imaging system and software into a miniaturized version of the prototype robot. The outcome will be a compact, low-cost system that will greatly improve the safety and accuracy of accessing veins.

Robot-Assisted Needle Guidance Aids Removal of Liver Tumors

Radiofrequency ablation (RFA) is a minimally invasive treatment that kills tumors with heat and can be a life-saving option for patients who are not eligible for surgery. However, broad use of FA has been limited because the straight paths taken by the needles that carry tumor-killing electrodes may damage lung or other sensitive organs. Also, large tumors require multiple needle insertions, which increases bleeding risk. To address the problem of tissue damage using straight needles, NIBIB-funded scientists are developing highly flexible needles that can be guided along controlled, curved paths through tissue, allowing the removal of tumors that are not accessible by a straight-line path. The technology combines needle flexibility with a 3D ultrasound guidance system that allows the doctor to correct the path of the needle to avoid unexpected obstacles as the needle advances toward the tumor. The device will ultimately increase the accuracy and reduce the damage to healthy tissue during tumor removal resulting in wider use of the technology for better patient outcomes.

Swallowable Capsule Identifies and Biopsies Abnormal Tissue in the Esophagus

Barrett's esophagus is a precancerous condition that requires repeated biopsies to monitor abnormal tissue. NIBIB-funded researchers are developing a swallowable, pill-sized device to improve the management and treatment of this condition. The unsedated patient can easily swallow the pill, which is attached to a thin tether made of cable and optic fiber. The device detects microscopic areas of the esophagus that may show evidence of disease and uses a laser to collect samples from the suspicious tissue – a technology known as "laser capture microdissection." The physician then retrieves the device from the patient without discomfort and the collected microsamples are examined for visual evidence of disease, as well as genetic analysis. This minimally invasive device improves patient comfort and provides a precise molecular profile of the biopsied regions, which helps the physician to better monitor and treat the disorder.

Chapter 32 | Advanced Therapies

Chapter Contents

Section 32.1 | Tissue Engineering and Regenerative Medicine

This section contains text excerpted from the following sources: Text beginning with the heading "What Are Tissue Engineering and Regenerative Medicine?" is excerpted from "NIBIB Tissue Engineering and Regenerative Medicine," National Institute of Biomedical Imaging and Bioengineering (NIBIB), November 2019; Text under the heading "Research Program" is excerpted from "Tissue Engineering & Regenerative Medicine Research Program," National Institute of Dental and Craniofacial Research (NIDCR), July 2018.

WHAT ARE TISSUE ENGINEERING AND REGENERATIVE MEDICINE?

Tissue engineering evolved from the field of biomaterials development and refers to combining scaffolds, cells, and biologically active molecules into functional tissues. The goal of tissue engineering is to assemble such fully functional constructs that restore, maintain, or improve damaged tissue or a whole organ. Skin and cartilage are examples of engineered tissue that have already been approved by the U.S. Department of Food and Drug Administration (FDA); however, currently, they have limited use in human patients.

Regenerative medicine is a broad field that includes tissue engineering but also incorporates the idea of self-healing – where the body uses its own systems, sometimes with help from added biological material from outside the body, to recreate cells or rebuild organs. The terms "tissue engineering" and "regenerative medicine" have become largely interchangeable, as the field hopes to focus on cure instead of treatment for complex, often chronic diseases.

The field continues to evolve. In addition to medical applications, nontherapeutic applications include using tissues as biosensors to detect biological or chemical threat agents and tissue chips that can be used to test the toxicity of an experimental medication.

HOW DO TISSUE ENGINEERING AND REGENERATIVE MEDICINE WORK?

Cells are the building blocks of tissue, but tissues are the basic unit of function in the body. Generally, groups of cells make and secrete their own support structures, called the "extra-cellular matrix." This matrix, or scaffold, does more than just support the cells; it also

379

acts as a relay station for various signaling molecules. Thus, cells receive messages from many sources that become available from the local environment. Each signal can start a chain of responses that determine what happens to the cell. By understanding how individual cells respond to signals, interact with their environment, and organize into tissues and organisms, researchers have been able to manipulate these processes to mend damaged tissues or even create new ones.

The process often begins with building a scaffold from a wide set of possible sources, from proteins to plastics. Once scaffolds are created, cells with or without a "cocktail" of growth factors can be introduced. If the environment is fertile, a tissue develops. In some cases, the cells, scaffolds, and growth factors are all mixed together at once, allowing the tissue to "self-assemble."

Another method to create new tissue uses an existing scaffold. The cells of a donor organ are stripped and the remaining collagen scaffold is used to grow new tissue. This process has been used to bio-engineer heart, liver, lung, and kidney tissue. This approach holds great promise for using scaffolding from human tissue discarded during surgery, combined with a patient's own cells to make customized organs that would not be rejected by the immune system.

HOW DO TISSUE ENGINEERING AND REGENERATIVE MEDICINE FIT IN WITH CURRENT MEDICAL PRACTICES?

Currently, tissue engineering plays a relatively small role in patient treatment. Supplemental bladders, small arteries, skin grafts, cartilage, and even a full trachea have been implanted in patients, but the procedures are still experimental and very costly. While more complex organ tissues such as the heart, lung, and liver tissue have been successfully recreated in the lab, they are a long way from being fully reproducible and ready to implant into a patient. These tissues, however, can be quite useful in research, especially in drug development. Using functioning human tissue to help screen medication candidates could speed up development, saving money and animals, and provide key tools for facilitating personalized medicine.

WHAT ARE NIBIB-FUNDED RESEARCHERS DEVELOPING IN THE AREAS OF TISSUE ENGINEERING AND REGENERATIVE MEDICINE?

Research supported by the National Institute of Biomedical Imaging and Bioengineering (NIBIB) includes development of new scaffold materials and new tools to fabricate, image, monitor, and preserve engineered tissues. Some examples of research in this area are described below.

- **Controlling stem cells through their environment.** For many years, scientists have searched for ways to control how stem cells develop into other cell types, in the hopes of creating new therapies. Two NIBIB researchers have grown pluripotent cells – stem cells that have the ability to turn into any kind of cell – in different types of defined spaces and found that this confinement triggered very specific gene networks that determined the ultimate fate for the cells. Most other medical research on pluripotent stem cells has focused on modifying the combination of growth solutions in which the cells are placed. The discovery that there is a biomechanical element to controlling how stem cells transform into other cell types is an important piece of the puzzle as scientists try to harness stems cells for medical uses.

- **Implanting human livers in mice.** NIBIB-funded researchers have engineered human liver tissue that can be implanted in a mouse. The mouse retains its own liver as well, and therefore its normal function, but the added engineered human liver can metabolize drugs in the same way humans do. This allows researchers to test susceptibility to toxicity and to demonstrate species-specific responses that typically do not show up until clinical trials. Using engineered human tissue in this way could cut down on the time and cost of producing new drugs, as well as allowing critical examinations of drug-drug interactions within a human-like system.

- **New hope for cartilage defects.** An NIBIB-funded tissue engineer has developed a biological gel that

381

can be injected into a cartilage defect following microfracture surgery to create an environment that facilitates regeneration. However, in order for this gel to stay in place within the knee, researchers also developed a new biological adhesive that is able to bond to both the gel as well as the damaged cartilage in the knee, keeping the newly regrown cartilage in place. The gel/ adhesive combo was successful in regenerating cartilage tissue following surgery in a recent clinical trial of fifteen patients, all of whom reported decreased pain at six months postsurgery. In contrast, the majority of microfracture patients, after an initial decrease in pain, returned to their original pain level within six months. This researcher worked in collaboration with another NIBIB grantee to image the patients who had undergone surgery enabling scientists to combine new, noninvasive methods to see the evolving results in real time.

- **Engineering mature bone stem cells.** Researchers funded by NIBIB completed the first published study that has been able to take stem cells all the way from their pluripotent – state to mature bone grafts that could potentially be transplanted in a patient. Previously, investigators could only differentiate the cells to a primitive version of the tissue which was not fully functional. Additionally, the study found that when the bone was implanted in immunodeficient mice there was no abnormal growth afterward – a problem that often occurs after implanting stem cells or bone scaffolds alone.

RESEARCH PROGRAM
Engineering Tissue Constructs

The National Institute of Dental and Craniofacial Research (NIDCR) encourages basic and translational research that takes advantage of advances in biology, chemistry, material science, nanotechnology, computer science, and engineering to develop tissue constructs that mimic structure and function of native oral and craniofacial tissues including bone, cartilage, skeletal muscle, vascular and neural components of craniofacial skeleton and temporomandibular joint, teeth, periodontal ligament, oral mucosa, and salivary glands. Areas of interest include but are not limited to:

- Cell-instructive and structural scaffolds, including biomimetic and nanotechnology-based scaffolds capable of delivering bioactive molecules at specific concentrations in a temporally and spatially defined fashion and confer external geometry, internal architecture, and mechanical properties to engineered constructs.
- Scaffolds fabricated from smart materials able to respond to environmental cues.
- Three-dimensional in vitro bioreactors, including nanotechnology and microfluidics-based bioreactors that recapitulate normal and pathological tissue development, structure, and function.
- Medium- and high-throughput assay systems, including nanotechnology and microfluidics-based microphysiological systems (a.k.a. tissue chips) for drug screening, studying mechanisms of disease, and other applications.
- Tissue and organ biofabrication or "printing" technologies that use layered manufacturing processes, such as rapid prototyping.
- Functional dynamic imaging of the dental and craniofacial tissues.
- Application of mechanical forces and electrical stimulation in shaping functional characteristics of engineered tissues.
- Isolation, characterization, expansion, and differentiation of stem and progenitor cells for engineering of dental, oral and craniofacial (DOC) tissues.
- Optimization, standardization, and side-by-side comparison and quality control of stem and progenitor cell sources for use in DOC tissue engineering and regeneration.

- Engineering of composite multitissue constructs, such as vascularized and innervated bone and skeletal muscle

Functional Integration of Engineered Constructs into Native Host Tissue

The NIDCR encourages research concerning functional and structural integration between the engineered tissue constructs and host DOC tissues. Areas of interest include but are not limited to:

- Optimization of grafting strategies of engineered tissue constructs
- Biocompatibility, immunogenicity, biotoxicity, and biodegradability of tissue engineering biomaterials and scaffolds in animal models, including preclinical large animal models
- Vascularization and innervation of grafted engineered constructs
- Augmentation of hierarchical intertissue interfaces in tooth, craniofacial skeleton, and temporomandibular joint
- Cell tracing approaches to monitor in vivo cell proliferation, differentiation, reprogramming, survival, and migration
- Small and large animal models to assess short- and long-term structural and functional integrity of engineered tissue constructs in vivo

Mechanistic Studies of DOC Tissue Damage and Regeneration

The NIDCR encourages research on cellular and molecular mechanisms of DOC tissue damage, degeneration, aging, and regeneration. Areas of interest include but are not limited to:

- Destruction and regeneration of the periodontium and inflammatory bone erosion associated with periodontal disease
- Distinct molecular and cellular mechanisms of intramembranous and endochondral bone regeneration

- Osteogenesis, angiogenesis, and matrix remodeling during bone regeneration
- Augmentation of craniofacial bone regeneration
- Characterization of in situ stem and progenitor populations and stem cell niches that contribute to tissue regeneration of DOC tissues
- Responses of fibrocartilage to injury and trauma.
- Dentin-pulp complex homeostasis, injury, regeneration, and other types of therapy
- Inflammation resolution, wound healing, connective tissue remodeling, and scarless wound healing
- Impact of biophysical forces on tissue damage and regeneration

Promoting Endogenous Host Tissue Healing and Regeneration

The NIDCR encourages research that takes advantage of advances in biology, chemistry, material science, nanotechnology, computer science, and engineering to facilitate regeneration of endogenous DOC tissues. This part of the program welcomes basic and translational research directed at patterning of host tissue microenvironment to resolve acute and chronic inflammation, to reduce tissue fibrosis, promote vascularization, innervation, and scarless wound healing. Areas of interest include but are not limited to:

- Targeted and controlled delivery, including temporal, spatial, and combinatorial delivery to tissues of therapeutic molecules, genes, and gene products that modify endogenous tissue microenvironment
- Scaffolds and biomolecules that guide self-organization of endogenous or exogenous cells into tissues in vivo.
- Recapitulation of structure and function of native stem cell niches in vivo
- Directed cell homing and migration and reprogramming in vivo

Section 32.2 | **Cartilage Engineering**

This section contains text excerpted from the following sources: Text in this section begins with excerpts from "Engineering Cartilage," National Institutes of Health (NIH), March 3, 2014. Reviewed June 2021; Text under the heading "How Engineered Cartilage Produces Anti-inflammatory Drug" is excerpted from "Engineered Cartilage Produces Anti-inflammatory Drug," National Institute on Aging (NIA), National Institutes of Health (NIH), February 24, 2021.

Researchers developed a 3-dimension (3-D) scaffold that guides the development of stem cells into specialized cartilage-producing cells. The approach could allow for the creation of orthopedic implants to replace cartilage, bone, and other tissues.

Cartilage is the slippery tissue that covers the ends of bones in a joint. In osteoarthritis (the most common type of arthritis), cartilage breaks down and wears away. Replacing cartilage in this and other situations have been a major goal in tissue engineering.

Cartilage contains water, collagen, proteoglycans, and chondrocytes. Collagens are fibrous proteins that serve as the building blocks of skin, tendon, bone, and other connective tissues. Proteoglycans, made of proteins and sugars, form strands that interweave with collagen to form a mesh-like structure. This structure called an "extracellular matrix," allows cartilage to flex and absorb shock. Chondrocytes, cells found throughout cartilage, produce and maintain the structure.

Creating replacements for musculoskeletal tissues is challenging. Stem cells have required extensive treatment in the lab with growth factors in order to develop (or differentiate) into suitable specialized cells. These cells then need to be placed into an appropriate 3-D structure. A team led by Drs. Farshid Guilak and Charles Gersbach at Duke University set out to create an artificial scaffold that could direct stem cells within to differentiate and form extracellular matrix. Their work was supported in part by the National Institute of Health's (NIH) National Institute of Arthritis and Musculoskeletal and Skin Diseases (NIAMS), National Institute on Aging (NIA), and an NIH Director's New Innovator Award.

The team used human mesenchymal stem cells, which are found in adult bone marrow. These cells can differentiate into different types of musculoskeletal cells. The scientists coated a

3-D woven scaffold with a compound that can secure viruses to a surface but still allow them to transfer genes into target cells. Lentiviruses were chosen to deliver the TGF-β3 (transforming growth factor β3) gene into the cells. TGF-β3 drives stem cells to become chondrocytes. After the viruses were attached to the structure, it was seeded with human mesenchymal stem cells and incubated in culture media.

Cells within the artificial scaffold successfully differentiated into chondrocytes within two weeks. Without any extra prompting, the cells created a cartilage-like extracellular matrix within four weeks. The results appeared online on February 18, 2014, in the *Proceedings of the National Academy of Sciences*.

"One of the advantages of our method is getting rid of the growth factor delivery, which is expensive and unstable, and replacing it with scaffolding functionalized with the viral gene carrier," Gersbach says. "The virus-laden scaffolding could be mass-produced and just sitting in a clinic ready to go. We hope this gets us one step closer to a translatable product."

This approach could allow for implants that restore function to a joint immediately and drive development of a mature, viable tissue replacement. The technique could also be applied to other kinds of tissues using other stem cells – or even a patient's own cells. However, further refinement will be needed before it could safely be used in the clinic.

HOW ENGINEERED CARTILAGE PRODUCES ANTI-INFLAMMATORY DRUG

Joints such as those in the knees and hands rely on cartilage tissue to keep the bones from rubbing together. Wear and tear over a lifetime can cause cartilage to break down. This leads to a condition called "osteoarthritis."

The symptoms of osteoarthritis can include joint pain, stiffness, and swelling. More than 30 million adults nationwide are living with the condition. Currently, no treatments exist to prevent or reverse its progression.

Researchers have been interested in growing new cartilage in the lab that could be implanted into joints. However, joints with arthritis contain many molecules that promote chronic inflammation. This inflammation, plus the physical stress produced by normal movement, can destroy replacement cartilage quickly.

A research team led by Dr. Farshid Guilak from Washington University in St. Louis has been testing whether cartilage cells could be engineered to protect themselves from inflammation. In a proof-of-concept study, the team altered cartilage cells from pigs to produce an anti-inflammatory molecule when stressed.

The study was funded in part by NIH's National Institute of Arthritis and Musculoskeletal and Skin Diseases (NIAMS), National Institute on Aging (NIA), and National Center for Advancing Translational Sciences (NCATS). Results were published on January 27, 2021, in *Science Advances.*

The researchers first identified a protein called "TRPV4" in the membrane of cartilage cells that senses alterations within cells under compression. They found that TRPV4 becomes activated by a change to the fluid in cells called "osmotic loading." The protein can also be triggered by mechanical forces.

The team showed that, in response, TRPV4 activates specific genetic pathways in cartilage cells associated with inflammation and metabolism. The researchers modified these genetic circuits to produce an anti-inflammatory molecule called "interleukin-1 receptor antagonist" (IL-1Ra). Cells with these circuits were then grown to form cartilage.

When exposed to either mechanical forces or osmotic loading, the engineered cells produced IL-1Ra. The timing and duration of production depended on which genetic circuit was used. This suggests that production could be customized by harnessing different cellular pathways that turn on and off at different times.

Finally, the researchers tested whether production of IL-1Ra could protect cartilage cells in an inflammatory environment, similar to that seen in osteoarthritis. They exposed the engineered cartilage to both an inflammatory molecule and osmotic loading for three days.

By the end of that period, cartilage that didn't produce IL-1Ra was breaking down. In contrast, cartilage that produced the molecule maintained its structure and strength.

These findings demonstrate the ability to engineer living tissue to produce its own therapeutic drugs. "We think this strategy could be a framework for doing what we might need to do to program cells to deliver therapies in response to a variety of medical problems," Guilak says.

Section 32.3 | Ortho-Bionomy: Painless Self-Care

When a physical injury disrupts the body's natural ability to heal, the body tries to adapt to the injury to the best of its ability. Yet, during this process, there is a possibility of creating even greater stress. Ortho-Bionomy® is a type of therapy that focuses on improving your posture and structural imbalances by means of gentle massage. The treatment helps ease muscle tension and pain without the use of medication or physical stressors in an effort to help the body to heal naturally. The practitioner uses gentle movements that position the body properly and manipulates specific trigger points in a manner that enables the body to self-correct its reflexes. The simplicity and gentleness of the ortho-bionomic techniques used by the practitioner reeducate the dysfunctional patterns stored in the body with the goal of restoring normal functioning. Ortho-Bionomy® therapy is based on the principle of allowing the body to heal itself.

ORIGIN OF ORTHO-BIONOMY®

Ortho-Bionomy® was invented by Dr. Arthur Lincoln Pauls, a Canadian-born British national who was an osteopath and martial arts instructor. He discovered the roots of Ortho-Bionomy® by observing the movements and energy flow of judo combined with his working knowledge of homeopathy. He believed that the body can regain its balance on its own when we work with it rather than against it, and avoiding using force. Ortho-Bionomy® is a combination of ortho, meaning "straight," bio, meaning "life," and nomy, meaning "pertaining to laws." The practitioner helps the body understand its own functioning by manipulating its physical and energetic patterns. The treatment is based on the belief that, when the structure of the body is positioned properly, one's overall well-being is enhanced due to improved circulation. Since this is a relatively new approach toward massage therapy, more research is required to validate its effectiveness for various ailments.

ORTHO-BIONOMY® SESSION

In a typical Ortho-Bionomy® session, the patient lies fully clothed on a massage table and identifies areas of bodily discomfort for the practitioner. The practitioner then applies brief compressions and subtle contacts to unlock tension and reduce stress. These techniques help break the cycle of pain and correct structural and physical dysfunctions of the body through compression or constriction of muscles to release tension, loosen joints, and improve overall functionality. This release of stress and tension relieves the body of pain and discomfort. Ortho-Bionomy® does not incorporate deep-tissue treatments as a regular therapeutic massage does but instead concentrates on gentle movements and slight manipulations of the limbs and joints to increase range of motion with the utmost care paid to the patient's comfort.

EFFECTS OF ORTHO-BIONOMY®

Ortho-Bionomy® is often used as an alternative to osteopathy, which uses stress to physically manipulate bones and muscles. Ortho-Bionomy® involves a gentler approach that is particularly helpful in cases in which the patient is emotionally and physically fragile, such as in the aftermath of an injury. The therapist helps strengthen the ability of the patient's body to self-regulate and heal by releasing stress from the body and correcting its structural imbalance.

Targeted outcomes for patients undergoing Ortho-Bionomy® treatment include:

- Dissolution of knots in the body's tissue
- Softening of tissue surrounding an injury

- Experiences of comfort and relaxation
- Changes to the body's temperature

The practitioner relies on verbal responses from the patient to ensure that techniques that best enable the body to return to its natural alignment are used. The practitioner may also teach the patient specific self-care release techniques that further assist in relieving pain and restoring function.

BENEFITS OF ORTHO-BIONOMY®

At least three Ortho-Bionomy® sessions are recommended for an improved outcome. Habitual movements or body stances may be altered after a physical injury and Ortho-Bionomy® helps to reinstate the body's natural function and performance over the course of these sessions. Sessions may also be used to improve a patient's posture in cases in which the body has been damaged by years of poor habitual movements and/or complications resulting from injuries sustained many years ago. Ortho-Bionomy® is commonly recommended when a patient has a low tolerance for pain since the technique uses no forceful movements or pressure and relies only on this noninvasive process of healing.

The benefits experienced as a result of Ortho-Bionomy® include:
- Better energy flow and relief from chronic pain
- Release of structural and muscular imbalances
- Relief from emotional tension and trauma-related symptoms
- Enhanced healing capacity
- A profound feeling of relaxation and comfort

Ortho-Bionomy® is also used to provide relief from conditions such as headaches, sports injuries, restricted movement (frozen shoulder), acute/chronic pain, and neuromuscular dysfunction (lower-back pain).

It is important to find a qualified practitioner with appropriate credentials to perform Ortho-Bionomy® treatment. The patient must also communicate specific needs and level of comfort with the practitioner prior to arranging and throughout each session.

References

1. Chrystele. "What Is Ortho-Bionomy?" Luxmama Club & ParentPrep, February 3, 2018.
2. "What Makes Ortho-Bionomy Different from All the Rest?" Zoee, February 1, 2002.
3. "OrthoBionomy® Unraveling the Mystery," Angelauriel. com, February 1, 2001.

Section 32.4 | Gene Therapy

This section contains text excerpted from the following sources: Text in this section begins with excerpts from "Gene Therapy," National Human Genome Research Institute (NHGRI), October 20, 2016. Reviewed June 2021; Text beginning with the heading "What Are Cells and Genes? How Do They Interact?" is excerpted from "What Is Gene Therapy? How Does It Work?" U.S. Food and Drug Administration (FDA), December 22, 2017. Reviewed June 2021; Text under the heading "Types of Gene Therapy" is excerpted from "What Is Gene Therapy?" U.S. Food and Drug Administration (FDA), July 25, 2018.

Gene therapy is an experimental form of treatment that uses gene transfer of genetic material into the cell of a patient to cure the disease. The idea is to modify the genetic information of the cell of the patient that is responsible for a disease, and then return that cell to normal conditions. Transfer of genetic material is done commonly by using viral vectors that use their own biological capacities to enter the cell and deposit the genetic material. Both inherited genetic diseases and acquired disorders can be treated with gene therapy. Examples of these disorders are primary immune deficiencies, where gene therapy has been able to fully correct the presentation of patients, and/or cancer, where the gene therapy is still at the experimental stage.

WHAT ARE CELLS AND GENES? HOW DO THEY INTERACT?

What is the relationship between cells and genes? Cells are the basic building blocks of all living things; the human body is composed of trillions of them. Within our cells, there are thousands of genes that provide the information for the production of specific proteins and enzymes that make muscles, bones, and blood, which in turn

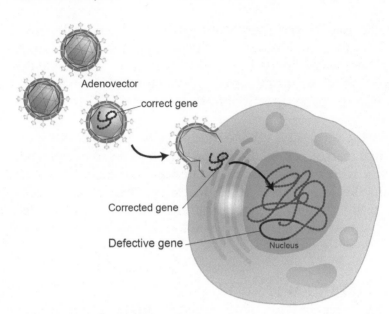

Figure 32.1. Illustration of Gene Therapy

support most of our body's functions, such as digestion, making energy and growing.

HOW GENE THERAPY WORKS

Sometimes the whole or part of a gene is defective or missing from birth, or a gene can change or mutate during adult life. Any of these variations can disrupt how proteins are made, which can contribute to health problems or diseases.

In gene therapy, scientists can do one of several things depending on the problem that is present. They can replace a gene that causes a medical problem with one that does not add genes to help the body fight or treat disease or turn off genes that are causing problems.

In order to insert new genes directly into cells, scientists use a vehicle called a "vector" which is genetically engineered to deliver the gene.

Viruses, for example, have a natural ability to deliver genetic material into cells, and therefore, can be used as vectors. Before a virus can be used to carry therapeutic genes into human cells, however, it is modified to remove its ability to cause infectious disease.

Gene therapy can be used to modify cells inside or outside the body. When it's done inside the body, a doctor will inject the vector carrying the gene directly into the part of the body that has defective cells.

In gene therapy that is used to modify cells outside of the body, blood, bone marrow, or another tissue can be taken from a patient, and specific types of cells can be separated out in the lab. The vector containing the desired gene is introduced into these cells. The cells are left, to multiply in the laboratory, and are then injected back into the patient, where they continue to multiply and eventually produce the desired effect.

TYPES OF GENE THERAPY

There are a variety of types of gene therapy products, including:

- **Plasmid DNA.** Circular DNA molecules can be genetically engineered to carry therapeutic genes into human cells.
- **Viral vectors.** Viruses have a natural ability to deliver genetic material into cells, and therefore some gene therapy products are derived from viruses. Once viruses have been modified to remove their ability to cause infectious disease, these modified viruses can be used as vectors (vehicles) to carry therapeutic genes into human cells.
- **Bacterial vectors.** Bacteria can be modified to prevent them from causing infectious disease and then used as vectors (vehicles) to carry therapeutic genes into human tissues.
- **Human gene-editing technology.** The goals of gene editing are to disrupt harmful genes or to repair mutated genes.
- **Patient-derived cellular gene therapy products.** Cells are removed from the patient, genetically modified (often using a viral vector), and then returned to the patient.

Section 32.5 | Light Therapy and Brain Function

This section includes text excerpted from "Shining a Healing Light on the Brain," Argonne National Laboratory (ANL), U.S. Department of Energy (DOE), March 24, 2021.

Scientists make pivotal discovery of method for wireless modulation of neurons with x-rays that could improve the lives of patients with brain disorders. The x-ray source only requires a machine like that found in a dentist's office.

Many people worldwide suffer from movement-related brain disorders. Epilepsy accounts for more than 50 million; essential tremor, 40 million; and Parkinson disease (PD), 10 million.

Relief for some brain disorder sufferers may one day be on the way in the form of a new treatment invented by researchers from the U.S. Department of Energy's (DOE) Argonne National Laboratory (ANL) and four universities. The treatment is based on breakthroughs in both optics and genetics. It would be applicable to not only movement-related brain disorders, but also chronic depression and pain.

This new treatment involves stimulation of neurons deep within the brain by means of injected nanoparticles that light up when exposed to x-rays (nanoscintillators) and would eliminate an invasive brain surgery currently in use.

"Our high-precision noninvasive approach could become routine with the use of a small x-ray machine, the kind commonly found in every dental office," said Elena Rozhkova, a lead author and a nanoscientist in Argonne's Center for Nanoscale Materials (CNM), a DOE Office of Science User Facility.

Traditional deep brain stimulation requires an invasive neurosurgical procedure for disorders when conventional drug therapy is not an option. In the traditional procedure, approved by the U.S. Food and Drug Administration (FDA), surgeons implant a calibrated pulse generator under the skin (similar to a pacemaker). They then connect it with an insulated extension cord to electrodes inserted into a specific area of the brain to stimulate the surrounding neurons and regulate abnormal impulses.

"The Spanish-American scientist José Manuel Rodríguez Delgado famously demonstrated deep brain stimulation in a

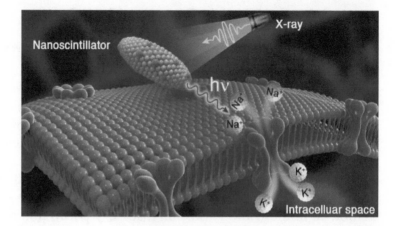

Figure 32.2. Illustration of Healing Light on the Brain

Artist's rendering shows x-rays striking radioluminescent nanoparticles in the brain, which emit red light that triggers a sodium (Na+) and potassium (K+) ion influx and thereby activates brain neurons.

bullring in the 1960s," said Vassiliy Tsytsarev, a neurobiologist from the University of Maryland and a co-author of the study. "He brought a raging bull charging at him to a standstill by sending a radio signal to an implanted electrode."

About 15 years ago, scientists introduced a revolutionary neuromodulation technology, "optogenetics," which relies on genetic modification of specific neurons in the brain. These neurons create a light-sensitive ion channel in the brain and, thereby, fire in response to external laser light. This approach, however, requires very thin fiberoptic wires implanted in the brain and suffers from the limited penetration depth of the laser light through biological tissues.

The team's alternative optogenetics approach uses nanoscintillators injected in the brain, bypassing implantable electrodes or fiberoptic wires. Instead of lasers, they substitute x-rays because of their greater ability to pass through biological tissue barriers.

"The injected nanoparticles absorb the x-ray energy and convert it into red light, which has significantly greater penetration depth than blue light," said Zhaowei Chen, former CNM postdoctoral fellow.

"Thus, the nanoparticles serve as an internal light source that makes our method work without a wire or electrode," added Rozhkova. Since the team's approach can both stimulate and quell targeted small areas, Rozhkova noted, it has other applications than brain disorders. For example, it could be applicable to heart problems and other damaged muscles.

One of the team's keys to success was the collaboration between two of the world-class facilities at Argonne: CNM and Argonne's Advanced Photon Source (APS), a DOE Office of Science User Facility. The work at these facilities began with the synthesis and multitool characterization of the nanoscintillators. In particular, the x-ray excited optical luminescence of the nanoparticle samples was determined at an APS beamline (20-BM). The results showed that the particles were extremely stable over months and upon repeated exposure to the high-intensity x-rays.

According to Zou Finfrock, a staff scientist at the APS 20-BM beamline and Canadian Light Source, "They kept glowing a beautiful orange-red light."

Next, Argonne sent CNM-prepared nanoscintillators to the University of Maryland for tests in mice. The team at the University of Maryland performed these tests over two months with a small portable x-ray machine. The results proved that the procedure worked as planned. Mice whose brains had been genetically modified to react to red light responded to the x-ray pulses with brain waves recorded on an electroencephalogram.

Finally, the University of Maryland team sent the animal brains for characterization using x-ray fluorescence microscopy performed by Argonne scientists. This analysis was performed by Olga Antipova on the Microprobe beamline (2-ID-E) at APS and by Zhonghou Cai on the Hard x-ray Nanoprobe (26-ID) jointly operated by CNM and APS.

This multi-instrument arrangement made it possible to see tiny particles residing in the complex environment of the brain tissue with a super-resolution of dozens of nanometers. It also allowed visualizing neurons near and far from the injection site on a microscale. The results proved that the nanoscintillators are chemically and biologically stable. They do not wander from the injection site or degrade.

"Sample preparation is extremely important in these types of biological analysis," said Antipova, a physicist in the x-ray Science Division (XSD) at the APS. Antipova was assisted by Qiaoling Jin and Xueli Liu, who prepared brain sections only a few micrometers thick with jeweler-like accuracy.

"There is an intense level of commercial interest in optogenetics for medical applications," said Rozhkova. "Although still at the proof-of-concept stage, we predict our patent-pending wireless approach with small x-ray machines should have a bright future."

Section 32.6 | Radiofrequency Thermal Ablation as Tumor Therapy

This section includes text excerpted from "Radiofrequency Thermal Ablation as Tumor Therapy," Clinical Center (CC), National Institutes of Health (NIH), May 6, 2020.

Recent developments in radiofrequency thermal ablation (RFA) have expanded the treatment options for certain oncology patients. Minimally invasive, image-guided therapy may now provide effective local treatment of isolated or localized neoplastic disease, and can also be used as an adjunct to conventional surgery, systemic chemotherapy, or radiation. RFA expands the medical application of heat, which for decades has been used as a cautery device to cut tissue. In the procedure, the tumors are located with ultrasound, computed tomography (CT), or magnetic resonance imaging (MRI) devices. Then, essentially the patient is turned into an electrical circuit by placing grounding pads on the thighs. A small needle-electrode with an insulated shaft and an uninsulated distal tip is inserted through the skin and directly into the tumor. Ionic vibration at the needle tip leads to frictional heat. After 10 to 30 minutes of contact with the tumor, the radiofrequency energy kills a 2.5- to 5-cm sphere. The dead cells are not removed, but become scar tissue and eventually shrink. RFA continues to play a time-tested, major role in the treatment of patients with painful osteoid osteomas in the bone and heart arrhythmias. In addition, RFA has been used to treat painful trigeminal neuralgia for 25 years. Today, the mainstream applications of RFA are increasing. In particular, this minimally invasive, percutaneous technique is showing promise as a treatment option for patients with primary or metastatic liver cancer.

Worldwide, primary liver cancer is the most common solid cancer, causing an estimated one million deaths annually. In the United States, 15,300 people were expected to be diagnosed with the disease in 2000, and 13,800 were expected to die. Hepatocellular carcinoma accounts for about 84 percent of primary liver cancers in the U.S. The number of people expected to die from colorectal carcinoma metastases to the liver is even greater than that of people expected to die from primary liver cancer. Twenty to 25 percent of patients with colorectal carcinoma liver metastases are eligible for surgery, and of those, the five-year survival rate is approximately 30 to 40 percent. RFA may provide a safe and effective option for patients with inoperable or recurrent liver cancer who have failed to respond to conventional methods. Given the lack of effective treatment options for the majority of patients with primary liver cancer and metastases to the liver, the oncology team should be aware of this relatively new treatment.

In addition to treatment of patients with liver cancers, clinical applications of RFA include treatment of kidney, adrenal, and prostate tumors; benign prostatic hyperplasia; painful or abnormal neural tissue; and painful soft tissue or bone masses that are unresponsive to conventional therapy.

Many times RFA can be an alternative to risky surgery, and sometimes it can change a patient from having an inoperable tumor to being a candidate for surgery. The procedure is proving useful as an adjunct to conventional treatments and as a palliative treatment. What's more, the cauterizing effect of the heated needle prevents excessive bleeding, leading to low complication rates. Although RFA may not be a magic bullet, it clearly can be a cure in some cases.

Multiple techniques have been studied and used to kill tumor cells. These techniques include laser, focused ultrasound, and microwave, as well as RFA, cryotherapy, and percutaneous ethanol injection (PEI). PEI has proven especially useful in treating primary liver tumors. In PEI, ethanol is injected directly into the tumor in multiple treatment sessions. Prospective, randomized clinical trials comparing PEI and RFA for the treatment of liver tumors are currently in progress. Cryotherapy is an ablation method that has been used primarily during open surgery, after mobilizing the liver. It has limited applications due to the size of the treatment probe, expense, and excessive complications, such as liver capsule fracture. Cryotherapy may be less effective and more prone to complications than RFA for liver tumors, although this is controversial. While these multiple technologies can each destroy tissue, RFA has emerged as safe, cheap, and predictable, and is becoming the treatment of choice for small but inoperable tumors of the liver.

Radiofrequency thermal ablation can usually be performed as an outpatient procedure under general anesthesia or conscious sedation. Alternatively, RFA may be performed laparoscopically or during open surgery.

Under light sedation, lidocaine or bupivacaine is administered subcutaneously at the needle entry site and down to the liver capsule. A needle is placed through the skin and into the tumor with imaging guidance. Treatment sessions of percutaneous RFA are easily monitored using real time ultrasound imaging, computed tomography, or magnetic resonance imaging. Most patients feel little pain during the procedure and go home the same day or the day after the procedure, usually with minimal to no pain or soreness, although there is a spectrum, and some patients will experience severe pain the day of the procedure.

During a 10- to 30-minute treatment session, nitrogen micro-bubbles gradually create a hyperechoic area on ultrasound that provides a rough estimation of the treated tissue, which is 2.5 to 5 cm per 10- to 30-minute treatment sphere. CT, MR imaging, or positron emission tomography (PET) imaging may provide more exquisite detail for follow-up verification of the treatment zone and for finding residual or recurrent neoplastic tissue. Although real time MR imaging and CT are available, they are not in widespread use. Ultrasound is a safe, common, and easy guidance method, although it is somewhat operator-dependent.

Once the needle has been properly positioned within the tumor, the tissue is heated. At temperatures exceeding 50 °C, cells are destroyed. To treat tumors of different sizes and shapes, the needle is available in different lengths and shapes of exposed tips.

Energy is transferred from the uninsulated distal tip of the needle to the tissue as current rather than as direct heat. The circuit is completed with grounding pads placed on the patient's thighs. As the alternating current flows to the grounding pads, it agitates ions in the surrounding tissue, resulting in frictional heat. The tissue surrounding the needle is desiccated, creating an oval or spherical lesion of coagulation necrosis, typically 2.5 to 5 cm in diameter for each 10- to 30-minute treatment. These spheres are added together in three dimensions to overlap and completely envelop the tumor. Ideally, the treated tissue will contain the entire tumor plus a variable rim of healthy tissue as a safety margin.

Failure to ablate the entire tumor with clean edges results in regrowth of the tumor. Depending on the size and configuration of new growth, the patient may or may not be suited for another treatment session. Over months to years, as the dead necrotic cells are reabsorbed and replaced by scar tissue and fibrosis, the size of the thermal lesion shrinks, although the remaining cells are ideally dead. The possibility of successful surgical resection may be augmented by decreasing the number of tumors. Treatment of a tumor in one lobe may broaden the surgical indications of a tumor in the other lobe. Due to the natural course of the disease, new or recurrent tumors may be suited for additional treatment sessions as well.

Various methods of increasing the volume of treated tissue have been explored. One type of ablation needle-electrode consists of a coaxial system or an expandable needle within a needle. The inner hooks are deployed once properly situated within the tumor. Different configurations allow for treatment of various shapes and locations of tumors. Another ablation system utilizes a triple parallel needle array, which synergistically increases the treated volume.

At temperatures exceeding 100 to 110 °C, the tissue surrounding the needle vaporizes. The gas from the vaporization insulates the area immediately around the needle, limiting energy deposition in the target zone and decreasing the volume of tissue treated. Overcooking or charring around the outside of the needle also insulates and causes incomplete destruction of target tissue remote from the needle, much like a hamburger cooked too fast on a grill, charred on the outside, and raw in the middle.

The deleterious effects of charring and vaporization may be decreased by monitoring temperature and/or impedance during treatment, and adjusting the current accordingly. The generators have computer chips or treatment algorithms to assist in optimizing this process. One system perfuses chilled saline within a closed-tip needle in order to deposit more energy without increasing the temperature. This system allows an increase in the lesion diameter while keeping the temperatures below the vaporization point.

At the end of a treatment session, the active needle is slowly retracted to heat and cauterize the needle pathway. This action prevents bleeding and tumor seeding of the needle track by destroying any cell that becomes attached to the needle or dislodged in the needle tract.

Three companies (RITA Medical Systems, Radionics, and RadioTherapeutics) market RFA systems. They currently have the FDA 510-K clearance for soft tissue ablation, and have or are pursuing FDA 510-K clearance for unresectable liver tumor ablation. Although it is in its infancy as a technique, RFA is no longer a completely experimental procedure.

LIVER CANCER AND RADIOFREQUENCY THERMAL ABLATION

Radiofrequency thermal ablation may be most effective in primary liver cancer (hepatocellular carcinoma or hepatoma). Primary tumors are often soft and encapsulated and usually occur in a cirrhotic liver, allowing for effective disbursement and retention of the heat. Although surgery and liver transplant are considered the only curative treatment for hepatocellular carcinoma, few patients are eligible. Eligibility criteria tend to vary by institution and physician. Contraindications include multiple tumors, decreased liver function, or multiple medical problems. While controlled, long-term studies of RFA have not been done, survival rates are likely to be similar to that of patients undergoing surgery or PEI treatment.

With a median follow-up of only 15 months, Curley and colleagues reported a 1.8 percent short-term recurrence rate following RFA of 169 tumors (median diameter 3.4 cm) in 123 patients with primary or metastatic liver cancer. RFA clearly can provide short-term local control of small, early, or focal liver cancer. The question remains if this finding of a low short-term recurrence rate will translate into prolonged survival. Extrapolation of data from the surgical literature for resection of solitary liver tumors suggests that successful local control may lead to prolonged survival. Combination therapies need to be further studied for impact upon survival as well.

Current studies are underway to evaluate the long-term efficacy of RFA for liver tumors. As yet, there have been no long-term, randomized studies, and the long-term benefits are thus somewhat speculative. Still, preliminary, short-term results are promising and suggest that this therapy can impact certain patients' survival.

TREATMENT FOR KIDNEY CANCER

Radiofrequency thermal ablation is being studied as a minimally invasive treatment for patients with kidney cancer. An effective, minimally invasive therapy could postpone kidney failure and prolong kidney function in patients with multiple or hereditary kidney cancer, such as von Hippel-Lindau disease, which causes multiple, recurrent, and diffuse tumors. RFA may also provide a useful option for patients who are not operative candidates or have solitary kidneys, multiple medical problems, or unresectable tumors.

Surgery for benign prostate hyperplasia and prostate cancer is not without morbidity. RFA may provide a safer option for removing abnormal prostate tissue, as well as predictably destroying the entire gland with a low complication rate to the adjacent rectum, sphincter, bladder base, and urethra.

Radiofrequency thermal ablation may also provide a method for alleviating pain that is unresponsive to conventional treatment, or to complement treatments that have a delayed response. For example, radiation therapy for painful bone metastases can average four weeks to show effect. Studies are underway to investigate the efficacy of RFA in the palliation of painful bone tumors and painful peripheral soft tissue tumors that are unresponsive or poorly responsive to conventional treatment. Preliminary data suggest that RFA may provide rapid pain relief for many tumors in the days following treatment and thus may decrease dependence on sedating painkillers.

Ablation of nerve and nerve ganglia continues to be used safely and effectively in the treatment of multiple pain syndromes, including trigeminal neuralgia, cluster headaches, chronic segmental thoracic pain, cervicobrachialgia, and plantar fasciitis.

Patients with functional or tumorous disorders of the brain, such as Parkinson disease (PD), and benign or malignant lesions may also be candidates for RFA, although it is experimental for brain tumors. One feasibility series on RFA for breast cancer in five patients suggests that it might play a role in select patient populations; however, this is also experimental.

WHAT ARE THE COMPLICATIONS?

Although RFA is relatively safe and minimally invasive, the benefits do not come without slight risks. The reported complication rate has been estimated at nearly 2 percent, and may include bleeding, effusion, fever, and infection. The proximity to vital structures may influence the risk for collateral damage. The risks are kept to a minimum by attention to detail as well as continuous monitoring of vital signs and oxygenation and preprocedural blood tests. Complications are usually managed nonoperatively.

The heating treatment inherent to RFA actually stops bleeding. The 14 to 17.5 gauge needles are very small; they are the same size needles used for biopsy, with the added benefits of cauterization and coagulation. The low rate of bleeding seen with RFA is likely the result of this cauterization effect, which is similar to electrocautery used to stop bleeding during surgery. This same treatment of the needle track should minimize the risk of needle-track seeding in the systems that are capable of cauterizing the track. The predictable nature of RFA allows for little collateral damage during treatments situated near vital structures. In fact, the "heat sink effect" actually preserves the vessels near a treatment area. However, with this effect, the inflow of "cool" blood at body temperature (cool relative to the cooked tissue) may impair the heating of the tumor cells closest to the vessels. The protected vessel often harbors an adjacent tumor that may regrow adjacent to large vessels.

Combining RFA therapy with chemoembolization can selectively block blood flow to a tumor, and thus may provide more effective treatment for larger tumors. Combining local radiation or local chemotherapy infusion with RFA could also be more effective than anyone treatment alone. Doxorubicin has been shown in mice to enhance the effects of RFA by increasing the volume of tumor treated. Early reports of combining RFA with chemotherapy infusion and chemoembolization should lead to larger studies of such combination therapies.

A wide variety of clinical applications for RFA are being developed. If a target can be seen with CT, MRI, or ultrasound, then a needle can be placed into it. If a needle can be placed, then the target tissue or tumor can be ablated and destroyed. If a clean margin is created, then the tumor will not recur at that site. Recent developments in RFA allow this treatment process to be done in a safe, predictable, and cheap fashion with low complication rates and minimal discomfort, on an outpatient basis. Further study is required to assess which patients will benefit from this new treatment, and most cancer patients will not be candidates due to the size or location of the tumor. Although long-term data have yet to be reported, early results suggest that RFA may prove to be an effective treatment option or adjunct for many oncology patients.

Part 5 | **Rehabilitation and Assistive Technologies**

Chapter 33 | **Rehabilitation Engineering**

WHAT IS REHABILITATION ENGINEERING?

Rehabilitation engineering is the use of engineering principles to 1) develop technological solutions and devices to assist individuals with disabilities and 2) aid the recovery of physical and cognitive functions lost because of disease or injury.

Rehabilitation engineers design and build devices and systems to meet a wide range of needs that can assist individuals with mobility, communication, hearing, vision, and cognition. These tools help people with day-to-day activities related to employment, independent living, and education.

Rehabilitation engineering may involve relatively simple observations of how individuals perform tasks and making accommodations to eliminate further injuries and discomfort. On the other end of the spectrum, rehabilitation engineering includes sophisticated brain-computer interfaces that allow an individual with a severe disability to operate computers and other devices simply by thinking about the task they want to perform.

Rehabilitation engineers also improve upon standard rehabilitation methods to regain functions lost due to congenital disorders, disease (such as stroke or joint replacement), or injury (such as limb loss) to restore mobility.

This chapter contains text excerpted from the following sources: Text beginning with the heading "What Is Rehabilitation Engineering?" is excerpted from "Rehabilitation Engineering," National Institute of Biomedical Imaging and Bioengineering (NIBIB), November 2016. Reviewed June 2021; Text beginning with the heading "Telephone-Based Rehab Programs" is excerpted from "Telephone-Based Rehab Program Helps People with Advanced Cancer Maintain Independence," National Cancer Institute (NCI), April 29, 2019.

HOW CAN FUTURE REHABILITATION ENGINEERING RESEARCH IMPROVE THE QUALITY OF LIFE FOR INDIVIDUALS?

Ongoing research in rehabilitation engineering involves the design and development of innovative technologies and techniques that can help people regain physical or cognitive functions. For example:

- Rehabilitation robotics, to use robots as therapy aids instead of solely as assistive devices. Smart rehabilitation robotics aid mobility training in individuals suffering from impaired movements, such as following a stroke.
- Virtual rehabilitation, which uses virtual reality simulation exercises for physical and cognitive rehabilitation. These tools are entertaining, motivate patients to exercise and provide objective measures, such as range of motion. The exercises can be performed at home by a patient and monitored by a therapist over the Internet (known as "telerehabilitation"), which offers convenience as well as reduced costs.
- Physical prosthetics, such as smarter artificial legs with powered ankles, exoskeletons, dexterous upper limbs, and hands. This is an area where researchers continue to make advances in design and function to better mimic natural limb movement and user intent.
- Advanced kinematics, to analyze human motion, muscle electrophysiology, and brain activity to more accurately monitor human functions and prevent secondary injuries.
- Sensory prosthetics, such as retinal and cochlear implants to restore some lost function to provide navigation and communication, increasing independence and integration into the community.
- Brain-computer interfaces, to enable severely impaired individuals to communicate and access information. These technologies use the brain's electrical impulses to allow individuals to move a computer cursor or a robotic arm that can reach and grab items, or send text messages.

- Modulation of organ function, as interventions for urinary and fecal incontinence and sexual disorders. Recent developments in neuromodulation of the peripheral nervous system offer the promise to treat organ function in the case of a spinal cord injury.
- Secondary disorder treatment, such as pain management

WHAT ARE NIBIB-FUNDED RESEARCHERS DEVELOPING IN THE AREA OF REHABILITATION ENGINEERING?

Promising research currently supported by the National Institute of Biomedical Imaging and Bioengineering (NIBIB) includes a wide range of approaches and technological development. Several examples are described below.

Navigation aids. Individuals who are blind require assistance to navigate through unfamiliar locations. Researchers are developing a cane that is enhanced with computer vision and vibration feedback. The cane uses advanced image processing to map the structure of a room, identify important features (door, stairs, obstacles), and create a navigation plan to guide the user towards his destination. It provides feedback in the form of either speech or vibrations through the handle.

Another group of researchers has developed a device that provides very low-resolution images to the user. The system consists of a retinal implant, a pair of glasses containing a small camera, and a cell phone-sized device to convert the camera's images into digital signals. The system provides electrical stimuli to the retina, which sends nerve impulses through the optic nerve to the brain. The resulting images observed by the user provide just enough information about the environment to navigate through a room and read large writing, such as street signs. The researchers are performing preclinical studies to attain the U.S. Food and Drug Administration's (FDA) approval to run a Phase I safety trial.

Restoring muscle control. People with spinal cord injuries have limited or no ability to control muscle groups below the site of the injury. This often requires assistive mobility devices (crutches, wheelchairs, or powered wheelchairs) and part- or full-time caregiver support. One research team is investigating a technological approach to bypass the injury. They have built a fully implantable system that uses a sensor to measure voluntary muscle contractions above the injury; the sensor, in turn, sends electrical signals to trigger muscle activity below the injury. The technology has enabled the restoration of standing, stepping, cycling, and hand grasp. Another research team is using electrical stimulus in conjunction with physical therapy to more effectively train the central nervous system to enhance the function of the few remaining neurons at the site of the injury. The team uses a completely noninvasive system to train the nervous system below the injury how to walk. This approach has improved walking speed long after the therapy has ended. Another approach uses implantable spinal cord stimulators, originally designed to reduce pain, to alter the neural activity in the spine to restore control of standing and stepping in patients. All of these teams are planning to attain the FDA's approval for Phase I safety trials.

Prosthesis control. Standard-of-care prostheses for amputees, while increasing in sophistication, lack the ability to reliably detect a user's fine motor commands. Several teams are developing technologies to more accurately record and transmit the user's intent to use their hands to grasp, grip or pinch by recording the electrical signals sent by the user. By implanting electrodes in the residual arm muscles, peripheral nerves, spinal cord, and brain, it is possible to detect these electrical signals, convert them into digital commands, and drive the motors in a hand prosthesis to significantly improve function. Researchers are fine-tuning the system for each limb as well as the different needs of each amputee. By exploring all of these approaches simultaneously, it should be possible to advance the state of the art faster. Several studies have the FDA's approval for clinical trials, and the others are still undergoing preclinical research prior to advancing to trial.

Closed-loop braces for limbs, spine. Traditional orthoses, or braces, were purely mechanical, passive devices to provide structural, postural, and functional characteristics of the musculoskeletal system. By incorporating electronic sensors, controllers, and motors, it is possible to greatly increase functional performance for users. One approach is to build an ankle-foot brace with a hydraulically adjustable stiffness to mimic the muscles and tendons in a healthy individual. This team is developing a child-size version of the device, which adjusts to maintain a proper fit as the child grows. Another approach is to develop a hydraulic system to use forces from a user's unimpaired or less-impaired limb to support motion by the impaired limb. And yet a third approach is to build an electromechanical control system capable of supporting a complete range of motion for individuals with thoracic/lumbar vertebrae that are compressed or crushed.

TELEPHONE-BASED REHAB PROGRAMS

A National Cancer Institute (NCI) funded clinical trial led by Dr. Cheville found that a 6-month physical rehabilitation program delivered by telephone modestly improved function and reduced pain for people with advanced cancer. The telerehabilitation program also reduced the time patients spent in hospitals and long-term care facilities, such as nursing homes.

"Overall, the study findings add to the growing evidence that low-tech interventions can effectively improve the delivery of supportive cancer care services," wrote Manali Patel, M.D., M.P.H., of the Stanford University School of Medicine, in a commentary on the study. Embracing these low-tech approaches "may be a smart move ... to improve patient-reported outcomes and keep patients at home," she concluded.

REMOTELY DELIVERED CARE

For the trial, dubbed COlchicine for acute PEricarditis (COPE), Dr. Cheville and her colleagues enrolled 516 adults (257 women and 259 men) with advanced-stage cancer and moderate functional impairment. People with moderate impairment can independently get around their home and, to a more limited extent, their communities, and manage activities of daily living (ADL), such as grocery shopping, but they do so with some difficulty. The average age of study participants was approximately 66 years of age.

To assess the value of a telerehabilitation program that addressed function and pain, patients eligible for the trial – all of whom had been seen at one of the three Mayo Clinic medical centers (in

Minnesota, Arizona, or Florida) were randomly assigned to one of three groups.

Those in the control group (group 1) continued their usual care and activities. Those in group 2 received an individualized telerehabilitation program delivered by a physical therapist with extensive experience in cancer rehabilitation – referred to as a "fitness care manager." They also received targeted rehabilitation to manage pain. Those in group 3 received the individualized telerehabilitation program plus medication-based pain management coordinated by a nurse.

At the time of enrollment, fitness care managers phoned group 2 and group 3 participants to discuss symptoms, identify goals, and discuss any physical impairments and barriers to staying active.

With supervision from a rehabilitation physician (Dr. Cheville), fitness care managers instructed patients in a simple set of strength training exercises using resistance bands and a walking program that used a pedometer to track steps. The fitness care managers monitored patients' progress and coordinated with their primary clinical team.

When needed, patients were referred to a local physical therapist to fine-tune their exercise programs or address physical impairments in consultation with the fitness care manager.

All participants were monitored for function, pain, and quality of life using short questionnaires that they could opt to answer either online or by telephone.

IMPROVEMENTS WITH TELEREHABILITATION
Over the six-month study period, group 2 participants (the telerehabilitation-only group) reported improvements in function, pain, and quality of life compared with patients in the control group.

The researchers expected that group 3 participants, who received telerehabilitation plus medication-based pain management, would see the greatest improvement in pain. But, to their surprise, pain control was similar in groups 2 and 3. Also, unexpectedly, telerehabilitation alone was most effective in improving function, and quality of life was not markedly better in group 3 than in the control group.

Telerehabilitation was associated with fewer and shorter hospitalizations, and hospitalized telerehabilitation participants were more likely than those in the control group to be discharged from the hospital to home, rather than to a long-term care facility.

Although the changes in function seen with telerehabilitation alone were modest, they were clinically meaningful, Dr. Cheville said.

"Even a small change can correlate with the ability to get in and out of a chair independently, go upstairs on your own, or get in and out of a car without help. These changes can make the difference between going home from the hospital rather than going to a nursing home," she said.

Chapter 34 | **Rehabilitation Medicine: Research Activities and Scientific Advances**

Through its intramural and extramural organizational units, the *Eunice Kennedy Shriver* National Institute of Child Health and Human Development (NICHD) supports and conducts a broad range of research projects that fall under the rehabilitation medicine umbrella, as well as research on conditions that cause disabilities.

INSTITUTE ACTIVITIES AND ADVANCES

Several NICHD organizational units support and conduct research related to rehabilitation medicine. Some of this research aims to establish an evidence base for the development of best practices; other activities aim to improve health outcomes related to specific diseases and conditions that cause disability, such as traumatic brain injury (TBI) and stroke.

The Institute's National Center for Medical Rehabilitation Research (NCMRR) fosters the development of scientific knowledge to enhance the health, productivity, independence, and quality of life of people with physical disabilities through basic and clinical research. The NCMRR also serves as the coordinating body for rehabilitation research across the National Institute of

This chapter includes text excerpted from "Rehabilitation Medicine: Research Activities and Scientific Advances," *Eunice Kennedy Shriver* National Institute of Child Health and Human Development (NICHD), November 4, 2020.

Health (NIH) and seeks collaborative opportunities with other NIH Institutes.

The NCMRR supports the development and application of devices to improve the human-environment interface and to restore or enhance an individual's capacity to function in his or her environment. This type of applied research and rehabilitation technology includes, but is not limited to, prosthetics, wheelchairs, biomechanical modeling, and other devices that aim to enhance mobility, communication, cognition, and environmental control.

The Center supports some of these activities through the Small Business Innovative Research (SBIR) and Small Business Technology Transfer (STTR) programs. For example, the NCMRR awarded funding to IntelliWheels, Inc. Policy, to develop ultra light weight, multigeared wheels for manual wheelchairs to give users increased mobility and independence. Another NICHD-funded SBIR grant involves development and testing of an instrumented glove for rehabilitation of individuals who have lost hand function from stroke. The glove requires the user to practice gripping movements by playing a computer game.

Through its research programs, the NCMRR addresses specific issues in rehabilitation medicine:

- The Behavioral Sciences and Rehabilitation Technologies (BSRT) program supports research related to development or redevelopment of emotional, cognitive, and physical processes and characteristics. This work includes interventions to encourage behavioral development in children with disabilities, as well as research on behavioral plasticity. The rehabilitative technology portion of the BSRT program supports research that applies bioengineering principles to developing assistive technology to help people with disabilities perform daily tasks and activities.

- Projects within the Biological Sciences and Career Development (BSCD) program support basic research on substrate responses to injury and on strategies to promote regeneration, plasticity, adaptation, and recovery. This research includes studies on

418

topics ranging from activity-mediated processes, such as treadmill training and constrained-use therapy, to genomic influences on outcomes and recovery. This program also includes research on secondary conditions, such as pain, depression, and cardiovascular dysfunction.

- Scientists supported by the Spinal Cord and Musculoskeletal Disorders and Assistive Devices (SMAD) program conduct research to develop rehabilitation technology for individuals with spinal cord injury (SCI) and musculoskeletal disorders such as cerebral palsy (CP), muscular dystrophy, multiple sclerosis (MS), arthritis, osteoporosis, and systemic lupus erythematosus (SLE).

A few advances by NCMRR-funded scientists are described below. Additional advances are available in the right column of this page.

- The NCMRR-funded scientists are currently working on major breakthroughs in walking technologies for lower-limb amputees. For example, at the University of Alabama, Tuscaloosa, a muscle-actuated robotic below-knee prosthesis is being developed that will give amputees a powered ankle joint capable of better meeting the demands of human locomotion than the passive ankle joints found in current prostheses. Scientists at Vanderbilt University are developing paired, coordinated robotic ankle and knee prostheses for bilateral transfemoral amputees. This will restore awareness and stability between the prostheses to enhance patients' ability to walk. At the University of Texas, scientists are studying the mechanics of falling in lower-limb amputees and designing rehabilitative interventions to prevent falls.
- Scientists supported in part by the NICHD, the National Institute of Biomedical Imaging and Bioengineering (NIBIB), the National Science Foundation, and the Defense Advanced Research

419

Projects Agency developed and implanted a wireless sensor into the brains of pigs and monkeys that recorded and transmitted information about brain activity for more than a year. The sensor could be used to study the brain's muscle and movement control mechanisms in animals that are able to interact more naturally with their environments. It could also eventually be used in patients with severe neurological impairment for wireless control of prosthetics that move with the power of thought, as well as in controlling motorized wheelchairs or other assistive technologies.

- Experts previously believed that recovery from TBI could occur only within a year after sustaining the injury. However, new findings from University of Texas at Dallas researchers indicate that a type of brain training called "gist-reasoning training" can improve cognitive performance months and even years after injury. Adolescents who experienced TBI at least 6 months prior to study enrollment completed eight, 45-minute training sessions over the course of a month. The gist-reasoning training involved reading texts and creating summaries and recalling important facts. Compared to a control group, the gist training group displayed significant improvement in several cognitive functions. The results suggest that this kind of cognitive training can be effective at improving brain functioning at 6 months and beyond the injury.

- Researchers supported in part by NICHD reported on results from an ongoing clinical trial of a brain-computer interface called "BrainGate" that allows paralyzed individuals to use their thoughts to control a robotic arm that makes reach-and-grasp movements. The published report documented the ability of a paralyzed study participant to reach for and sip from a drink with no assistance. The article reported on several other tasks that the participants were able to complete. While the device requires additional testing before it can be widely used in paralyzed patients, it could eventually represent a way to restore some level of everyday function in these individuals.

In addition to NCMRR, the several other NICHD components also address rehabilitation medicine research, including (but not limited to):

In the Division of External Research (DER), the Intellectual and Developmental Disabilities Branch (IDDB) sponsors research and research training intended to prevent and ameliorate a variety of intellectual and developmental disabilities. These efforts include support of national research networks and programs that include some rehabilitation medicine-related work: Autism Centers of Excellence (ACE) program, the *Eunice Kennedy Shriver* Intellectual & Developmental Disabilities Research Centers (EKS-IDDRCs), the Fragile X Syndrome Research Center (FXSRC) program, and the Paul D. Wellstone Muscular Dystrophy Specialized Research Centers (MDSRCs).

The DIR program on Pediatric Imaging and Tissue Sciences develops and evaluates noninvasive imaging methods for assessing normal development, screening, diagnosis, and prognosis of diseases, disorders, and disabilities in pediatric populations. Studies include both basic and applied explorations of the science of tissues, physics, and imaging. The program's Section on Tissue Biophysics and Biomimetics invents, develops, and implements novel quantitative in vivo methods for imaging tissues and organs. For example, an ongoing study uses multimodal magnetic resonance imaging to evaluate cerebral reorganization caused by various rehabilitation approaches in children with cerebral palsy and TBI. Another line of investigation examines plasticity changes after rehabilitation in military personnel affected by TBI.

Chapter 35 | Vision and Hearing Loss

Section 35.1 | Low Vision and Blindness Rehabilitation

This section includes text excerpted from "Vision Research: Needs, Gaps, and Opportunities," National Eye Institute (NEI), August 2012. Reviewed June 2021.

Low vision is an impairment to vision that hampers one's ability to function in daily life. Low vision is not correctable with medical or surgical therapies, spectacles, or contact lenses. Although low vision most often includes loss of sharpness or acuity, there may also be reduced field of vision, abnormal light sensitivity, distorted vision, or loss of contrast. Visual impairment can range from mild to severe, including total blindness or functional blindness where no useful vision remains. Although important advances have been made in treating and preventing eye diseases and disorders that cause visual impairment, many remain incurable. According to the World Health Organization (WHO), about 314 million people have visual impairment worldwide, of which 45 million are blind. Conservative estimates suggest that there are at least 3.6 million Americans have visual impairment of which more than one million are legally blind.

Low vision may occur as a result of birth defects, injury, aging, or as a complication of the disease. More than two-thirds of people with visual impairment are older than 65 years of age, where the leading causes are age-related macular degeneration, glaucoma, diabetic retinopathy, cataract, and optic nerve atrophy. Visual impairment in the elderly decreases independence increases the risk of falls and fractures, and often leads to isolation and depression. Visual impairment also affects infants and children, due to conditions, such as retinopathy of prematurity, deficits in the visual centers of the brain, juvenile cataract, and retinal abnormalities. These conditions can severely impair a child's quality of life and can have major consequences on educational advancement and future opportunities for employment. Visual impairment treatment and rehabilitation is an important component of visual healthcare in the United States. Ophthalmologists and optometrists who specialize in low vision may choose from an assortment of specialized eyewear, filters, magnifiers, adaptive equipment, closed-circuit television systems, independent living aids, and may offer training and counseling to patients. Although assistive devices and services do not cure visual disorders, research in this field leads to improved devices and new approaches designed to enhance the quality of life for millions of individuals with visual impairment.

RECENT PROGRESS IN LOW VISION AND BLINDNESS REHABILITATION
Assistive Technology

Because most content on the Internet is displayed visually, several new applications are geared to interpret this content for users with visual impairment, such as dynamic pin displays for online braille and tactile graphics. Recent advances in computing power and image-processing have revolutionized applications for individuals with visual impairment. Screen-magnifying and screen-reading software are widely deployed so that computers and smartphones are now accessible to users who have low vision and are blind, without the need for costly third-party software accessories. The latest generation of smartphones has stimulated the development of innovative products to aid individuals with visual impairment. These include flexible image magnifiers, mobile optical character recognition, bar code readers, and indoor wayfinding aids. In the past few years, research and development of global positioning system-based navigation aids for people with visual impairment have refined commercially available products.

Behavioral and Neuroscience Basic Research

When we move around our environment, in our mind's eye, we construct a picture of the world around us. This picture, or cognitive map, is attributed to a neural network thought to be located in the medial temporal brain area. The parietal area of the brain is closely tied to the accrual of perceptual information. The interaction between the parietal and temporal regions may explain how ongoing perceptual input leads to the formation of cognitive maps and has implications for understanding how individuals with visual impairment learn different strategies for orienting and navigating.

426

Following pathological insult to retina or brain, perceptual training techniques have been examined using videogames.

Behavioral studies have demonstrated that extensive practice can improve visual sensitivity. Infants with congenital cataracts or other treatable eye conditions experience visual deprivation during a period of robust visual development. Studies of these children are finding that once vision is restored, substantial functional and organizational changes in the visual cortex occur; whether the same holds true later in life is an actively debated topic. This neuroplasticity can now be studied noninvasively with functional magnetic resonance imaging. These findings regarding plasticity hold promise for informing vision rehabilitation efforts. Different areas of the brain respond to different types of perceptual stimuli (vision, touch, sound). Perception depends on integrating this multisensory information. Research shows that normally sighted, as well as individuals with visual impairment, recruit the visual cortex when interpreting tactile or auditory information. The functional roles of such cross-modal activations are not well understood, but are hot topics of current research and may provide the neural basis for sensory substitution, where perceptual processing for one sensory modality is largely replaced for another.

Implications of Vision Loss

With an increased understanding of the interdependence of physical and mental health, vision loss has been shown to be an independent predictor of depression. Depression (both major depressive disorders and subthreshold depression) affects roughly one-third of older adults with vision loss, which is similar to rates found among medically ill populations and those with other chronic conditions. In individuals with visual impairment, depression further exacerbates functional disability in everyday activities. Thus, visual impairment has been found to have widespread negative effects on quality of life, and psychological and social well-being.

Quality of Life

Quality-of-life (QOL) issues are gaining increased attention in vision impairment and rehabilitation research. With the development of standardized metrics (e.g., NEI Visual Functioning Questionnaire), quality-of-life measurements complement objective measures of visual function. Furthermore, there is a growing recognition that quality of life is a multidimensional concept that includes financial status, employment, physical and mental health, social relationships, and recreation and leisure time activities.

Activities of Daily Living

Research on activities of daily living (ADL) includes reading, mobility, and orientation in lab settings and real-world environments. Recent research has focused on the complicated visual environment encountered in the real world to appreciate how normally sighted and individuals with visual impairment process a visually rich environment. Extensive work relating reading to basic processes in visual perception (e.g., eye movement behavior during visual search) in sighted and individuals with visual impairment subjects has provided a solid theoretical foundation for developing improved rehabilitation regimens. There has been significant progress in understanding visually guided behavior in natural settings. Using wavelet-based sensors to capture basic sensory information akin to a crude visual system, researchers are able to model which visual cues are needed to help individuals orient themselves in a complicated environment. In addition, real-world studies that elucidate the challenges that the individuals with visual impairment experience in complex public transportation environments, and evaluate technologies that enhance safe and efficient street crossings in demanding urban environments, have provided important data. The development of objective measures of abilities to function in daily life has added to the understanding of the capacity for function and adds dimensions to research beyond self-reporting of difficulties with function.

Sight-Recovery Procedures

An impressive array of sight-recovery procedures are being studied in clinical trials, including retinal prostheses, gene therapy, and stem cell transplants. There are also global health initiatives increasing access to established therapies, such as cataract surgery or corrective lenses, to communities in developing countries that would otherwise remain individuals with visual impairment. There is an opportunity to study the behavioral and psychosocial impact of site recovery as well as implications for rehabilitation and neurodevelopment.

NEW MOBILE ASSISTIVE TECHNOLOGIES

For individuals with visual impairment, smartphone applications, commonly known as "apps," are emerging as important tools for everyday functioning and independence. The National Eye Institute (NEI) funded researchers are developing apps to assist individuals to maneuver around obstacles, read, and recognize faces and objects. For example, researchers are developing products that will allow the visually impaired to use smartphone cameras for identifying packaged food content and prices at the grocery store by scanning the barcodes on the package labels. Another app scans money to determine bill denominations, which provides confidence to the user for transactions at the cash register. Several assistive devices also are under development for the home or the workplace. For example, researchers are developing an app that immediately converts an image of the clock on a microwave oven or the temperature setting on a thermostat into an audio report on the phone's speaker. Indoor wayfinding systems use scannable signs or other locators so that the visually impaired can navigate unfamiliar locations.

For outdoor navigation, researchers are developing apps to capture images of intersections and analyze them to identify crosswalks, curbs, and the status of "Walk/Do not Walk" signs in real time. Others are creating services that provide subscribers with on-demand assistance, where a caller describes a situation or snaps a picture of an item, and an offsite assistant immediately calls back and describes the scene or item to the subscriber. The latest mobile technologies have opened up seemingly unlimited possibilities for assisting the visually impaired, and NEI remains committed to supporting the development of these and other cutting-edge technologies.

NEEDS AND OPPORTUNITIES IN LOW VISION AND BLINDNESS REHABILITATION
Understanding Visual Impairment

- Investigate multisensory processes and cross-modal plasticity. Determine whether cross-modal plasticity associated with visual deprivation differs from normal multisensory interactions. Determine the organizing principles and limits that exist for cross-modal plasticity. Determine the informational requirements of a task that affect whether a remaining sensory modality (e.g., touch) can substitute for the absence of sight. Further research using neural network approaches, behavioral, and neuropsychological methods are necessary to inform effective sensory substitution and improve rehabilitation efforts.

- Characterize variation in spatial cognition, important for many tasks, such as navigation. Spatial cognitive abilities vary widely. Normally sighted individuals with poor spatial cognition may be able to compensate through parallel processing using visual areas of the brain as well as perspective-free cognitive maps. In severe visual impairment, such compensation is limited or impossible, so the consequences of poor spatial cognition (whether innate or through lack of spatial cognitive experience) could be much more profound for the visually impaired than for the normally sighted.

- Determine spatial cognitive abilities of individuals with visual impairment to determine the extent to which nonvisual cues contribute to spatial cognition and how the contribution of nonvisual cues can be enhanced to improve spatial cognition under conditions of visual impairment.

- Understand the use of multisensory spatial representations, or cognitive maps, in learning strategies and whether learning strategies change with cross-modal plasticity. Does visual impairment result in fundamentally different learning strategies and does this differ by age?

Screening and Testing

- Design and validate tests of visual perception. Early detection of visual deficits will improve outcomes, but such tests can be used to benchmark outcomes of rehabilitative treatments. Sensitive, efficient testing is important to refine rehabilitation therapies and reduce burden on patients and clinicians.
- Create and validate vision tests relevant for the tasks of daily living. Eye charts that test letter acuity are not sufficient to characterize functional vision for people with visual impairment. Eye charts of high-contrast patterns are not useful or predictive for a majority of the visual tasks of daily living, which involve dynamic inputs of objects and scenes with varying color and contrast.
- Develop and standardize tests for evaluating more complex visually intensive behavior, such as reading, face recognition, mobility, and driving. Such tests will be useful in determining disability and progress toward rehabilitative goals.
- Develop testing specific to various patient populations. Nonverbal methods for testing vision (e.g., visual fields, retinal function) in special populations (children, neurological patients) are an important, yet unaddressed, area. In addition, developmental testing of children with visual impairment, particularly pre- or nonverbal children, is limited, as current tests require vision to accomplish some or many of the tasks (e.g., stack blocks; match figures). Even motor milestones are affected by vision impairment, but details of how this occurs are unknown, and standards for normal development for children with visual impairment are unknown.

Assistive Device Technology

- Develop new technology to improve access to Internet, print, graphic display, and navigation resources. Some areas require specialized technology innovation (such as online braille and tactile graphics, specialized embossers, and braille software), but there are also opportunities for developing new assistive devices and products by modifying devices, such as mobile phones, global-positioning system, accelerometers, and speech engines. Success in the visually impaired community depends on optimizing format and delivery methods, particularly for elderly, individuals with cognitive impairment, or individuals who are technologically naïve.

- Use models of eccentric vision (using peripheral retina when central field is dysfunctional) to translate technology developed for sighted users to users with visual impairment. Additionally, basic science on navigation, limited vision use, and multimodal perception can inform new assistive device development. For instance, a fundamental question concerns the limits of sensory substitution: Conveying visual information via auditory and tactile means has proven difficult. Normally, visual recognition of an embossed line drawing is trivial, but using either auditory or tactile means is challenging. Even when sensory substitution succeeds, only fairly simple visual information can be conveyed via these other modalities. A better understanding of the key aspects of visual information that are difficult to convey via other modalities could clearly inform the development of assistive technologies. Furthermore, studies of the effectiveness of these technologies are needed.

Visual Prostheses

- Determine critical parameters for continued improvement of prostheses. The visual prostheses are now being tested in patients. Different approaches include obtaining visual information (detected by a camera) to electrically stimulate the visual system (retina, or the visual cortex). Another relies on sensory substitution (e.g., encoding visual information into sensations on the tongue). In using a prosthesis, certain questions need to be resolved, for example, given a person's state of vision and what tasks can be done. If synchrony between modalities is required, how is one modality affected when the other input is degraded?

- Understand the level of acceptable visual enhancement using prosthetics. This can be determined using models of low vision, such as low-quality images, to determine how much information is necessary for particular visual tasks. 'Low quality' indicates low resolution, reduced fields, poor color contrast, and more generally, any other image quality decrement that can be associated with low vision. Although normally sighted humans use high visual acuity to perform tasks, such as face recognition, experiments with highly degraded images suggest that many of these skills are exceptionally robust in spite of acuity reductions. Such results could inform prosthesis design engineering and serve as feasibility criteria – if a planned neural prosthesis can only offer a low-resolution image, is it worth implantation? What kinds of visual abilities will it be able to support?

Rehabilitation and Improving Public Health

- Define heterogeneity of visually impaired populations. Within the legally blind/low vision population, there is heterogeneity with respect to visual function, even within a particular disease group. Advanced age is an important variable, ultimately affecting vision in almost all adults. Visual disorders are also associated with concussions and neurocognitive disorders that are not well understood. Studying how behavior and neural processing are altered and differ across the spectrum of visual impairment will improve our understanding of the sources of the heterogeneity and in personalizing rehabilitative efforts.
- Understand the causes and consequences of cortical reorganization in the blind. Several studies have demonstrated that blindness causes visual areas to respond to auditory and tactile stimuli. However, the behavioral consequences of the plasticity are not

yet clear. Determine if rehabilitative processes can improve functional plasticity. Determine whether such reorganization affects visual learning if sight is restored. Recent studies on establishing sight in individuals who were previously blind provide opportunities to investigate neuroplasticity and how the brain adapts to new visual input (anatomically and functionally). Determining which visual skills can be acquired, as well as how these changes correlate with age and extent of visual deprivation, will inform the prospects for recovery.

- Develop and test rehabilitation models and training paradigms. Low vision and blindness rehabilitation models continue to evolve. Interventions that are multimodal, multidisciplinary, and address functional and emotional aspects uniquely related to low vision, blindness, loss of vision, and vision restoration hold particular promise. These include findings from basic psychophysical research (e.g., training visual skills to develop a preferred retinal locus in central vision loss or for the use of a visual prosthetic), research on psychosocial implications of vision impairment (e.g., the mechanisms by which visual impairment leads to reduced quality of life), and developing training for prevention and adaptation strategies (e.g., lifestyle changes).

- Create and standardize performance-based outcome assessments as well as quality of life or other self-reported measures for low-vision interventions, whether they are prosthetic devices, assistive devices, or multidisciplinary rehabilitative strategies.

- Compare the effectiveness of rehabilitation approaches using randomized, controlled clinical trials. Rehabilitation currently lacks standardized methods and outcome assessments. Agreement on protocol and instrumentation will enable large-scale, multisite clinical trials.

- Identify comorbidities that interact with vision impairment and their influence on rehabilitation outcomes, and integrate visual rehabilitation models into subacute rehabilitation inpatient units. Poor vision hampers rehabilitation in a variety of age-related conditions (e.g., stroke, falls, hip fracture). Specialized rehabilitation needs for the visually impaired as they age (e.g., arthritis for life-long cane users), as well as for individuals with age-related vision loss, are not understood. Needs can vary depending on environment (e.g., nursing home residents) and comorbidities (e.g., wheelchair user; individuals who are deaf or hard of hearing).

RETINAL IMPLANTS FOR VISION RESTORATION

While working to prevent blindness and to restore natural vision, NEI also supports the development of retinal prostheses, also known as "retinal implants." Second Sight Medical Products, Inc., supported in part by NEI and by the U.S. Department of Energy (DOE), has engineered the Argus II Retinal Prosthesis System, which provides limited sight to people blinded by retinitis pigmentosa (RP), a genetic eye disease that causes gradual loss of the retina's light-sensing photoreceptor cells. Argus II consists of a video camera mounted on a pair of glasses, which captures and wirelessly transmits electrical signals through a 60-electrode grid surgically attached to the retina. The array bypasses the diseased photoreceptor machinery and directly activates the retinal ganglion cells that bring visual information to the brain. A clinical trial that included 30 RP patients equipped with the Argus II system showed that not only did the device not hinder the performance of participants with residual vision, it improved participants' ability to identify shapes, detect motion, locate objects, walk along a white line, and in the best cases, read large letters.

Although tested in RP patients, Argus II may be suitable for other conditions that damage the photoreceptors but leave the eye's neural networks intact, including AMD. Second Sight is currently developing a newer version of the device that uses a 256-electrode array that promises greater visual resolution. In 2011, Argus II became the 8 millionth patent issued by the U.S. Patent Office and it is now on the market in Europe. Other NEI-funded projects use complementary technologies. The Boston Retinal Implant Project is developing a device with external parts small enough to fit on the sclera – the outer wall of the eye. Another prosthetic device captures images with a video camera and then converts them into pulsed near-infrared light. Special glasses worn by the user project the near-infrared light through the eye and onto photodiodes implanted beneath the retina, which then convert the light into electrical signals that stimulate optic neurons. NEI-funded researchers are working to overcome technical barriers to retinal prostheses. They are adapting new nanotechnology to visual prostheses, expanding knowledge of how devices interact with neurons, and developing neurotransmitter-based prostheses.

Section 35.2 | Artificial Retina

This section includes text excerpted from documents published by two public domain sources. Text under the headings marked 1 are excerpted from "Overview of the Artificial Retina Project," U.S. Department of Energy (DOE), May 15, 2018; Text under the heading marked 2 is excerpted from "How the Artificial Retina Works," U.S. Department of Energy (DOE), May 15, 2018.

OVERVIEW OF THE ARTIFICIAL RETINA PROJECT[1]

The U.S. Department of Energy (DOE) Artificial Retina Project was a multi-institutional collaborative effort to develop and implant a device containing an array of microelectrodes into the eyes of people blinded by retinal disease. The ultimate goal was to design a device to help restore limited vision that enables reading, unaided mobility, and facial recognition.

The device is intended to bypass the damaged eye structure of those with retinitis pigmentosa and macular degeneration. These diseases destroy the light-sensing cells (photoreceptors, or rods and cones) in the retina, a multilayered membrane located at the back of the eye.

HISTORY OF THE ARTIFICIAL RETINA PROJECT[1]

The DOE project builds on the foundational work of its leader, Mark Humayun at the Doheny Eye Institute (DEI) of the University of Southern California (USC). In a breakthrough operation performed in 2002, a team led by Humayun successfully implanted the first device of its kind – an array containing 16 microelectrodes – into the eye of a patient who had been blind for more than 50 years. Since then, more than 30 additional volunteers around the world have had first- or second-generation (60-electrode) devices implanted. These devices enable patients to distinguish light from dark and localize large objects.

HOW DOES THE ARTIFICIAL RETINA WORK?[2]

Normal vision begins when light enters and moves through the eye to strike specialized photoreceptor (light-receiving) cells in the retina called "rods and cones." These cells convert light signals to electric impulses that are sent to the optic nerve and the brain. Retinal diseases, such as age-related macular degeneration and retinitis pigmentosa destroy vision by annihilating these cells.

With the artificial retina device, a miniature camera mounted in eyeglasses captures images and wirelessly sends the information to a microprocessor (worn on a belt) that converts the data to an electronic signal and transmits it to a receiver on the eye. The receiver sends the signals through a tiny, thin cable to the microelectrode array, stimulating it to emit pulses. The artificial retina device thus bypasses defunct photoreceptor cells and transmits electrical signals directly to the retina's remaining viable cells. The pulses travel to the optic nerve and, ultimately, to the brain, which perceives patterns of light and dark spots corresponding to the electrodes stimulated. Patients learn to interpret these visual patterns.

INTEGRATING REVOLUTIONARY DOE TECHNOLOGIES FOR USEFUL VISION[1]

Achieving the quantum improvements in the resolution needed for useful vision requires the integration of revolutionary technologies, such as those developed at DOE national laboratories. In 1999, the Doheny group began collaborating with researchers at DOE's Oak Ridge National Laboratory (ORNL), who also were working on approaches for restoring sight to the blind. Shortly thereafter they began to evaluate technologies at several other national laboratories as well.

To speed the design and development of better models, in 2004 Doheny and DOE (including six of its national laboratories), two additional universities, and Second Sight™ Medical Products, Inc. (a private-sector company), signed a Cooperative Research and Development Agreement (CRDA). Under the agreement, the institutions jointly share intellectual property rights and royalties from their research. This spurs progress – freeing the researchers to share details of their work within the collaboration.

MODELS IN TESTING AND DEVELOPMENT OF ARTIFICIAL RETINA PROJECT[1]
Model 1 (Argus™ I)
The Model 1 device [developed by Second Sight™ Medical Products, Inc. (SSMP)] was implanted in six blind patients between 2002 and 2004, whose ages ranged from 56 to 77 at the time of implant and all of whom have retinitis pigmentosa. The device consists of a 16-electrode array in a one-inch package that allows the implanted electronics to wirelessly communicate with a camera mounted on a pair of glasses. It is powered by a battery pack worn on a belt. This implant enables patients to detect when lights are on or off, describe an object's motion, count individual items, and locate objects in their environment. To evaluate the long-term effects of the retinal implant, five devices have been approved for home use.

Model 2 (Argus™ II)
The smaller, more compact Model 2 retinal prosthesis (developed by SSMP with DOE contributions) is currently undergoing clinical trials to evaluate its safety and utility. This model is much smaller, contains 60 electrodes, and surgical implant time has been reduced from the 6 hours required for Model 1 to 2 hours.

Model 3
The Model 3 device, which will have more than 200 electrodes, has undergone extensive design and fabrication studies at the DOE

438

national laboratories and is ready for preclinical testing. The new design uses more advanced materials than the two previous models and has a highly compact array. This array is four times more densely packed with metal contact electrodes and required wiring connecting to a microelectronic stimulator. Simulations and calculations indicated that the 200+ electrode device should provide improved vision for patients.

Section 35.3 | Cochlear Implants: Different Kind of Hearing Aid

This section includes text excerpted from "What Is a Cochlear Implant?" U.S. Food and Drug Administration (FDA), February 4, 2018.

WHAT IS A COCHLEAR IMPLANT?

A cochlear implant is an implanted electronic hearing device, designed to produce useful hearing sensations to a person with severe-to-profound nerve deafness by electrically stimulating nerves inside the inner ear.

These implants usually consist of two main components:
- The externally worn microphone, sound processor, and transmitter system
- The implanted receiver and electrode system, which contains the electronic circuits that receive signals from the external system and send electrical currents to the inner ear

Currently made devices have a magnet that holds the external system in place next to the implanted internal system. The external system may be worn entirely behind the ear or its parts may be worn in a pocket, belt pouch, or harness.

WHO USES COCHLEAR IMPLANTS

Cochlear implants are designed to help severely to profoundly deaf adults and children who get little or no benefit from hearing aids.

Even individuals with severe or profound "nerve deafness" may be able to benefit from cochlear implants.

WHAT DETERMINES THE SUCCESS OF COCHLEAR IMPLANTS

Many things determine the success of implantation. Some of them are:

- How long the patient has been deaf – as a group, patients who have been deaf for a short time do better than those who have been deaf a long time
- How old they were when they became deaf – whether they were deaf before they could speak
- How old they were when they got the cochlear implant – younger patients, as a group, do better than older patients who have been deaf for a long time
- How long they have used the implant
- How quickly they learn
- How good and dedicated their learning support structure is
- The health and structure of their cochlea – the number of nerve (spiral ganglion) cells that they have
- Implanting variables, such as the depth and type of implanted electrode and signal processing technique
- Intelligence and communicativeness of patient

HOW DOES A COCHLEAR IMPLANT WORK?

A cochlear implant receives sound from the outside environment, processes it, and sends small electric currents near the auditory nerve. These electric currents activate the nerve, which then sends a signal to the brain. The brain learns to recognize this signal and the person experiences this as hearing.

The cochlear implant somewhat simulates natural hearing, where sound creates an electric current that stimulates the auditory nerve. However, the result is not the same as normal hearing.

WHY ARE THERE DIFFERENT KINDS OF IMPLANTS?

Current thinking is that the inner ear responds to sound in at least two separate ways.

One theory, the place theory, says the cochlea responds greater to a simple tone at one place along its length. Another theory is that the ear responds to the timing of the sound.

Researchers, following the place theory, devised implants that separated the sound into groups. For example, they sent the lower pitches to the area of the cochlea where it seemed more responsive to lower pitches. And they sent higher pitches to the area more responsive to high pitches. Thus, they used several channels and electrodes spaced out inside the cochlea. Since there were also timing theories, researchers devised implants that made the sound signals into pulses to see if the cochlea would respond better to various kinds of pulses.

Most modern cochlear implants are versatile, in that they are somewhat capable of being adjusted to respond to sound in various ways. Audiologists try a variety of adjustments to see what works best with a particular patient.

Chapter 36 | **Robotics in Rehabilitation**

Chapter Contents

Section 36.1 | Cybernetics

Cybernetics uses technology to study different parts of regulatory systems, such as their structures, control mechanisms, and limitations. Cybernetic approaches allow a deeper understanding of the functions and processes within systems that can receive, collect, store, process, and retrieve data, which can later be used for system control.

Cybernetics has a broad scope that includes studying mechanical, biological, social, or cognitive systems in the environment. Cybernetics finds its most significant use in closed-loop signaling systems. A closed-loop signaling system is one where the action and the reaction occur within the same system. In the system, a generated action produces a resulting change that alters the system environment. Cybernetics is involved in models or systems that have a monitoring entity that compares the system's internal processes at different times with a standard flow of action and a controller that alters the system's behavior accordingly to maintain normal function.

Norbert Wiener proposed the term "cybernetics" and defined it as the science and study of control and communication in organisms and machines. Cybernetics can be closely related to the physiology of the animal nervous system, where the controller is the brain, and the eyes are the monitors. Feedback is a crucial part of a closed-loop signaling system where the monitor sends information to the controller, which issues instructions based on the received data. Cybernetics' earliest application was in prosthetic limbs where human control systems were studied to help the construction of artificial limbs that could be connected with the brain.

FIELDS OF APPLICATION
Cybernetics influences various fields such as:
- Game theory
- Artificial intelligence

- Philosophy
- System theory
- Architecture
- Perceptual control
- Prosthetics and rehabilitation
- Robotics
- Bioinformatics

CYBERNETICS IN REHABILITATION

As cybernetics finds uses in different fields, one crucial use that has been studied in recent years is its application in prosthetic limb attachments as part of rehabilitation. Gait rehabilitation is one of the prominent applications of cybernetic rehabilitation. Sometimes, as a result of experiencing a stroke or partial paralysis, individuals can lose normal body balance, which can affect gait while walking. Cognitive therapy and cybernetics can be combined based on human mechatronic systems to provide gait rehabilitation therapy. Adaptive rehabilitation therapy can include various technologies such as medical electronics and robotic assistive devices. Cybernetics for gait rehabilitation can be found in a gait enhancing shoe, working as a passive device that functions and adapts over varying terrains to help the patient walk better. Other research avenues include the study of cybernetics in upper-limb rehabilitation that can help patients who have lost mobility in their arm muscles due to stroke-induced paralysis. Cybernetic rehabilitation involves a human-machine-human approach with a cybernetic interface platform for biological signals of motor skills and the learning of such skills. This kind of rehabilitation involves four components:

- The physiotherapist
- The cybernetic interface platform
- The rehabilitation robot such as the attached prosthetic
- The patient

Different types of robotic rehabilitation devices use cybernetics to help with artificial limb attachments and movements. They are classified according to the interface with the user as end-effector devices and exoskeletal devices.

- End-effector devices are used for upper-limb interface and gait training. Some examples include the HapticWalker and the G-EO system.
- Exoskeletal devices act directly on the joints and are more complex to construct as they must mirror the limb they are working upon for maximum efficiency. Specific examples are ARMin, MGA for the arm, AnkleBot, and LOPES for the leg.

References

1. Laut, J., et al. "The Present and Future of Robotic Technology in Rehabilitation," Current Physical Medicine and Rehabilitation Reports, November 19, 2016.
2. "Cybernetics," Techopedia, June 2020.
3. "Cybernetics," Britannica, March 14, 2021.

Section 36.2 | Prosthetic Engineering

This section includes text excerpted from "Prosthetic Engineering: Overview," Center for Limb Loss and Mobility (CLiMB), U.S. Department of Veterans Affairs (VA), March 30, 2017. Reviewed June 2021.

The aim is to improve prosthetic prescription by investigating the efficacy of prosthetic components used in current clinical practice and by developing novel approaches to improve the current standard of care. The amputee-centric research encompasses improving patient mobility and comfort and preventing injury. Support for this research (2000 to present) includes funding from the U.S. Department of Veterans Affairs (VA) Rehabilitation Research and Development Service and the National Institutes of Health (NIH).

MOBILITY RESEARCH
Disturbance Response in Amputee Gait

Errors in foot placement while avoiding obstacles and maneuvering in the household and community environments may lead to

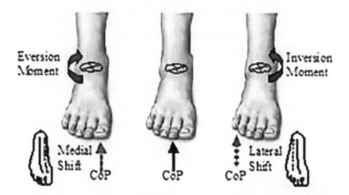

Figure 36.1. Eversion and Inversion Movement Model

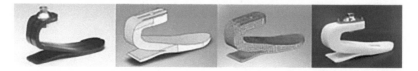

Figure 36.2. Models of Foot Stiffness

falls and injuries. This research aims to develop an ankle that can invert and evert and thereby control the center of pressure under the prosthetic foot; enhancing balance and stability of lower limb amputees.

Foot-Ankle Stiffness

Many ambulatory lower limb amputees exhibit fatigue, asymmetrical gait, and the inability to walk at varying speeds. A rapid prototyping approach is used to fabricate feet of varying stiffness for exploring the effects of foot stiffness on amputee gait.

Turning Gait

Turning corners and maneuvering around obstacles are essential abilities for a successful community and household ambulation. The aim of this research is to test the efficacy of a compliant torque adapter in the pylons of transtibial amputees.

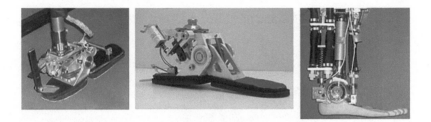

Figure 36.3. Three Different Propulsion Test Devices

Energy Storage and Release

Many ambulatory lower limb amputees exhibit fatigue, asymmetrical gait, and the inability to walk at varying speeds. Several approaches aimed at providing the propulsive forces necessary to alleviate these problems are being developed and tested.

Stochastic Resonance

Stochastic resonance (sub-threshold vibration) may enhance peripheral sensation sufficiently to result in improved postural stability and locomotor function. This research explores the application of this phenomenon to the residual limb and intact plantar surface of diabetic lower limb amputees.

Research in Robotics and Biomechanics

Dr. Aubin's research spans robotics and biomechanics with applications in health and mobility. He motivates his research by engaging with patients and stakeholders to understand shortcomings in the areas of rehabilitation, prosthetics, orthotics, and physical therapy. Dr. Aubin strives to address these unmet patient and caregiver needs by establishing multidisciplinary research teams that leverage state-of-the-art technologies in robotics, neuroscience, and computational intelligence. Dr. Aubin's research goal is to develop and utilizes novel sensors, algorithms, assistive powered devices, and robotic tools that can augment human performance and/or improve mobility and function for those affected by diseases, age, or trauma.

Biologically Informed Robotics

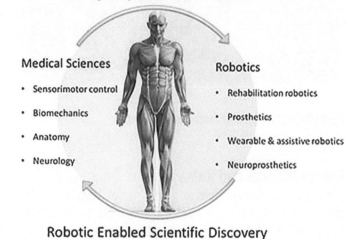

Medical Sciences

- Sensorimotor control
- Biomechanics
- Anatomy
- Neurology

Robotics

- Rehabilitation robotics
- Prosthetics
- Wearable & assistive robotics
- Neuroprosthetics

Robotic Enabled Scientific Discovery

Figure 36.4. Work Flow of Robotics and Biomechanics

Smart Cane System

People with pain or arthritis in their knee often walk with a cane to reduce knee pain and to improve or maintain their mobility. Increased pressure on the knee joint likely causes knee arthritis and reducing the pressure on the knee joint may slow the progression of arthritis. Walking with a cane reduces the pressure inside the knee joint, but only if the cane supports 10 percent to 20 percent of a person's weight. Many people may not be using their cane in the best way they can because they do not know how much force (percent of their body weight) they are putting on the cane when they walk. In this study the researchers are looking at how using a computerized cane that beeps or vibrates (such as a cell phone) when a certain amount of force is applied to it might help people learn to more effectively use a cane. It is also examining how walking with a cane changes the pressure in the knee joint. It is hypothesized that giving the user biofeedback, a sound or vibration signal from the cane will help them apply the optimal amount of force on the cane. The secondary hypothesis is that increased cane loading will result in a decrease in knee joint pressure.

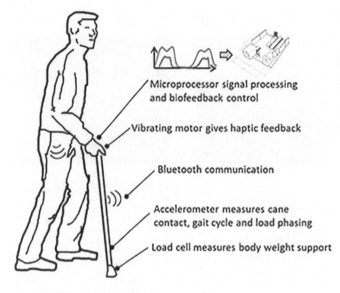

Figure 36.5. Smart Cane System

Sensory Feedback for Prosthetic Limbs

It has long been recognized that restoring movement function after amputation is a priority. We are now entering an era in which restoration of sensation may be possible as well through the use of smart sensorized prosthetic devices and haptic feedback. Researchers are working on understanding how feedback of forces and events on the foot – for example, the placement of the prosthetic foot as the user is walking downstairs – can lead to improved function.

INJURY PREVENTION RESEARCH
Vacuum Suspension Systems

Many amputees live with an ill-fitting socket and can experience limb pistoning within the socket, which in turn may result in skin irritation, tissue breakdown, discomfort, and reduction inactivity. The aims of this research are to characterize the response of the lower residual limb to a vacuum suspension system and to measure changes in limb volume with a structured light scanning system.

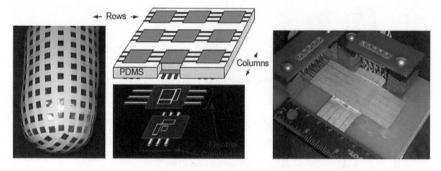

Figure 36.6. Distributed Sensing Images

Socket Systems and Tissue O$_2$

Limb health and wound healing capacity is closely related to the amount of oxygen present in limb tissues. Using the fiber-optic video-oximetry imaging system, the aim is to discover if the prosthetic prescription can influence residual limb tissue oxygenation during both rest and gait.

Distributed Sensing

The goal of the proposed project is to develop enabling sensing technology based on a flexible array and to build a prototype of a prosthetic liner with distributed, unimodal field sensing capability. The specific aims include:

- The design of the flexible sensing array for measurement of moisture, temperature, pressure, and shear stress
- Integration of this array into a prosthetic liner/ socket
- Testing of device performance

Torsional Prosthesis

This research seeks to develop a prosthetic limb whose torsional characteristics can adapt depending on the activity. The goal is to reduce torsional stresses and the incidence of residual limb injuries.

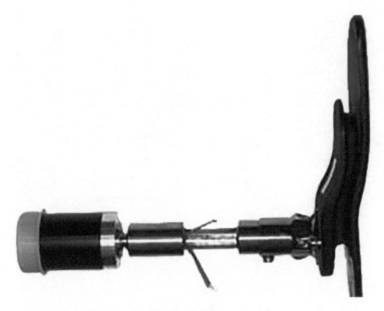

Figure 36.7. Prosthetic Limb with Torsional Characteristics

PATIENT COMFORT RESEARCH
Thermal Comfort

Lower-limb amputations often experience discomfort related in part to higher skin temperatures within their prosthetic socket. Research has found prosthetic liners and sockets are excellent insulators that can retain heat. Activity can cause a dramatic increase in skin temperature within the prosthesis requiring substantially long periods of inactivity to restore resting state temperatures. Current work involves developing active cooling systems and embedded sensor networks to monitor skin temperature.

Evaporative Cooling and Perspiration Removal

Amputees often complain about uncomfortably warm residual limb skin temperatures and the accumulation of perspiration within their prosthesis. This research will discover if a novel evaporative cooling system can provide ameliorate these problems.

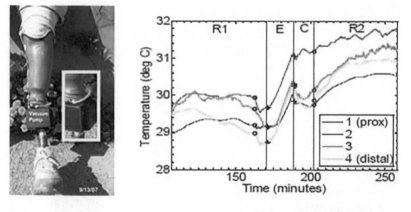

Figure 36.8. Evaporating Cooling System

Section 36.3 | **New Robotic Wheelchair**

This section includes text excerpted from "A Multipurpose Robotic Wheelchair and Rehabilitation Device for the Home," National Institute of Standards and Technology (NIST), December 14, 2020.

It is said that "today, approximately 10 percent of the world's population is over 60 years of age; by 2050 this proportion will have more than doubled" and "the greatest rate of increase is amongst the oldest old, people 85 years of age and older." She follows by adding that this group is subject to both physical and cognitive impairments more than younger people. These facts have a profound impact on how the world will maintain the elderly independent as long as possible from caregivers. Both physical and cognitive diminishing abilities address the body and the mental process of knowing, including aspects such as awareness, perception, reasoning, intuition, and judgment. Assistive technology for the mobility impaired includes the wheelchair, lift aids, and other devices, all of which have been around for decades. However, the patient typically or eventually requires assistance to use the device; whether it is someone to push them in a wheelchair, to lift them from the bed to a chair or to the toilet, or for guiding them through cluttered areas. With fewer caregivers and more elderly, there is a need for improving these devices to provide them independent assistance.

There has been an increasing need for wheelchairs over time. L.H.V. van der Woude states that mobility is fundamental to health, social integration, and individual well-being of humans. Henceforth, mobility must be viewed as being essential to the outcome of the rehabilitation process of wheelchair dependent persons and to their successful (re-)integration into society and to a productive and active life. Thrun said that, if possible, rehabilitation to relieve the dependence on the wheelchair is ideal for this type of patient to live a longer, healthier life. Van der Woude continues stating that many lower limb disabled subjects depend upon a wheelchair for their mobility. Estimated numbers for Europe and the United States are respectively 2.5 million and 1.25 million. The quality of the wheelchair, the individual work capacity, the functionality of the wheelchair/user combination, and the effectiveness of the rehabilitation program do indeed determine the freedom of mobility.

Just as important as wheelchairs are the lift devices and people who lift patients into wheelchairs and other seats, beds, automobiles, etc. The need for patient lift devices will also increase as generations get older. When considering if there is a need for patient lift devices, several references state the positive, for example:

"The question is, what does it cost not to buy this equipment? A back injury can cost as much as $50,000, and that's not even including all the indirect costs. If a nursing home can buy these lifting devices for $1,000 to $2,000, and eliminate a back injury that costs tens of thousands of dollars, that is a good deal," 1 in every 3 nurses becomes injured from the physical exertion put forth while moving nonambulatory patients; costing their employers $35,000 per injured nurse. 1 in 2 nonambulatory patients fall to the floor and become injured when being transferred from a bed to a wheelchair.

"Nursing and personal care facilities are a growing industry where hazards are known and effective controls are available," said the Occupational Safety and Health Administration (OSHA) Administrator John Henshaw. "The industry also ranks among the highest in terms of injuries and illnesses, with rates about 2 1/2 times that of all other general industries..."

"Already today there are over 400,000 unfilled nursing positions causing health-care providers across the country to close wings or risk negative outcomes. Over the coming years, the declining ratio of working age adults to elderly will further exacerbate the shortage. In 1950 there were eight adults available to support each elder 65+, today the ratio is 5:1 and by 2020 the ratio will drop to three working age adults per elder person."

In 2005, the National Institute of Standards and Technology (NIST) Intelligent Systems Division (ISD) began the Healthcare Mobility Project to target this staggering healthcare issue of patient lift and mobility. The ISD researchers looked at currently available technology through a survey of patient lift and mobility devices. That report showed that there is need for technology that includes mobility devices that can lift and maneuver patients to other seats and technology that can provide for rehabilitation to help the patient become independent of the wheelchair.

An additional area investigated in the survey was intelligent wheelchairs. The NIST has been studying intelligent mobility for the military, transportation, and the manufacturing industry for nearly 30 years through the Intelligent Control of Mobility Systems (ICMS) Program. Toward a standard control system architecture and advanced 3-D imaging technologies, as being researched within the ICMS Program, and applying them to intelligent wheelchairs, the NIST has begun outfitting the Home Lift, Position and Rehabilitation (HLPR) Chair with computer controls. Although throughout the world there are or have been many research efforts in intelligent wheelchairs, including: and many others, the authors could find no sources applying standard control methods nor the application of the most advanced 3-D imagers prototyped today to intelligent wheelchairs. Therefore, NIST began developing the HLPR Chair to investigate these specific areas of mobility, lift, and rehabilitation, as well as advanced autonomous control.

THE HLPR CHAIR STRUCTURE AND MOBILITY DESIGN

The HLPR Chair prototype, shown in Figure 36.9, is based on a manual, steel, inexpensive, off-the-shelf, and sturdy forklift. The

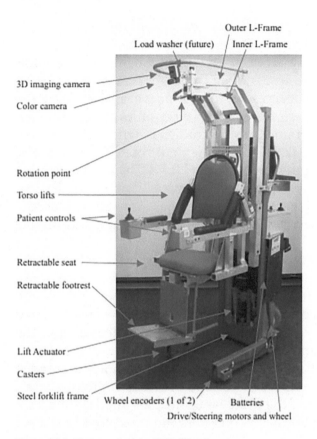

3D imaging camera

Color camera

Load washer (future)

Outer L-Frame

Inner L-Frame

Rotation point

Torso lifts

Patient controls

Retractable seat

Retractable footrest

Lift Actuator

Casters

Steel forklift frame

Wheel encoders (1 of 2)

Batteries

Drive/Steering motors and wheel

Figure 36.9. Photograph of the HLPR Chair Prototype

forklift includes a U-frame base with casters in the front and rear and a rectangular vertical frame. The lift and chair frame measures 58 cm (23 in) wide by 109 cm (43 in) long by 193 cm (76 in) high (when not in the lift position) making it small enough to pass through even the smallest, typically 61 cm (24 in) wide x 203 cm (80 in) high, residential bathroom doors. The HLPR Chair frame could be made lighter with aluminum instead of steel.

The patient seat/stand mechanism is a double, nested and inverted L-shape where the outer L is a seat base frame that provides a lift and rotation point for the inner L seat frame. The L frames are made of square, aluminum tubing welded as shown in the photograph. The outer L is bolted to the lift device while the

457

inner L rotates with respect to the seat base frame at the end of the L as shown in Figure 36.9. The frames rotation point is above the casters at the very front of the HLPR Chair frame to allow for outside wheelbase access when the seat is rotated π rad (180°) and is the main reason access to other seats is available. Drive and steering motors, batteries and control electronics along with their aluminum support frame provide counterweight for the patient to rotate beyond the wheelbase. When not rotated, the center of gravity remains near the middle of the HLPR Chair. When rotated to π rad (180°) with a 136 kg (300 Lb.) patient on board, the center of gravity remains within the wheelbase for safe seat access. Patients who are severely overweight would require additional counterweight.

The HLPR Chair is powered similarly to typical powered chairs on the market. Powered chairs include battery-powered, drive and steer motors. However, the HLPR Chair has a tricycle design to simplify the need to provide steering and drive linkages and provide for a more vertical and compact drive system design. The drive motor is mounted perpendicular to the floor and above the drive wheel with chain drive to it. The steering motor is coupled to an end cap on the drive motor and provides approximately π rad (180°) rotation of the drive wheel to steer the HLPR Chair. The front of the robot has two casters mounted to a U-shaped frame.

The prototype drive motor is geared such that its high speed drives a chain-driven wheel providing further speed reduction. HLPR Chair speed is 0.7 m/s (27 in/s). While this is sufficient speed for typical eldercare needs, a more powerful motor can replace the drive motor for additional speed.

Steering is a novel single wheel design hard stopping the wheel at just beyond π rad (180°) for safety of the steering system. Steering is reverse Ackerman controlled as joystick left rotates the drive wheel counterclockwise and joystick right rotates the drive wheel clockwise. The steering rotation amount can be limited by the amount of drive speed so as not to roll the frame during excessive speed with large steering rotation. The navigation and control of the vehicle under this novel rear wheel steer and drive is currently under study and will be described in later publications.

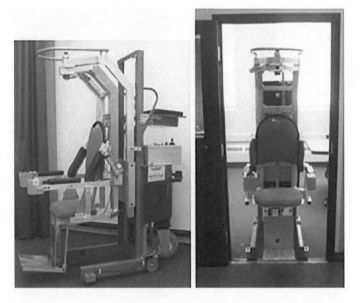

Figure 36.10. Photographs of the HLPR Chair in the Mobility Configuration Showing the Side View (Left) and Front View Relative to a Typical Doorway (Right)

For access to the HLPR Chair and for mobility, the HLPR Chair is lowered as shown in Figure 36.10. A seat belt or harness will be required for eldercare occupant safety. For access/exit to/from the HLPR Chair, the footrest can be retracted beneath the seat. For mobility, the footrest is deployed to carry the feet. Also, manually rotated feet pads can be deployed to provide a wider footrest. When retracted, the footrest pads automatically rotate within the footrest volume.

PATIENT LIFT

Patient lift is designed into the HLPR Chair to allow user access to high shelves or other tall objects while seated. The HLPR Chairs' patient lift (see Figure 36.11) is approximately 1 m (36 in) to reach what a typical, standing 2 m (6 ft) tall person could reach. This is a distinct advantage over marketed chairs and other concepts. The additional height comes at no additional cost of frame and only minimally for actuator cost.

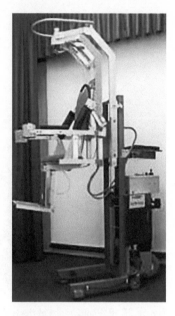

Figure 36.11. HLPR Chair Prototype
Shown in the Patient Lift Position

Lift is achieved by a 227 kg (500 Lbs.) max. lift actuator that can support 681 (1500 Lbs.) statically on the HLPR Chair prototype. The actuator can be replaced with a higher capacity unit if needed. The actuator connects to a lift plate with a steel chain that is fix-mounted at one end to the HLPR Chair frame and to the lift plate at the other end. The actuator pushes up on a sprocket of which the chain rolls over providing 1 m (36 in) lift with only a 0.5 m (18 in) stroke actuator. The outer L-frame is then bolted to the lift plate. Rollers mounted to the lift plate roll inside the HLPR Chair vertical C-channel frame.

PLACEMENT ON OTHER SEATS

It is estimated that 1 in 3 nurses or caregivers will develop back injuries. Most injuries occur because the patient is relatively heavy to lift and access to them is difficult when attempting to place the patient onto another seat. Wheelchair dependents have difficulty

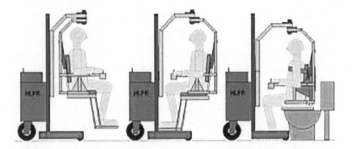

Figure 36.12. Graphic Showing the Concept of Placing a Patient onto a Toilet or Chair with the HLPR Chair

The patient drives to the target seat (left), manually rotates near or over the seat (middle) while the torso lifts support the patient and the seat retracts, and then is lowered onto the seat – toilet, chair or bed (right).

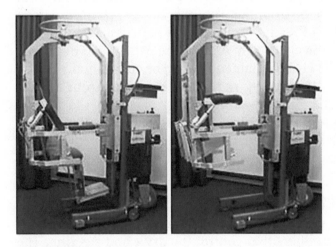

Figure 36.13. Photographs of the HLPR Chair in the Same Positions as in the Center and Right

moving from a seat to their wheelchair and back without a caregivers help or other lift mechanisms. The HLPR Chair was designed with the patient lift, as explained previously, to not only access tall objects, but to also pick up and place the patient in other chairs, on toilets, and on beds.

Figure 36.12 shows the concept of placing a patient onto a toilet. Figure 36.13 (left) shows the HLPR Chair prototype in the rotated

461

position and Figure 36.13 (right) shows it in the torso support position similar to the Figure 36.12 (center and right) graphic.

To place a HLPR Chair user on another seat, they can drive to, for example, a toilet, seat, or bed. Once there, the HLPR Chair rotates the footrest up and beneath the seat, and the patients feet are placed on the floor personally or by a caregiver. The HLPR Chair inner L-frame can then be rotated manually with respect to the chair frame allowing the patient to be above the toilet. Padded torso lifts then lift the patient from beneath her/his arm joints similar to crutches. The seat, with the footrest beneath, then rotates from horizontal to vertical behind the patients back clearing the area beneath the patient to be placed on the toilet, seat, bed, etc.

Once the person is placed on a toilet, the HLPR Chair can remain in the same position to continue supporting them from potential side, back or front fall. However, when placing a person onto a chair, the HLPR Chair must lift the patient and the patient manually rotates the chair from around the patient and out of the patients space. The HLPR Chair could then be conceptually driven from the seat location, using radio frequency or through voice commands, to a charging or waiting location and out of the patients view. When requesting to be picked up again, the patient could conceptually call the HLPR Chair remotely and have it return to the same pick up location and reverse the seat placement procedure.

MANUAL CONTROL

The HLPR Chair controls include a joystick that sends drive controls to power amplifiers that control the drive and steering. The patient lift actuator is also controlled with the same type power amplifier through a rocker switch. A lever switch is used to control seat and footrest retraction or deployment. The footrest, seat and torso lift actuators are direct controlled switched forward and reverse from the battery through momentary rocker switches. Actuators for the footrest and each torso lift have 8cm (3 in) stroke while the seat includes a 31 cm (12 in) actuator to rotate it from seated to behind the back and vice versa.

Behind the seat and frame and above the drive/steer wheel is the electronics box that houses the controls for the HLPR Chair while also providing a "Nurse" or caregiver control panel that duplicates the patient controls at the seat. The Nurse control panel (see Figure 36.14) includes all the control functions for a nurse or caregiver to drive or lift a dependent patient. Control redundancy is designed into the HLPR Chair to also allow a caregiver to quickly gain control of the device as needed. A "Nurse/Patient" switch on the Nurse control panel allows switching between the rear (Nurse) controls and the chair (Patient) controls.

TOWARDS AUTONOMOUS CONTROL

Recently, the HLPR Chair was modified (see figure 36.14) to include encoders, attached between its' frame and front caster wheels, a computer and computer interface electronics. The encoder design included adapting a shaft to one side of each caster wheel, passing it through a bearing attached to the frame and to an encoder. Although the encoder and housing add an additional 2.5 cm (1 in) to each side of the base, the overall HLPR Chair base width is still within the chair-frame width and therefore, within the overall HLPR Chair width of 58 cm (23 in). The encoders provide 3600 pulses per revolution allowing relatively fine measurement over a 12.7 cm (5 in) diameter caster wheel or approximately 90 pulses/cm (230 pulses/in) of linear travel. The relatively high measurement accuracy of the wheels will support development of accurate path planning and control algorithms for the HLPR Chair.

Included in the "Nurse" control panel is a computer/manual switch. While switched in manual mode, all of the "Nurse" – labeled (rear) controls on the box or on the "Patient" – labeled (chair) can be used. While in computer control, drive and steer are controlled by an onboard computer. The computer is currently a personal computer (PC) laptop interfacing to off-the-shelf input/output (I/O) devices housed in the box beneath the PC and connected through a universal serial bus (USB) interface. This design was chosen as a simple developer interface to the HLPR Chair prototype knowing that the computer and its interfaces can be significantly reduced in size as future commercial versions are designed. Software drivers for the HLPR Chair drive and steer control were written in C++ under the Linux operating system.

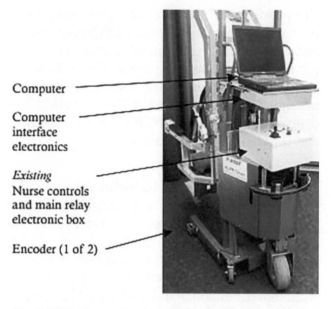

Computer

Computer
interface
electronics

Existing
Nurse controls
and main relay
electronic box

Encoder (1 of 2)

Figure 36.14. Photograph of the HLPR Chair with Recently Added Front Wheel Encoders, Development Computer and Interface Electronics, and Advanced 3D Imaging Camera and Color Camera

This low level control is now ready to add planned HLPR Chair navigation and obstacle avoidance control. NIST and the University of Delaware (UD) are teaming to use the NIST standard software control architecture for intelligent machines called "4 dimensional/ real-time control system" (4D/RCS) and UD's robot behavior generation. NIST has recently applied 4D/RCS to a Defense Advanced Research Project Agency (DARPA) Project called "Learning Applied to Ground Robots" (LAGR). The 4D/RCS structure developed for LAGR is shown in figure 36.15. The basic premise of the 4D/RCS columns of boxes are to sense the environment around the robot (left column), to place the sensed information into a world model (middle column), then plan and generate appropriate navigational paths and input these paths into the robot actuators in real time (right column). The horizontal rows of 4D/RCS boxes stack from a servo level control (bottom row) to grouped pixels, a lower resolution map, and a higher level planner (top row).

The authors plan to adopt this standard control architecture on the HLPR Chair so that advanced 3D imagers, such as the ones shown in figure 36.14, and robust control algorithms can be plug-and-played to address the variety of patient mobility controls that may be needed. An earlier version (from the one pictured in figure 36.14, 3D imaging camera was mounted on an early version of the HLPR Chair and a control algorithm was developed and tested. Results of this test, as explained in, clearly show detected obstacles in the vehicle path and a planned path around the obstacles.

PATIENT REHABILITATION

The HLPR Chair enhances patient rehabilitation through a load sensor and control on the lift actuator, as described in. The authors designed rehabilitation into the HLPR Chair to allow, for example, stroke patients to keep their legs active without supporting the entire load of the patient's body weight. The patient, once lifted, could walk while supported by the HLPR Chair driving at a slow walking pace towards regaining leg control and eliminating the need for a wheelchair.

To accomplish rehabilitation, the HLPR Chair includes, as explained in the Placement on Other Seats section, footrest and seat rotate behind the patient while she/he is lifted with torso lifts. However, instead of being placed low on a seat, the patient lift continues to move uplifting the patient as they move their legs beneath them to standing position. The HLPR Chair's open U-frame base allows access to the floor directly beneath the patient for standing. Figure 36.16 shows a photograph of the prototype in this configuration and a concept of how the HLPR Chair can be used for patient rehabilitation.

Additionally, the patient can be continuously monitored with a load washer at the L-frames rotation point. The patient could adjust the amount of load she/he wishes to place onto their legs and on the floor by rotating a dial on the controls from 0 to 100 percent. Load control is a future concept to be applied to the HLPR Chair prototype in the next several months.

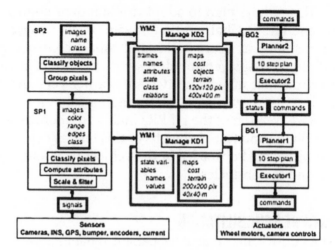

Figure 36.15. NIST 4D/RCS 2-Level, Hierarchical Control Architecture Developed for the DARPA LAGR Project and Planned for Implementation on the HLPR Chair

FUTURE RESEARCH

The HLPR Chair was designed to be a revolutionary patient lift and mobility system for wheelchair dependents, the elderly, stroke patients, and others desiring or even requiring personal mobility and lift access. The system shows promise for moving these groups of patients into the work force and removing the burden placed on the healthcare industry. The system has been prototyped to show the basic concept of such a patient lift and mobility system. The HLPR Chair was built to demonstrate its' relatively inexpensive capabilities to the healthcare industry and to build on its capabilities with robust controls for mobility and rehabilitation in the near-term.

Autonomous mobility control using the 4D/RCS standard control architecture and advanced 3D imagers is planned for a next step while teaming with the University of Delaware under a federal grant. Force loading for rehabilitation of patient legs will also be studied in the near term. Collaborations for proving the service capabilities and evaluating performance of the HLPR Chair to the healthcare industry are being pursued and expected in the near future.

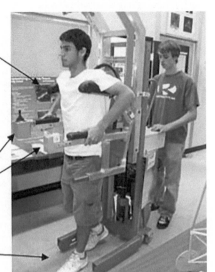

Padded Torso
Lifts for under
arms

Seat and
Footrest are
retracted behind
patient.

Accessible
controls

Open frame
base for walking

Figure 36.16. Photograph of the HLPR Chair Prototype in the Rehabilitation/Walking Configuration. Summer Interns (Alex Page and Robert Vlacich) Demonstrate the Patient and Nurse Configuration as Part of Their Official Duties

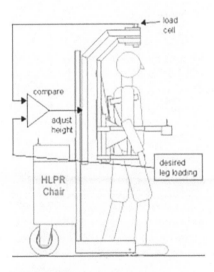

Figure 36.17. Graphic Showing the Concept of How the HLPR Chair Can Be Used for Patient Rehabilitation and Incorporate Future Legs Load Control

Chapter 37 | Electrical Signals and Stimulations

Chapter Contents

Section 37.1 | BrainGate

This section includes text excerpted from "Composing Thoughts: Mental Handwriting Produces Brain Activity That Can Be Turned into Text," National Institutes of Health (NIH), May 12, 2021.

Scientists have developed a brain-computer interface (BCI) designed to restore the ability to communicate in people with spinal cord injuries and neurological disorders, such as amyotrophic lateral sclerosis (ALS). This system has the potential to work more quickly than previous BCIs, and it does so by tapping into one of the oldest means of communications we have – handwriting.

The study, published in *Nature,* was funded by the National Institutes of Health's Brain Research Through Advancing Innovative Neurotechnologies® (BRAIN) Initiative as well as the National Institute of Neurological Disorders and Stroke (NINDS) and the National Institute on Deafness and Other Communication Disorders (NIDCD), both part of the NIH.

Researchers focused on the part of the brain that is responsible for fine movement and recorded the signals generated when the participant attempted to write individual letters by hand. In doing so, the participant, who is paralyzed from the neck down following a spinal cord injury, trained a machine-learning computer algorithm to identify neural patterns representing individual letters. While demonstrated as a proof of concept in one patient so far, this system appears to be more accurate and more efficient than existing communication BCIs and could help people with paralysis rapidly type without needing to use their hands.

"This study represents an important milestone in the development of BCIs and machine learning technologies that are unraveling how the human brain controls processes as complex as communication," said John Ngai, Ph.D., director of the NIH BRAIN Initiative. "This knowledge is providing a critical foundation for improving the lives of others with neurological injuries and disorders."

When a person becomes paralyzed due to spinal cord injury, the part of the brain that controls movement still works. This means that, while the participant could not move their hand or arm to write, their brain still produced similar signals related to the intended movement. Similar BCI systems have been developed to restore motor function through devices, such as robotic arms.

"Just think about how much of your day is spent on a computer or communicating with another person," said study co-author Krishna Shenoy, Ph.D., a Howard Hughes Medical Institute (HHMI) Investigator and the Hong Seh and Vivian W. M. Lim Professor at Stanford University. "Restoring the ability of people who have lost their independence to interact with computers and others is extremely important, and that is what is bringing projects like this one front and center."

First, the participant was asked to copy letters that were displayed on the screen, which included the 26 lower-case letters along with some punctuation: ">" which was used as space, and "~" which was used as a "full stop." At the same time, implanted electrodes recorded the brain activity from approximately 200 individual neurons that responded differently while he mentally "wrote" each individual character. After a series of training sessions, the BCI's computer algorithms learned how to recognize neural patterns corresponding to individual letters, allowing the participant to "write" new sentences that had not been pointed out before, with the computer displaying the letters in real time.

"This method is a marked improvement over existing communication BCIs that rely on using the brain to move a cursor to "type" words on a screen," said Frank Willett, Ph.D., an HHMI Research Scientist at Stanford University and the study's lead author. "Attempting to write each letter produces a unique pattern of activity in the brain, making it easier for the computer to identify what is being written with much greater accuracy and speed."

Using this system, the participant was able to compose sentences and communicate with others at a speed of about 90 characters per minute, comparable to someone of a similar age typing on a smartphone. In contrast, "point-and-click" interfaces have only achieved about 40 characters per minute.

This system also provides a level of flexibility that is crucial to restoring communication. Some studies have gone as far as attempting direct thought-to-speech BCIs that, while promising, are currently limited by what is possible through recordings from the surface of the brain which averages responses across thousands of neurons.

"Right now, other investigators can achieve about a 50-word dictionary using machine learning methods when decoding speech," said Dr. Shenoy. "By using handwriting to record from hundreds of individual neurons, we can write any letter and thus any word which provides a truly 'open vocabulary' that can be used in almost any life situation."

For individuals who are paralyzed or living with "locked-in syndrome" due to brainstem stroke or late-stage ALS, the ability to communicate is largely or even completely lost without technological intervention. While preliminary, the technologies being developed here offer the potential to help those who have completely lost the ability to write and speak.

"Communication is central to how we function in society," said Debara L, Tucci, M.D., M.S., M.B.A, director, NIDCD. "In today's world of internet-based communication, people with severe speech and physical impairments can face significant communication barriers and, potentially, isolation. We hope these findings will encourage commercial development of this latest BCI technology."

In the future, Dr. Shenoy's team intends to test the system on a patient who has lost the ability to speak, such as someone with advanced ALS. In addition, they are looking to increase the number of characters available to the participants (such as capital letters and numbers).

The clinical trial, called "BrainGate," a collaboration of internationally recognized laboratories, universities, and hospitals working to advance brain-computer interface technologies, is testing the safety of BCIs that directly connect a person's brain to a computer. The study was a collaboration between Dr. Shenoy's and Jaimie Henderson, M.D.'s research group at Stanford University, Leigh Hochberg, M.D., Ph.D. from Brown University, Massachusetts General Hospital, and Providence VA and sponsor-investigator of the BrainGate trial. Dr. Henderson at Stanford University also performed the surgery to place the necessary electrodes.

"Thanks to the pioneering spirit of the participants in BrainGate, we are able to gain new insights into human brain function, which could lead to the creation of systems that will help others with paralysis," said Dr. Hochberg.

Section 37.2 | Noninvasive Spinal Cord Stimulation for Paralysis

This section includes text excerpted from "Reversing 21 Years of Chronic Paralysis via Non-invasive Spinal Cord Neuromodulation: A Case Study," National Center for Biotechnology Information (NCBI), May 20, 2020.

Millions of patients are suffering from paralysis worldwide following traumatic spinal cord injury (SCI), and an estimated 768,473 new patients are adding to this number each year. Although there is no complete recovery from paralysis yet, recent groundbreaking studies on epidural electrical stimulation (eES) of the lumbosacral spinal cord have successfully restored voluntary control of paralyzed limbs full weight-bearing standing and over-ground stepping in chronic motor-complete SCI patients when combined with extensive physical therapy and motor-training. However, eES of the spinal cord requires surgical implantation of a neurostimulator and associated stimulation electrodes into the patient, which may cause complications.

Transcutaneous electrical stimulation (tES) is a noninvasive neuromodulation method to activate neural circuits via electric current between a pair of stimulating electrodes placed onto the skin. The tES to SCI patients has recently demonstrated successful activation of motor pools of distal muscles, facilitation for standing, and inducing stepping-like movements in a gravity-neutral position. However, tES has not yet exhibited full restoration of voluntary movements of paralyzed limbs, independent full-weight-bearing standing, or bipedal stepping without any assistance in paralyzed patients. Herein a chronic SCI patient with lower-extremity monoplegia, who had been wheelchair-bound for the last 21 years since a traumatic cervical cord injury following a traffic accident, regained full volitional movements of her paralyzed leg, independent standing, and squatting after 16 consecutive weeks

(52 sessions) of weight-bearing standing and assisted stepping training with noninvasive spinal cord stimulation (tES).

Recent landmark studies have demonstrated that the application of invasive epidural electrical neuromodulation (eES) to spinal cord networks caudal to the spinal lesion dramatically improves motor control in patients with SCI when combined with activity-based therapies, such as massed practice and treadmill training. However, activity-based therapies alone showed no benefit to the functional recovery of these patients. Furthermore, in no case have any of the studies observed in an animal or human experiments after complete paralysis to be able to train. Apparently, a paralyzed nervous system cannot be trained if it cannot be activated. In the present study, using noninvasive electrical stimulation and motor training, we have demonstrated significant improvements in motor function recovery including volitional control of the pelvic limb, independent standing, and squatting of a patient with cervical cord injury who had been paralyzed for more than 21 years. In this study, we tested two tES parameters at spinal segments near the target lumbosacral spinal cord region to detect the recruitment of the patient's lower limb motor pools in a resting condition. With rigorous analysis of MEP in the lower limbs, we found that shorter burst duration (100 μsec) caused more homogeneous recruitment of motor pools than longer burst duration (1 msec) used in previous studies. Our patient also preferred shorter to longer tES burst, perhaps, because of having better sensation of the paretic areas during shorter tES bursts. Further research is warranted to better understand the relation between burst duration and the functional connection.

Although recent transcutaneous spinal cord stimulation studies have shown improvement of trunk control during sitting and self-assisted standing in individuals with SCI, this is the first study to show that tES can facilitate volitional movements in the completely paralyzed leg of a SCI patient after just 16 weeks of stimulation and training. This finding is comparable with previous research using invasive epidural electrical stimulation on a motor complete paraplegic patient regaining volitional movements of lower limbs after stimulation and training. Furthermore, the impacts of tES on our patient's full leg extension and flexion movements were similar to the findings in previous epidural stimulation studies. The improved leg extension facilitated our patient to control her knees to prevent buckling during standing. Similar to a previous study, our patient became less dependent on the stimulation to control her legs as the training progressed.

In this study, substantial flexor and extensor movements of both legs occurred even in the absence of spinal stimulation after around 32 treatment sessions. To the best of our knowledge, the only study that matches the chronic effect of stimulation was reported by Gerasimenko et al., where it was observed that the magnitude of bilateral rhythmic motions of the lower limbs was similar regardless of the presence or absence of the stimulation. In the present study, it was noted that coactivations of different muscle groups were obvious during the transition from sitting to standing and vice versa. However, this is almost a universal phenomenon following spinal cord injury, differing only in the degrees of abnormality of coactivations. Prior research has shown that neuromodulation of the lumbosacral enlargement via tES increases the electromyography (EMG) activity in lower-extremity muscles in SCI patients during treadmill and robot-assisted locomotion. However, in the current study, tES exhibited little improvement in our patient's bipedal walking. Furthermore, increasing either burst duration or stimulation intensity did not facilitate walking. A previous study also found that higher levels of stimulation interfere with the robustness of the stepping pattern.

After 52 sessions of tES and motor training, our patient regained full volitional movements of her paralyzed leg, as well as independent standing and squatting. Following this treatment, the total lower extremity motor score of her left leg improved significantly from a fully paralyzed condition. This was the most significant recovery since her injury 21 years ago. Cessation of tES and training for 6 weeks did not cause the motor scores to return to the baseline level. The fact that the score was still significantly higher compared to the baseline suggests some level of permanency of recovery possibly through neuroplasticity. There was, however, no noticeable post-treatment change in the spasticity of the lower limbs as measured by the Modified Ashworth Scale (MAS) scores. In particular, MAS scores of the bilateral lower limbs were 1+.

Blood pressure and resting heart rate at seated position did not change significantly throughout the study. Other posttreatment autonomic functions, such as bladder and bowel control were similar to those at baseline. Some trunk control might have improved over the course of the study as after tES training the patient was able to sit in a more upright position on command, however, we did not quantify such functional recovery. The patient did not experience any pain throughout the treatment period, and there was no significant change in tactile sensation, although improved pin-prick sensation was reported at the end of the study.

This single case study highlights the possibility of using tES as a promising noninvasive intervention to restore the physical functions of individuals with chronic paralysis following a SCI. In the present case, we reported several novel results, in particular, the level of recovery achieved after 21 years of complete paralysis in one leg and severe paralysis in the other, and the ability regained by the patient to voluntarily generate movements of such a magnitude. A recent epidural electrical stimulation study has demonstrated significant autonomic and some motor function recoveries without simultaneous physical training in chronic SCI patients. However, no noninvasive stimulation has yet been investigated on the sole effects of electrical stimulation on functional recovery without physical training.

Despite the promising results, the current study has some limitations. First, the current findings may not be generalized to other patients with SCI. Future research with larger sample sizes is warranted to confirm the positive outcomes. Second, it remains unclear whether the position of the stimulation electrodes may have effects on the treatment results. Future studies should be conducted to identify the optimal electrode locations. Furthermore, the mechanism underlying the recovery remains unclear. Future mechanistic studies should be conducted to understand the functional mechanisms of such recovery, which can help determine the optimal stimulation parameters for the best treatment outcomes for these patients.

Chapter 38 | **Physical Therapists of the Future**

Stroke, caused by death of brain cells as a result of blockage of a blood vessel supplying the brain (ischemic stroke) or bleeding into or around the brain (hemorrhagic stroke), is a serious medical emergency. Stroke can result in death or substantial neural damage and is a principal contributor to long-term disabilities. According to the World Health Organization (WHO) estimates, 15 million people suffer stroke worldwide each year. Although technology advances in healthcare, the incidence of stroke is expected to rise over the next decades. The expense on both caring and rehabilitation is enormous which reaches $34 billion per year in the U.S. More than half of stroke survivors experience some level of lasting hemiparesis or hemiplegia resulting from the damage to neural tissues. These patients are not able to perform daily activities independently and thus have to rely on human assistance for basic activities of daily living (ADL) such as feeding, self-care, and mobility.

The human hands are very complex and versatile. Researches show that the relationship between the distal upper limb (i.e., hand) function and the ability to perform ADL is stronger than the other limbs. The deficit in hand function would seriously impact the quality of patients' life, which means more demand is needed on the hand motor recovery. However, although most patients get reasonable motor recovery of proximal upper extremity according to relevant research findings, recovery at distal upper extremity has been limited due to low effectivity. There are two main reasons for challenges facing the recovery of the hand. First, in movement, the

This chapter includes text excerpted from "Hand Rehabilitation Robotics on Poststroke Motor Recovery," National Center for Biotechnology Information (NCBI), November 2, 2017. Reviewed June 2021.

hand has more than 20 degree of freedom (DOF) which makes it flexible, thus being difficult for therapist or training devices to meet the needs of satiety and varied movements. Second, in function, the area of cortex in correspondence with the hand is much larger than the other motor cortex, which means a considerable amount of flexibility in generating a variety of hand postures and in the control of the individual joints of the hand. However, to date, most researches have focused on the contrary, lacking of individuation in finger movements. Better rehabilitation therapies are desperately needed.

Robot-assisted therapy for poststroke rehabilitation is a new kind of physical therapy, through which patients practice their paretic limb by resorting to or resisting the force offered by the robots. For example, the MIT-Manus robot uses the massed training approach by practicing reaching movements to train the upper limbs; the Mirror Image Movement Enabler (MIME) uses the bilateral training approach to train the paretic limb while reducing abnormal synergies. Robot-assisted therapy has been greatly developed over the past three decades with the advances in robotic technology such as the exoskeleton and bioengineering, which has become a significant supplement to traditional physical therapy. For example, compared with the therapist exhausted in training patients with manual labor, the hand exoskeleton designed by Wege et al. can move the fingers of patients dexterously and repeatedly. Besides, some robots can also be controlled by a patient's own intention extracted from biosignals such as electromyography (EMG) and electroencephalograph (EEG) signals. These make it possible to form a closed-loop rehabilitation system with the robotic technology, which cannot be achieved by any conventional rehabilitation therapy.

Existing reviews of hand rehabilitation robotics on poststroke motor recovery are insufficient, for most studies research on the application of robot-assisted therapy on other limbs instead of the hand. Furthermore, current reviews focus on either the hardware design of the robots or the application of specific training paradigms, while both of them are indispensable to an efficient hand rehabilitation robot. The hardware system makes the foundation of the robots' function, while the training paradigm serves as the real functional parts in the motor recovery that decides the effect of rehabilitation training. These two parts are closely related to each other.

AN OVERVIEW OF HAND REHABILITATION ROBOTICS
Robot-assisted poststroke therapy for the upper extremity dates back to the 1990s. It has been greatly developed over the past decades with the progress in robotic technology and has been a significant supplement to traditional physical therapy. The hand rehabilitation robots were first designed to do heavy labor work as a better replacement for human therapists. These early robots focus on the design of structure, actuator, method of control, and so forth to achieve a robotic hand that is more adaptive to the motion characteristics of bones and joints and meets the needs of rehabilitation more effectively.

Now, hand rehabilitation robotics has been greatly developed with the rapid development of neurosciences and clinic knowledge, which makes the design of hand rehabilitation robotics for post-stroke rehabilitation become more complex for involving multidisciplinary knowledge such as anatomy, neurosciences, cognitive and learning science, and rich experience in the clinic. Apart from the robots themselves, knowledge of stroke patients' differences, rehabilitation theories, and evaluation are all essential for the design of an effective hand rehabilitation robot.

Subject Differences
Motor impairment of stroke patients differs from person to person, and states and conditions vary in the course of recovery. Factors such as types of muscle state (e.g., atony or hypermyotonia), phases of stroke (chronic, acute, or subacute), and levels of stroke (from mild-to-severe stroke) should all be taken into consideration for individualized treatment. For example, patients with atony cannot use the assistive robots that require residual motion ability or too many sets of force training which may cause abnormal motion modalities. The benefits of using hand rehabilitation robotics are

that the robotic technology can be used to quantify and track motor behaviors or biosignals for individual patients, thus rehabilitation robotics can represent the sophisticated method existing today for precisely driving therapeutic engagement and measuring precise outcomes. Lacking consideration of the difference between subjects may greatly decrease the efficacy of robot-assisted therapy.

Theories for Rehabilitation

Although current theories underlying motor recovery are insufficient, a few of existing rehabilitation theories are still instructive and significant for the application of robot-assisted therapy. The three main popular directions are the theories of neurophysiology, neurodevelopment, and motor learning. The neurophysiology mechanism, such as the plasticity and compensatory function, is the theoretical basis of poststroke motor recovery. The neuro-developmental treatment (NDT), or the Bobath concept, which mostly formed from clinical experience, focuses on normalizing muscle tone and movement patterns in order to improve recovery of the hemiparetic side and inspire training strategies such as continuous passive motion and constraint-induced therapy. The learning theories, such as the Hebbian learning or motor relearning which instructed many strategies including goal-oriented training, active training with all kinds of feedbacks, are the current trend in hand rehabilitation robotics. Although there is not much specific convincing evidence for these strategies, many applications in cooperation with the robotic hand have been practically used in rehabilitation and have achieved some good results.

Application of Hand Rehabilitation Robotics

The application of hand rehabilitation robotics is to achieve effective rehabilitation by making a serial of decisions on the designing of both hardware system and the training paradigm. For designs that focus on the hardware system, they solve problems such as the safety issues of mechanism and the portability or flexibility of devices. For example, Wege et al. adopt an across joint linkage structure to solve the joint coordination problem, while a finger can be flexibly controlled with four degrees of freedom. In et al. design an underactuation jointless exoskeleton that can be safe in motion and light in weight. For designs that focus on the paradigm, they deal with the interaction between humans and robots to promote motor relearning. For example, Ueki et al. and Sarakoglou et al. develop a system that provides the feedback of real-time state in virtual reality (VR) scene, to enrich the perception of motion in training; Sarakoglou et al., Hu et al., and Ramos et al. study the hand rehabilitation robot, respectively, controlled by patients' own force signal, EMG signal, and an EEG signal, to generate patient participation in training. For a hand rehabilitation robot system, hardware system and the training paradigm are both essential and dependent on each other.

Evaluation of Treatments

The evaluation of rehabilitation robotics reflects the recovery effects of human functions, which makes it imperative for a complete design. There are varied ways on evaluating the robots in current researches, including the performance on improving range of motion (ROM) of joints, the velocity of motion, the force exerting to hands, and the executing of functional tasks. A set of classic clinical scales is also used to evaluate the design by measuring the recovery of stroke patients. The most frequently used scales include the Arm Research Assessment Test (ARAT), Fugl-Meyer Assessment (FMA), and Motor Activity Log (MAL). It should be focused on the evaluation of rehabilitation robotics that is different from traditional robots, because of the special clinical applications. To the validation before clinical use, therapy has to follow the principle of evidence-based medicine (EBM), which indicates that many results of current research are collected to demonstrate the usefulness. For example, a surprising finding from the results of independent researches shows the usefulness of current hand rehabilitation robots while research under the principle of EBM gives weak demonstration for the usefulness. It might be explained by the small sample sizes and low quality of the experiment that limits the supportive evidence in the current research of hand rehabilitation robotics. That shows the reason why the validation of robots, especially the designing of more standard randomized controlled trials (RCTs) with large-scale samples and high quality, is so imperative for rehabilitation robotics.

CLASSIFICATION OF HAND REHABILITATION ROBOTS

There exist many kinds of ways for the classification of hand rehabilitation robots, some of which follow the convention in mechanical design (focus on the hardware system), while others follow the convention in rehabilitation (which focus on the training paradigms). In fact, each of these ways of classification has its own value, and they are dependent on each other. For example, the hardware system depends on the basic abilities of rehabilitation robotics (e.g., possible movements and feedback information), while the training paradigms are the main functional components in the recovery (e.g., the application of specific rehabilitation theories).

Hardware System

The hardware system is the foundation of hand rehabilitation robots. It decides the possible types of motion the robots can offer to the patients and the possible signals the robots can obtain from patients. The hardware system can be classified in detail in a mechanical classification. However, here, the classification is made in cruder categorization for highlighting several most important aspects in the design of hand rehabilitation robots. The hardware systems are divided into aspects including types of robots, the actuations, types of transmission, and sensors.

Robot Type

Existing hand rehabilitation robots can be divided into two main types according to the alignment of the device and the user: the end effector and the exoskeleton. The end effector is external to the patients' body while the exoskeleton is worn by human beings.

END EFFECTOR

The end effector is external to the body of patients, and it provides required force to the end of the user's extremity to help or resist the motion. For example, the AMADEO robotic system designed by an Austrian is already a commercial product. After fastening, the finger supports the finger tips and thumb, and bending and stretching movements can be performed followed the slider. The HandCARE is another end effector designed by Dovat et al., in which each finger is attached to an instrumented cable loop allowing force control and a predominantly linear displacement. The end effector provides force without considering the individual joint motions of the patients' limbs, which bring problems such as the limited range of motion and the dead point issues. Furthermore, the end effector is not portable for being external to the human body, which limited the practical use in clinic.

EXOSKELETON

Different from the end effector, exoskeleton device can be worn on the body of patients. The joint and links of the robot have direct correspondence with the human joints and limbs, respectively. For example, Ho et al. develop a wearable hand rehabilitation robot that offers 2 DOFs for each finger; Chiri et al. designed the HANDEXOS which is low in overall size and light weight. This portability of exoskeleton makes it a good choice for stroke rehabilitation, especially for patients in the later period of stroke when they can train themselves at home. Although there are problems such as the robot axes have to be aligned with the anatomical axes of the hand, the exoskeleton robots are widely used in rehabilitation robotics and have been greatly developed these years. The mention of functional degrees of freedom (fDOF) which offers a method for using less complex actuation strategies to simplify the complex multi-DOF movements and the development of soft-bodied robots both promote the application of exoskeleton robotics. In et al. designed the underactuated jointless robots that are very light in weight. Now, the exoskeleton robots have been the trend of hand rehabilitation robots in poststroke rehabilitation.

Actuation

The function of actuation is to transform different kinds of energy to actuate the motion of robots. There are five kinds of actuation:

elector motor, hydraulic, pneumatic, pneumatic muscle, and human muscle. Although there are still some other kinds of actuation such as the piezoelectric and the shape memory alloy which are promising for being thin and lightweight, they are not mentioned here for either being limited by their own technical dilemma in practical application or just being theoretical design.

ELECTRICAL MOTOR

The electrical motor is almost the most widely used actuation in design of hand rehabilitation robots because they are easily available, reliable, and easy to control and with high precision. For example, the HANDEXOS designed by Chiri A et al. is actuated by the force transmitted for DC motor to a Bowden cable; the exoskeleton hand robotic training device designed by Ho et al. is actuated by micro linear electrical motor. The general performance in the torque-velocity space makes the electrical motor useful in applications such as hand rehabilitation robots where variability in control strategies is sought-after. The might disadvantage of the electrical motor is that the rigid structure of electrical motor might bring safety problems. Nevertheless, the electrical motor can be controlled in torque, which makes the actuator able to get the information of the robots without the need for extra sensors.

PNEUMATIC

The pneumatic actuators are used much less than the electrical motor in hand rehabilitation robots, such as the ASSIST designed by Sasaki et al. This actuator has advantages such as less requirement of maintenance and can be stopped under a load without causing damages. Although problems such as noise can be overcome by using precompressed air storage, the problem of size cannot be settled because the air storage chamber is necessary. Thus, the pneumatic actuator might better be used for systems with lower mobility.

The development of pneumatic artificial muscle makes the actuation another choice. The pneumatic muscle made of rubber inner tube with a shell can inflate or contract. For example, the commercial hand rehabilitation robotic system produced by Kinetic Muscles Inc. (USA) is actuated by air muscle actuator. There is also another kind of pneumatic muscle, namely, the bending type pneumatic muscle. For example, the pneumatic rubber muscle was designed by Noritsugu et al. The disadvantage of pneumatic actuation is that the actuators are difficult to control for its time variability and nonlinear.

HYDRAULIC

The hydraulic actuators are very good in performance such as can generate higher torque compared with the electric or pneumatic systems and can be controlled in high precision and frequency. But, the requirement of a wider space to accommodate the oil trans-mitting pipes and conduits makes the hydraulic actuators seldomly used in hand rehabilitation robots.

CONTRALATERAL EXTREMITY

The contralateral extremity can be thought as an actuation too. The hand rehabilitation robots actuated by the bilateral limb are usually used in the robotic system applying the bilateral training strategies. The robots for the impaired hand can be directly actuated by the force offered by the healthy extremity or indirectly actuated in a synchronized control by the signal obtained from the healthy hand. To date, only the latter one has been researched. For example, Rahman et al. designed the bilateral therapeutic hand device, in which the exoskeleton was worn on the impaired moves according to the data from the glove worn on the healthy hand.

HUMAN MUSCLE

The human muscle on the impaired hand can be activated by functional electrical stimulation (FES) to complete the motion of impaired hand the same as robotic actuation. Moreover, some applications combine it with the robotic actuator for rehabilitation. Thus, the human muscle can be classified as a kind of actuation in a broad sense here. Rong et al. have proposed an FES and robotic glove rehabilitation robotic hand that better realizes the recovery of hand function through the balance of FES and robot. Researchers often stimulate FES with processed EMG signals or EEG that are produced from patients' spontaneous motor to contain spontaneous motor.

OTHERS

Other designs that corresponded with the active training modalities may not provide actuations, but totally actuated by patients' own hand; this means for a high requirement to patients' residual motor abilities. Another compromised choice is the use of spring as actuation, in which the spring offers force to compensate the effect of hypermyotonia.

Transmission

The function of transmission is to transform the motion of actuator into a desired direction to complete the execution of a hand's motion. Most of these are a consequence of the choices of actuator or the mechanism.

LINKAGE

Linkages are popular choices in the hand rehabilitation robot system, the same as in the traditional mechanical design. The linkages are light, convenient, and can be easily controlled in a given trajectory. On the one hand, the problem of coincidence of the rotational axis can be settled by using the cross-joint structure. On the other hand, the complexity of device can be reduced according to the concept of fDOF by using the linkage structure. For example, Fontana et al. designed the cross-joint exoskeleton that uses the virtual joints to avoid misalignment; the mechanisms designed by Wege et al. adopt a linkage structure connecting the adjacent finger segments, and Fiorilla et al. designed the 2-finger hand exoskeleton that adopts the concept of fDOF to simplify the structure. The redundancy can be eliminated by this structure while offers an easy way to control the movement.

CABLE

The cable is also frequently used as the transmission in the hand rehabilitation robots, including the pulley cable and Bowden cable. The pulley requires continuous tension to maintain traction on the pulleys, which limits the use. On the other hand, the Bowden cable is better for its cable conduit and is flexible. Disadvantages are the variable and high-friction force caused by the curve. For example, the cable actuated finger exoskeleton (CAFE) designed by Jones et al. and the HandCARE designed by Dovat et al. adopt the pulley cable. These devices can be easily controlled by force while not so convenient in usage. The robot designed by Wege et al. adopts the Bowden cable to control the motion of fingers independently. In fact, this robot combined both the cable and the linkage structure. Cables are similar to the muscle of the hand, so it might be an effective tool for the hand rehabilitation robotic system. The jointless exoskeleton designed by In et al. is a good application of this concept.

Sensor

Although the hand rehabilitation robot system has some effects just according to the continuous passive motion (CMP) concept, the participation of patients seems to be more effective in the rehabilitation system. This makes the sensor very important in the hand rehabilitation robot system. The sensor detects information of human to offer feedbacks or control signals to the human or robots. The sensors are classified by the types of detected signals.

PHYSICAL SIGNAL

The sensors detecting physical signals such as the force and position (or motion) are the most used sensors in the robot system of hand rehabilitation. The function of force or position signal is to provide the physical state of the hand such as the exerted force of motion or the bending angle of the finger. For example, the sensing and force-feedback exoskeleton (SAFE) robotics was designed by Ben-Tzvi et al., in which an optical position sensor and strain gauges are set to detect the motion and force signal.

BIOELECTRICAL SIGNAL

The other kinds of sensors detecting the bioelectrical signals such as the EEG or EMG signals are also frequently used in the hand rehabilitation robot system. The function of the bioelectrical signal is to reflect the motion intention of humans, which can be used as the controlling signals of robots. The EEG and EMG signals are the most representative signal obtained from the brain or muscle, since other possible but inconvenient signals such as the magnetic resonance imaging (MRI) signal are not listed here. Examples are SAFE that uses the EEG cap to detect the EEG signal from the brain and the robot designed by Hu et al. that uses several EMG electrodes arranged on the extensor digitorum muscle and abductor pollicis brevis muscle.

Chapter 39 | **Assistive Devices**

Chapter Contents

Section 39.1 | Rehabilitative and Assistive Technology: Overview

This section includes text excerpted from "Rehabilitative and Assistive Technology," *Eunice Kennedy Shriver* National Institute of Child Health and Human Development (NICHD), October 24, 2018.

Rehabilitative and assistive technology refers to tools, equipment, or products that can help people with disabilities successfully complete activities at school, home, work, and in the community. Disabilities are disorders, diseases, health conditions, or injuries that affect a person's physical, intellectual, or mental well-being and functioning. Rehabilitative and assistive technologies can help people with disabilities function more easily in their everyday lives and can also make it easier for a caregiver to care for a person with disabilities. The term "rehabilitative technology" refers to aids that help people recover their functioning after injury or illness. "Assistive technologies" may be as simple as a magnifying glass to improve vision or as complex as a digital communication system.

Some of these technologies are made possible through rehabilitative engineering research, which applies engineering and scientific principles to study how people with disabilities function in society. It includes studying barriers and designing solutions so that people with disabilities can interact successfully in their environments.

Eunice Kennedy Shriver National Institute of Child Health and Human Development (NICHD) houses the National Center for Medical Rehabilitation Research (NCMRR), which is charged with advancing scientific knowledge on disabilities and rehabilitation, while also providing vital support and focus for the field of medical rehabilitation to help ensure the health, independence, productivity, and quality of life of all people. Through the NCMRR, NICHD supports the development and testing of rehabilitative and assistive technologies, with a focus on physical rehabilitation.

WHAT ARE SOME TYPES OF ASSISTIVE DEVICES AND HOW ARE THEY USED?

Some examples of assistive technologies are:

- Mobility aids, such as wheelchairs, scooters, walkers, canes, crutches, prosthetic devices, and orthotic devices.
- Hearing aids to help people hear or hear more clearly.
- Cognitive aids, including computer or electrical assistive devices, to help people with memory, attention, or other challenges in their thinking skills.
- Computer software and hardware, such as voice recognition programs, screen readers, and screen enlargement applications, to help people with mobility and sensory impairments use computers and mobile devices.
- Tools such as automatic page-turners, book holders, and adapted pencil grips to help learners with disabilities participate in educational activities.
- Closed captioning to allow people with hearing problems to watch movies, television programs, and other digital media.
- Physical modifications in the built environment, including ramps, grab bars, and wider doorways to enable access to buildings, businesses, and workplaces.
- Lightweight, high-performance mobility devices that enable persons with disabilities to play sports and be physically active.
- Adaptive switches and utensils to allow those with limited motor skills to eat, play games, and accomplish other activities.
- Devices and features of devices to help perform tasks such as cooking, dressing, and grooming; specialized handles and grips, devices that extend reach, and lights on telephones and doorbells are a few examples.

WHAT ARE SOME TYPES OF REHABILITATIVE TECHNOLOGIES?

Rehabilitative technologies and techniques help people recover or improve function after injury or illness. Examples include the following:

- **Robotics.** Specialized robots help people regain and improve function in arms or legs after a stroke.

- **Virtual reality (VR).** People who are recovering from an injury can retrain themselves to perform motions within a virtual environment.
- **Musculoskeletal modeling and simulations.** These computer simulations of the human body can pinpoint underlying mechanical problems in a person with a movement-related disability. This technique can help improve assistive aids or physical therapies.
- **Transcranial magnetic stimulation (TMS).** TMS sends magnetic impulses through the skull to stimulate the brain. This system can help people who have had a stroke recover movement and brain function.
- **Transcranial direct current stimulation (tDCS).** In tDCS, a mild electrical current travels through the skull and stimulates the brain. This can help recover movement in patients recovering from stroke or other conditions.
- **Motion analysis.** It captures video of human motion with specialized computer software that analyzes the motion in detail. The technique gives health-care providers a detailed picture of a person's specific movement challenges to guide proper therapy.

Some devices incorporate multiple types of technologies and techniques to help users regain or improve function. For example, the BrainGate project, which was partially funded by NICHD through the NCMRR, relied on tiny sensors being implanted in the brain. The user could then think about moving their arm, and a robotic arm would carry out the thought.

HOW DOES REHABILITATIVE TECHNOLOGY BENEFIT PEOPLE WITH DISABILITIES?

Rehabilitative technology can help restore or improve function in people who have developed a disability due to disease, injury, or aging. Appropriate assistive technology often helps people with disabilities compensate, at least in part, for a limitation.

For example, assistive technology enables students with disabilities to compensate for certain impairments. This specialized technology promotes independence and decreases the need for other support.

Rehabilitative and assistive technology can enable individuals to:
- Care for themselves and their families
- Work
- Learn in typical school environments and other educational institutions
- Access information through computers and reading
- Enjoy music, sports, travel, and the arts
- Participate fully in community life

Assistive technology also benefits employers, teachers, family members, and everyone who interacts with people who use the technology.

As assistive technologies become more commonplace, people without disabilities are benefiting from them. For example, people for whom English is a second language are taking advantage of screen readers. Older individuals are using screen enlargers and magnifiers.

The person with a disability, along with her or his caregivers and a team of professionals and consultants, usually decide which type of rehabilitative or assistive technology would be most helpful. The team is trained to match particular technologies to specific needs to help the person function better or more independently. The team may include family doctors, regular and special education teachers, speech-language pathologists, rehabilitation engineers, occupational therapists, and other specialists, including representatives from companies that manufacture assistive technology.

What Conditions May Benefit from Assistive Devices?

Some disabilities are quite visible, while others are "hidden." Most disabilities can be grouped into the following categories:
- **Cognitive disability.** Intellectual and learning disabilities/disorders, distractibility, reading disorders, inability to remember or focus on large amounts of information.

- **Hearing disability.** Hearing loss or impaired hearing.
- **Physical disability.** Paralysis, difficulties with walking or other movements, inability to use a computer mouse, slow response time, difficulty controlling movement.
- **Visual disability.** Blindness, low vision, color blindness.
- **Mental conditions.** Posttraumatic stress disorder (PTSD), anxiety disorders (AD), mood disorders, eating disorders, psychosis.

Hidden disabilities are those that might not be immediately apparent when you look at someone. They can include visual impairments, movement problems, hearing impairments, and mental-health conditions.

Some medical conditions may also contribute to disabilities or may be categorized as hidden disabilities under the Americans with Disabilities Act (ADA). For example, epilepsy; diabetes; sickle cell conditions; human immunodeficiency virus/acquired immunodeficiency syndrome (HIV/AIDS); cystic fibrosis; cancer; and heart, liver, or kidney problems may lead to problems with mobility or daily function and may be viewed as disabilities under the law. The conditions may be short term or long term; stable or progressive; constant or unpredictable; and changing, treatable, or untreatable. Many people with hidden disabilities can benefit from assistive technologies for certain activities or during certain stages of their diseases or conditions.

People who have spinal cord injuries (SCIs), traumatic brain injury (TBI), cerebral palsy (CP), muscular dystrophy (MD), spina bifida, osteogenesis imperfecta (OI), multiple sclerosis (MS), demyelinating diseases, myelopathy, progressive muscular atrophy (PMA), amputations, or paralysis often benefit from complex rehabilitative technology. The assistive devices are individually configured to help each person with her or his own unique disability.

Section 39.2 | **Assistive Devices for Communication**

This section includes text excerpted from "Assistive Devices for People with Hearing, Voice, Speech, or Language Disorders," National Institute on Deafness and Other Communication Disorders (NIDCD), November 12, 2019.

WHAT ARE ASSISTIVE DEVICES?

The terms assistive device or assistive technology can refer to any device that helps a person with hearing loss or a voice, speech, or language disorder to communicate. These terms often refer to devices that help a person to hear and understand what is being said more clearly or to express thoughts more easily. With the development of digital and wireless technologies, more and more devices are becoming available to help people with hearing, voice, speech, and language disorders communicate more meaningfully and participate more fully in their daily lives.

WHAT TYPES OF ASSISTIVE DEVICES ARE AVAILABLE?

Health professionals use a variety of names to describe assistive devices:

- Assistive listening devices (ALDs) help amplify the sounds you want to hear, especially where there is a lot of background noise. ALDs can be used with a hearing aid or cochlear implant to help a wearer hear certain sounds better.
- Augmentative and alternative communication (AAC) devices help people with communication disorders to express themselves. These devices can range from a simple picture board to a computer program that synthesizes speech from text.
- Alerting devices connect to a doorbell, telephone, or alarm that emits a loud sound or blinking light to let someone with hearing loss know that an event is taking place.

WHAT TYPES OF ASSISTIVE LISTENING DEVICES ARE AVAILABLE?

Several types of assistive listening devices (ALDs) are available to improve sound transmission for people with hearing loss. Some are designed for large facilities such as classrooms, theaters, places of worship, and airports. Other types are intended for personal use in small settings and for one-on-one conversations. All can be used with or without hearing aids or a cochlear implant. ALD systems for large facilities include hearing loop systems, frequency-modulated (FM) systems, and infrared systems.

Hearing Loop

Hearing loop (or induction loop) systems use electromagnetic energy to transmit sound. A hearing loop system involves four parts:

- A sound source, such as a public address system, microphone, or home TV or telephone
- An amplifier
- A thin loop of wire that encircles a room or branches out beneath carpeting
- A receiver worn in the ears or as a headset

Amplified sound travels through the loop and creates an electromagnetic field that is picked up directly by a hearing loop receiver or a telecoil, a miniature wireless receiver that is built into many hearing aids and cochlear implants. To pick up the signal, a listener must be wearing the receiver and be within or near the loop. Because the sound is picked up directly by the receiver, the sound is much clearer, without as much of the competing background noise associated with many listening environments. Some loop systems are portable, making it possible for people with hearing loss to improve their listening environments, as needed, as they proceed with their daily activities. A hearing loop can be connected to a public-address system, a television, or any other audio source. For those who do not have hearing aids with embedded telecoils, portable loop receivers are also available.

FM Systems

FM systems use radio signals to transmit amplified sounds. They are often used in classrooms, where the instructor wears a small microphone connected to a transmitter and the student wears the receiver, which is tuned to a specific frequency, or channel. People who have a telecoil inside their hearing aid or cochlear implant may also wear a wire around the neck (called a "neckloop") or behind their aid or implant (called a "silhouette inductor") to convert the signal into magnetic signals that can be picked up directly by the telecoil. FM systems can transmit signals up to 300 feet and are able to be used in many public places. However, because radio signals are able to penetrate walls, listeners in one room may need to listen to a different channel than those in another room to avoid receiving mixed signals. Personal FM systems operate in the same way as larger-scale systems and can be used to help people with hearing loss follow one-on-one conversations.

Infrared Systems

Infrared systems use infrared light to transmit sound. A transmitter converts sound into a light signal and beams it to a receiver that is worn by a listener. The receiver decodes the infrared signal back to sound. As with FM systems, people whose hearing aids or cochlear implants have a telecoil may also wear a neckloop or silhouette inductor to convert the infrared signal into a magnetic signal, which can be picked up through their telecoil. Unlike induction loop or FM systems, the infrared signal cannot pass through walls, making it particularly useful in courtrooms, where confidential information is often discussed, and in buildings where competing signals can be a problem, such as classrooms or movie theaters. However, infrared systems cannot be used in environments with too many competing light sources, such as outdoors or in strongly lit rooms.

Personal Amplifiers

Personal amplifiers are useful in places in which the above systems are unavailable or when watching TV, being outdoors, or traveling in a car. About the size of a cell phone, these devices increase sound levels and reduce background noise for a listener. Some have directional microphones that can be angled toward a speaker or other source of the sound. As with other ALDs, the amplified sound can be picked up by a receiver that the listener is wearing, either as a headset or as earbuds.

WHAT TYPES OF AUGMENTATIVE AND ALTERNATIVE COMMUNICATION DEVICES ARE AVAILABLE FOR COMMUNICATING FACE TO FACE?

The simplest AAC device is a picture board or touch screen that uses pictures or symbols of typical items and activities that make up a person's daily life. For example, a person might touch the image of a glass to ask for a drink. Many picture boards can be customized and expanded based on a person's age, education, occupation, and interests.

Keyboards, touch screens, and sometimes a person's limited speech may be used to communicate desired words. Some devices employ a text display. The display panel typically faces outward so that two people can exchange information while facing each other. Spelling and word prediction software can make it faster and easier to enter information.

Speech-generating devices go one step further by translating words or pictures into speech. Some models allow users to choose from several different voices, such as female or male, child or adult, and even some regional accents. Some devices employ a vocabulary of prerecorded words while others have an unlimited vocabulary, synthesizing speech as words are typed in. Software programs that convert personal computers into speaking devices are also available.

WHAT AUGMENTATIVE AND ALTERNATIVE COMMUNICATION DEVICES ARE AVAILABLE FOR COMMUNICATING BY TELEPHONE?

For many years, people with hearing loss have used text telephone, or telecommunications devices, called "teletypewriter" (TTY) or "telecommunications device for the deaf" (TDD) machines, to communicate by phone. This same technology also benefits people with speech difficulties. A TTY machine consists of a typewriter keyboard that displays typed conversations onto a readout panel or printed on paper. Callers will either type messages to each other over the system or, if a call recipient does not have a TTY machine, use the national toll-free telecommunications relay service at 711 to communicate. Through the relay service, a communications assistant serves as a bridge between two callers, reading typed messages aloud to the person with hearing while transcribing what is spoken into type for the person with hearing loss.

With today's new electronic communication devices, however, TTY machines have almost become a thing of the past. People can place phone calls through the telecommunications relay service using almost any device with a keypad, including a laptop, personal digital assistant, and cell phone. Text messaging has also become a popular method of communication, skipping the relay service altogether.

Another system uses voice recognition software and an extensive library of video clips depicting American Sign Language to translate a signer's words into text or computer-generated speech in real time. It is also able to translate spoken words back into sign language or text.

Finally, for people with mild-to-moderate hearing loss, captioned telephones allow you to carry on a spoken conversation, while providing a transcript of the other person's words on a read-out panel or computer screen as backup.

WHAT TYPES OF ALERTING DEVICES ARE AVAILABLE?

Alerting or alarm devices use sound, light, vibrations, or a combination of these techniques to let someone know when a particular event is occurring. Clocks and wake-up alarm systems allow a person to choose to wake up to flashing lights, horns, or a gentle shaking.

Visual alert signalers monitor a variety of household devices and other sounds, such as doorbells and telephones. When the phone rings, the visual alert signaler will be activated and will vibrate or flash a light to let people know. In addition, remote receivers placed around the house can alert a person from any room. Portable vibrating pagers can let parents and caretakers know when a baby is crying. Some baby monitoring devices analyze a baby's cry and light up a picture to indicate if the baby sounds hungry, bored, or sleepy.

WHAT RESEARCH IS BEING CONDUCTED ON ASSISTIVE TECHNOLOGY?

The National Institute on Deafness and Other Communication Disorders (NIDCD) funds research into several areas of assistive technology, such as those described below.

- Improved devices for people with hearing loss.
- NIDCD-funded researchers are developing devices that help people with varying degrees of hearing loss communicate with others. One team has developed a portable device in which two or more users type messages to each other that can be displayed simultaneously in real time. Another team is designing an ALD that amplifies and enhances speech for a group of individuals who are conversing in a noisy environment.
- Improved devices for nonspeaking people.
  - **More natural synthesized speech.** The NIDCD-sponsored scientists are also developing a personalized text-to-speech synthesis system that synthesizes speech that is more intelligible and natural sounding to be incorporated in speech-generating devices. Individuals who are at risk of losing their speaking ability can prerecord their own speech, which is then converted into their personal synthetic voice.
  - **Brain–computer interface research.** A relatively new and exciting area of study is called "brain–computer interface" research. The NIDCD-funded scientists are studying how neural signals in a person's brain can be translated by a computer to help someone communicate. For example, people with amyotrophic lateral sclerosis (ALS, or Lou Gehrig disease) or brainstem stroke lose their ability to move their arms, legs, or body. They can also become locked-in, where they are not able to express words, even though they are able to think and reason normally. By implanting electrodes

503

on the brain's motor cortex, some researchers are studying how a person who is locked-in can control communication software and type out words simply by imagining the movement of her or his hand. Other researchers are attempting to develop a prosthetic device that will be able to translate a person's thoughts into synthesized words and sentences. Another group is developing a wireless device that monitors brain activity that is triggered by visual stimulation. In this way, people who are locked in can call for help during an emergency by staring at a designated spot on the device.

Section 39.3 | Hearing Aids

This section includes text excerpted from "Hearing Aids," U.S. Food and Drug Administration (FDA), January 15, 2021.

More than 35 million children and adults in the United States have some degree of hearing loss. Hearing loss can have a negative effect on communication, relationships, school/work performance, and emotional well-being. However, hearing loss does not have to restrict your daily activities. Properly fitted hearing aids and aural rehabilitation (techniques used to identify and diagnose hearing loss, and implement therapies for patients who are hard of hearing, including using amplification devices to aid the patient's hearing abilities), can help in many listening situations. Aural rehabilitation helps a person focus on adjusting to their hearing loss and the use of their hearing aids. It also explores assistive devices to help improve communication. Most people who are hearing-impaired will need two hearing aids as both ears may be affected by hearing loss, though some people may only need one hearing aid.

This section includes information on the difference between hearing aids, intended for use by people with hearing loss, and

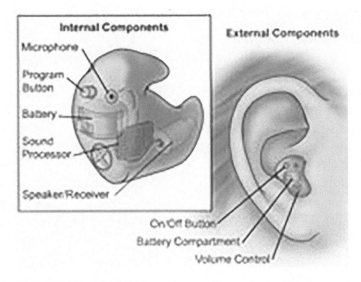

Figure 39.1. Hearing Aid Device

sound amplifiers for consumers with no hearing loss who want to make environmental sounds louder for recreational use. While the U.S. Food and Drug Administration (FDA) regulates hearing aids, which are medical devices, it does not consider sound amplifiers to be medical devices when labeled for recreational or other use by individuals with normal hearing. However, certain safety regulations related to sound output levels still apply to these products.

The President's Council of Advisors on Science and Technology (PCAST), and the National Academies of Sciences (NAS), Engineering and Medicine issued reports recommending ways to improve the access and affordability of hearing aids. The FDA considered these recommendations along with input from the public and has issued the "Immediately in Effect Guidance Document: Conditions for Sale for Air-Conduction Hearing Aids" guidance document. The FDA issued this guidance to communicate that it does not intend to enforce certain conditions for sale applicable to hearing aids for users 18 years of age or older.

TYPES OF HEARING AIDS
What Are Hearing Aids?

Hearing aids are sound-amplifying devices designed to aid people who have a hearing impairment.

Most hearing aids share several similar electronic components, including a microphone that picks up sound; amplifier circuitry that makes the sound louder; a miniature loudspeaker (receiver) that delivers the amplified sound into the ear canal; and batteries that power the electronic parts.

Hearing aids differ by:

- Design
- Technology used to achieve amplification (i.e., analog versus digital)
- Special features

Some hearing aids also have earmolds or earpieces to direct the flow of sound into the ear and enhance sound quality. The selection of hearing aids is based on the type and severity of hearing loss, listening needs, and lifestyle.

What Are the Different Styles of Hearing Aids?

Behind-the-ear (BTE) aids. Most parts are contained in a small plastic case that rests behind the ear; the case is connected to an earmold or an earpiece by a piece of clear tubing. This style is often chosen for young children because it can accommodate various earmold types, which need to be replaced as the child grows. Also, the BTE aids are easy to be cleaned and handled and are relatively sturdy.

"Mini" BTE (or "on-the-ear") aids. A new type of BTE aid called the "mini BTE" (or "on-the-ear") aid. It also fits behind/on the ear, but is smaller. A very thin, almost invisible tube is used to connect the aid to the ear canal. Mini BTEs may have a comfortable earpiece for insertion ("open fit"), but may also use a traditional earmold. Mini BTEs allow not only reduced occlusion or "plugged up" sensations in the ear canal, but also increase comfort, reduce feedback and address cosmetic concerns for many users.

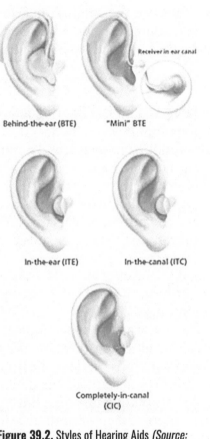

Figure 39.2. Styles of Hearing Aids *(Source: National Institute on Deafness and Other Communication Disorders (NIDCD)/National Institutes of Health (NIH).)*

In-the-ear (ITE) aids. All parts of the hearing aid are contained in a shell that fills in the outer part of the ear. The ITE aids are larger than the in-the-canal and completely-in-the-canal aids (see Figure 39.2), and for some people may be easier to handle than smaller aids.

In-the-canal (ITC) aids and completely-in-the-canal (CIC) aids. These hearing aids are contained in tiny cases that fit partly or completely into the ear canal. They are the smallest hearing aids available and offer cosmetic and some listening advantages. However, their small size may make them difficult to handle and adjust for some people.

What Is the Difference between Analog and Digital Hearing Aids?

Analog hearing aids make continuous sound waves louder. These hearing aids essentially amplify all sounds (e.g., speech and noise) in the same way. Some analog hearing aids are programmable. They have a microchip that allows the aid to have settings programmed for different listening environments, in a quiet place, such as at a library, or at a noisy place such as at a restaurant, or at a large area such a soccer field. The analog programmable hearing aids can store multiple programs for various environments.

As the listening environment changes, hearing aid settings may be changed by pushing a button on the hearing aid. Analog hearing aids are becoming less and less common.

Digital hearing aids have all the features of analog programmable aids, but they convert sound waves into digital signals and produce an exact duplication of sound. Computer chips in digital hearing aids analyze speech and other environmental sounds. The digital hearing aids allow for more complex processing of sound during the amplification process which may improve their performance in certain situations (e.g., background noise and whistle reduction). They also have greater flexibility in hearing aid programming so that the sound they transmit can be matched to the needs for a specific pattern of hearing loss. Digital hearing aids also provide multiple program memories. Most individuals who seek hearing help are offered a choice of only digital technology these days.

What Are Some Features for Hearing Aids?

Hearing aids have optional features that can be built in to assist in different communication situations. For example:

- Directional microphone may help you converse in noisy environments. Specifically, it allows sound coming from a specific direction to be amplified to a greater level compared to sound from other directions. When the directional microphone is activated, sound coming from in front of you (as during a face-to-face conversation) is amplified to a greater level than sound from behind you.

- T-coil (Telephone switch) allows you to switch from the normal microphone setting to a "T-coil" setting in order to hear better on the telephone. All wired telephones produced today must be hearing aid compatible. In the "T-coil" setting, environmental sounds are eliminated, and sound is picked up from the telephone. This also turns off the microphone on your hearing aid so you can talk without your hearing aid "whistling."

- The T-coil works well in theaters, auditoriums, houses of worship, and other places that have an induction loop or FM installation. The voice of the speaker, who can be some distance away, is amplified significantly more than any background noise. Some hearing aids have a combination "M" (Microphone)/"T" (Telephone) switch so that, while listening with an induction loop, you can still hear nearby conversation.

- Direct audio input allows you to plug in a remote microphone or an FM assistive listening system, connect directly to a TV, or connect to other devices such as your computer, a CD player, tape player, radio, etc.

- Feedback suppression helps suppress squeals when a hearing aid gets too close to the phone or has a loose-fitting earmold.

The more complicated features may allow the hearing aids to best meet your particular pattern of hearing loss. They may improve their performance in specific listening situations; however, these sophisticated electronics may significantly add to the cost of the hearing aid as well.

HEARING AIDS AND CELLPHONES
What Is That Buzzing Noise in Your Cell Phone?

People who wear hearing aids or have implanted hearing devices may experience some difficulties when trying to use cell phones. That buzzing noise you hear is interference due to radiofrequency (RF) emissions from your phone. RF interference does not occur for all combinations of digital wireless telephones and hearing aids. However, when interference does occur, the buzzing sound can make understanding speech difficult, communication over cell phones annoying, and, in the worst case, render the cell phone unusable for the hearing aid user.

Fortunately, the compatibility of cell phones and hearing aids is improving. Some cell phones have lower radiofrequency emissions or use different technologies that can reduce the unwanted effects on hearing aids.

What Should You Look for in a Cell Phone?

Rules set by the Federal Communications Commission (FCC) make it easier for you to choose a cell phone right for you. The FCC requires cell phone manufacturers to test and rate their wireless handsets' hearing aid compatibility using the American National Standards Institute (ANSI) C63.19 standard. These ratings give an indication of the likelihood that a cell phone may interfere with hearing aids; the higher the rating, the less likely the cell phone-hearing aid combination will experience undesired interference.

Labeling on the outside packaging of cell phones will tell you if they are hearing aid compatible (HAC). Hearing aid users should read and understand these ratings when choosing a cell phone.

What Do These Ratings Mean?

Cell phones that are rated "good" or "excellent" for use with hearing aids set in microphone (M) mode will have a rating of M3 or M4. The higher the "M" rating, the less likely you will experience interference when the hearing aid is set in the microphone mode while using the cell phone.

Cell phones are also rated with hearing aids or cochlear implants that have a T-coil. Those rated "good" or "excellent" for use with hearing aids set in T-coil mode will have a rating of T3 or T4. The higher the "T" rating, the less likely you will experience interference when the hearing aid is set in the T-coil mode while using the cell phone.

Hearing aid manufacturers also use a rating system from the same ANSI standard. The hearing aid ratings and the cell phone ratings should be combined to help identify combinations that will provide you with a positive experience. So, a hearing aid rated M2 and a wireless device rated M3 with a combined rating of 5 and would likely provide "normal" use. A ratings combination of 6 would likely provide "excellent performance." Every individual's hearing aid technology and settings are unique; therefore, these ratings do not guarantee performance.

Because these HAC ratings do not guarantee performance, you should "try before you buy" any wireless device if possible. You should try different brands and models to see which phone works best for you. Also, be sure to closely examine the return policy for the device and the service provider's policy on early termination of contracts before signing up for service.

OTHER PRODUCTS AND DEVICES TO IMPROVE HEARING
Assistive Listening Devices
Assistive listening devices (ALDs) or assistive listening systems include a large variety of devices designed to help you hear sounds in everyday activities. ALDs are available in some public places such as auditoriums, movie theaters, houses of worship, and meeting rooms.

ALDs can be used to overcome the negative effects of distance, poor room acoustics, and background noise. To achieve this purpose, many ALDs consist of a microphone near the source of the sound and a receiver near the listener. The listener can usually adjust the volume of the receiver as needed. Careful microphone placement allows the level of the speaker's voice to stay constant regardless of the distance between the speaker and the audience. The speaker's voice is also heard clearly over room noises such as chairs moving, fan motors running, and people talking.

ALDs can be used with or without hearing aids.

Table 39.1. Difference between Hearing Aids and Cochlear Implants

Hearing Aids	Cochlear Implants
Hearing aids are indicated for individuals with all degrees of hearing loss (from mild to profound).	Cochlear implants are indicated only for individuals with severe-profound hearing loss.
Most hearing aids are not implanted (although some bone-conduction hearing aids have an implanted component).	Cochlear implants are composed of both internal (implanted) and external components. A surgical procedure is needed to place the internal components.
In hearing aids, sound is amplified and conveyed through both the outer and middle ear and finally to the sensory receptor cells (hair cells) in the inner ear. The hair cells convert the sound energy into neural signals that are picked up by the auditory nerve.	Cochlear implants bypass the outer and middle ears, and the damaged hair cells and replace their functions by converting sound energy into electrical energy that directly stimulates the auditory nerve.

Cochlear Implants

A cochlear implant is an implanted electronic device that can produce useful hearing sensation by electrically stimulating nerves inside the inner ear. Cochlear implants currently consist of two main components:

- External component, comprised of an externally worn microphone, sound processor, and transmitter system
- Internal component, comprised of an implanted receiver and electrode system, which contains the electronic circuits that receive signals from the external system and send electrical signals to the inner ear.

Cochlear implants are different from hearing aids in some aspects:

Implantable Middle Ear Hearing Devices

Implantable middle ear hearing devices (IMEHDs) help increase the transmission of sound to the inner ear. IMEHDs are small implantable devices that are typically attached to one of the tiny bones in the middle ear. When they receive sound waves, IMEHDs vibrate and directly move the middle ear bones. This creates sound vibrations in the inner ear, which helps you to detect the sound. This device is generally used for people with sensorineural hearing loss.

Bone-Anchored Hearing Aids

A bone-anchored hearing aid (BAHA), such as a cochlear implant, has both implanted and external components. The implanted component is a small post that is surgically attached to the skull bone behind your ear. The external component is a speech processor which converts sound into vibrations; it connects to the implanted post and transmits sound vibrations directly to the inner ear through the skull, bypassing the middle ear. BAHAs are for people with middle ear problems (usually a mixed hearing loss) or who have no hearing in one ear.

Personal Sound Amplification Products

Personal sound amplification products (PSAPs), or sound amplifiers, increase environmental sounds for nonhearing impaired consumers. Examples of situations when these products would be used include hunting (listening for prey), bird watching, listening to a lecture with a distant speaker, and listening to soft sounds that would be difficult for normal hearing individuals to hear (e.g., distant conversations, performances). PSAPs are not intended to be used as hearing aids to compensate for hearing impairment.

Section 39.4 | Mobility Aids

This section includes text excerpted from "Wheelchairs, Mobility Aids, and Other Power-Driven Mobility Devices," ADA.gov, U.S. Department of Justice (DOJ), January 31, 2014. Reviewed June 2021.

People with mobility, circulatory, respiratory, or neurological disabilities use many kinds of devices for mobility. Some use walkers, canes, crutches, or braces. Some use manual or power wheelchairs or electric scooters. In addition, advances in technology have given rise to new devices, such as Segways®, that some people with disabilities use as mobility devices, including many veterans injured while serving in the military. And more advanced devices will inevitably be invented, providing more mobility options for people with disabilities.

This article is designed to help title II entities (state and local governments) and title III entities (businesses and nonprofit organizations that serve the public) (together, "covered entities") understand how the new rules for mobility devices apply to them. These rules went into effect on March 15, 2011.

Covered entities must allow people with disabilities who use manual or power wheelchairs or scooters, and manually powered mobility aids such as walkers, crutches, and canes, into all areas where members of the public are allowed to go.

Covered entities must also allow people with disabilities who use other types of power-driven mobility devices into their facilities unless a particular type of device cannot be accommodated because of legitimate safety requirements. Where legitimate safety requirements bar accommodation for a particular type of device, the covered entity must provide the service it offers in alternate ways if possible.

The rules set out five specific factors to consider in deciding whether or not a particular type of device can be accommodated.

WHEELCHAIRS

Most people are familiar with the manual and power wheelchairs and electric scooters used by people with mobility disabilities. The term "wheelchair" is defined in the new rules as "a manually-operated or power-driven device designed primarily for use by an individual with a mobility disability for the main purpose of indoor or of both indoor and outdoor locomotion."

OTHER POWER-DRIVEN MOBILITY DEVICES

Some people with mobility disabilities have begun using less traditional mobility devices such as golf cars or Segways®. These devices are called "other power-driven mobility devices" (OPDMDs) in the rule. OPDMD is defined in the new rules as "any mobility device powered by batteries, fuel, or other engines that are used by individuals with mobility disabilities for the purpose of loco-motion, including golf cars, electronic personal assistance mobility devices such as the Segway® PT, or any mobility device designed to operate in areas without defined pedestrian routes, but that is not a wheelchair." When an OPDMD is being used by a person with a mobility disability, different rules apply under the ADA than when it is being used by a person without a disability.

CHOICE OF DEVICE

People with disabilities have the right to choose whatever mobility device best suits their needs. For example, someone may choose to use a manual wheelchair rather than a power wheelchair because it enables her to maintain her upper body strength. Similarly, someone who is able to stand may choose to use a Segway® rather than a manual wheelchair because of the health benefits gained by standing. A facility may be required to allow a type of device that is generally prohibited when being used by someone without a dis-ability when it is being used by a person who needs it because of a mobility disability. For example, if golf cars are generally prohibited in a park, the park may be required to allow a golf car when it is being used because of a person's mobility disability, unless there is a legitimate safety reason that it cannot be accommodated.

REQUIREMENTS REGARDING MOBILITY DEVICES AND AIDS

Under the new rules, covered entities must allow people with disabilities who use wheelchairs (including manual wheelchairs, power wheelchairs, and electric scooters) and manually-powered mobility aids such as walkers, crutches, canes, braces, and other similar devices into all areas of a facility where members of the public are allowed to go.

In addition, covered entities must allow people with disabilities who use any OPDMD to enter the premises unless a particular type of device cannot be accommodated because of legitimate safety requirements. Such safety requirements must be based on actual risks, not on speculation or stereotypes about a particular type of device or how it might be operated by people with disabilities using them.

- For some facilities – such as a hospital, a shopping mall, a large home improvement store with wide aisles, a public park, or an outdoor amusement park – covered entities will likely determine that certain classes of OPDMDs being used by people with disabilities can be accommodated. These entities must allow people with disabilities to use these types of OPDMDs in all areas where members of the public are allowed to go.
- In some cases, even in facilities such as those described above, an OPDMD can be accommodated in some areas of a facility, but not in others because of legitimate safety concerns. For example, a cruise ship may decide that people with disabilities using Segways® can generally be accommodated, except in constricted areas, such as passageways to cabins that are very narrow and have low ceilings.
- For other facilities – such as a small convenience store, or a small town manager's office – covered entities may determine that certain classes of OPDMDs cannot be accommodated. In that case, they are still required to serve a person with a disability using one of these devices in an alternate manner if possible, such as providing curbside service or meeting the person at an alternate location.

Covered entities are encouraged to develop written policies specifying which kinds of OPDMDs will be permitted and where and when they will be permitted, based on the following assessment factors.

ASSESSMENT FACTORS

In deciding whether a particular type of OPDMD can be accommodated in a particular facility, the following factors must be considered:

- The type, size, weight, dimensions, and speed of the device;
- The facility's volume of pedestrian traffic (which may vary at different times of the day, week, month, or year);
- The facility's design and operational characteristics (e.g., whether its business is conducted indoors or outdoors, its square footage, the density and placement of furniture and other stationary devices, and the availability of storage for the OPDMD if needed and requested by the user);
- Whether legitimate safety requirements (such as limiting speed to the pace of pedestrian traffic or prohibiting use on escalators) can be established to permit the safe operation of the OPDMD in the specific facility; and
- Whether the use of the OPDMD creates a substantial risk of serious harm to the immediate environment or natural or cultural resources or poses a conflict with federal land management laws and regulations.

It is important to understand that these assessment factors relate to an entire class of device types, not to how a person with a disability might operate the device. All types of devices powered by fuel or combustion engines, for example, may be excluded from indoor settings for health or environmental reasons but may be deemed acceptable in some outdoor settings. Also, for safety reasons, larger electric devices such as golf cars may be excluded from narrow or crowded settings where there is no valid reason to exclude smaller electric devices such as Segways®.

Based on these assessment factors, the Department of Justice (DOJ) expects that devices such as Segways® can be accommodated in most circumstances. The Department also expects that, in most circumstances, people with disabilities using ATVs and other combustion engine-driven devices may be prohibited indoors and in outdoor areas with heavy pedestrian traffic.

POLICIES ON THE USE OF OPDMDS

In deciding whether a type of OPDMD can be accommodated, covered entities must consider all assessment factors and, where appropriate, should develop and publicize rules for people with disabilities using these devices. Such rules may include:

- Requiring the user to operate the device at the speed of pedestrian traffic
- Identifying specific locations, terms, or circumstances (if any) where the devices cannot be accommodated
- Setting out instructions for going through security screening machines if the device contains technology that could be harmed by the machine
- Specifying whether or not storage is available for the device when it is not being used

CREDIBLE ASSURANCE

An entity that determines it can accommodate one or more types of OPDMDs in its facility is allowed to ask the person using the device to provide credible assurance that the device is used because of a disability. If the person presents a valid, state-issued disability parking placard or card or a state-issued proof of disability, that must be accepted as credible assurance on its face. If the person does not have this documentation but states verbally that the OPDMD is being used because of a mobility disability, that also must be accepted as credible assurance, unless the person is observed doing something that contradicts the assurance. For example, if a person is observed running and jumping, that may be evidence that contradicts the person's assertion of a mobility disability.

However, it is very important for covered entities and their staff to understand that the fact that a person with a disability is able to walk for a short distance does not necessarily contradict a verbal assurance – many people with mobility disabilities can walk but need their mobility device for longer distances or uneven terrain. This is particularly true for people who lack stamina, have poor balance, or use mobility devices because of respiratory, cardiac, or neurological disabilities. A covered entity cannot ask people about their disabilities.

STAFF TRAINING

Ongoing staff training is essential to ensure that people with disabilities who use OPDMDs for mobility are not turned away or treated inappropriately. Training should include instruction on the types of OPDMDs that can be accommodated, the rules for obtaining credible assurance that the device is being used because of a disability, and the rules for the operation of the devices within the facility.

Chapter 40 | Space Technologies in the Rehabilitation of Movement Disorders

More than 50 years have passed since the first human space-flight. As the duration of the flights has increased considerably, and amount of in-orbit activities has become greater, the need to maintain healthy bones and muscles in space has become more critical. Bones and muscles rely on performing daily activities in the presence of Earth's gravity to stay healthy. In space, traditional Earth-based methods to maintain bones and muscles, such as physical exercise, are challenging due to constraints that include such factors as crew time and vehicle size.

To meet these challenges, specialists from the Institute of Biomedical Problems in Russia and their commercial partner, Zvezda, developed the Penguin suit to provide loading along the length of the body (axial loading) in a way that compensates for the lack of daily loading that the body usually experiences under the Earth's gravity. The first testing of the suit in space was performed in 1971 aboard the Salyut-1 station. Now the Penguin suit is actively used on the International Space Station as a regular component of the Russian countermeasure system of health maintenance.

This chapter includes text excerpted from "Space Technologies in the Rehabilitation of Movement Disorders," National Aeronautics and Space Administration (NASA), November 19, 2015. Reviewed June 2021.

Since the early 1990s, Professor Inessa Kozlovskaya and her team at the Institute of Biomedical Problems in Russia have implemented the use of this axial loading suit in clinical rehabilitation practice. The clinical version of the Penguin suit, the Adeli, was developed at the Institute of Pediatrics Russian Academy of Science under the leadership of Professor Ksenia Semyonova and is used for the comprehensive treatment of cerebral palsy (CP) in children. The treatment method is focused on restoring functional links of the body through a corrective flow of sensory information to the muscles, thereby improving the health of the tissues being loaded. This results in the correction of walking patterns and stabilization of balance in a relatively short period of time, including for those CP children with deep motor disturbances. The Adeli suit was licensed in 1992 and has been continuously developed since. These methods have become one of the most popular and widely used in Russian medical clinics for rehabilitation of children with infantile cerebral paralysis.

New methods were also developed for patients undergoing motor rehabilitation after stroke and brain trauma. Paralytic and paretic alterations of motor functions that are the most frequent after-effects of these diseases typically lead to significant limitations in motor and social activity of these patients, decrease their functional abilities and obstruct their rehabilitation. Given all of the complexities and importance of the rehabilitation of these patients, another clinical modification of the Penguin suit was developed called the "Regent suit." The complex effect of the Regent suit on the body is based on an increase of the axial loading on skeletal structures and an increase in resistive loads on muscles during movement, which results in an increase of sensory information to the nervous system that is important for counteracting the development of pathological posture and for normalization of vertical stance and walking control. The Regent suit is effectively used at the early stage of rehabilitation for patients having movement disorders after cerebrovascular accident and cranium-brain traumas.

The clinical studies of the efficacy of the Regent suit in the rehabilitation of motor disorders in patients with limited lesions of the central nervous system were performed in acute and chronic studies with the participation of hundreds of stroke and brain trauma patients in the hospital No 83 Federal Medical- Biological Agency of Russia under leadership of professor Sergey Shvarkov, and in the Center of Speech Pathology and Neurorehabilitation (CSPN) under leadership of Professor Vicktor Shklovsky. The efficacy of the suit in patients with poststroke hemiparesis was assessed at the Scientific Center of Neurology under leadership of professor Ludmila Chernikova. These studies have shown that use of the suit results in a significant decrease in paresis and spasticity in the lower leg muscle groups, as well as an improvement of sensitivity in distal parts of lower limbs, and an overall improvement of locomotor functions. The positive effect on high mental functions was noticed at the same time, namely, an improvement of speech characteristics, an increase of active vocabulary, and an improvement in the patient's ability to recognize objects.

The use of the Regent suit is a complex, drug-free approach to the treatment of motor disorders. The method is closely related to the natural function of walking, activates all of the muscles involved in posture and spatial orientation, and is very safe. It allows for shorter treatment time, can be used both under hospital and outpatient conditions, and allows for a wide range of adjustments that allow individualized rehabilitation programs based on uniqueness of the neurological deficit and functional abilities of each patient. The Regent suit is applied in 43 medical institutions in Russia and abroad, and the results related to using both the Adeli and Regent suits are based on numerous observations and clinical studies.

Part 6 | Health Information Technology and Its Future

Chapter 41 | **Understanding Health Information Technology**

Chapter Contents

Section 41.1 | Basics of Health Information Technology

This section contains text excerpted from the following sources: Text in this section begins with excerpts from "What Is Health IT?" HealthIT.gov, Office of the National Coordinator for Health Information Technology (ONC), May 2, 2019; Text beginning with the heading "Patient Consent Decisions" is excerpted from "Health Information Technology," HealthIT.gov, Office of the National Coordinator for Health Information Technology (ONC), September 19, 2018.

Health IT, shorthand for "health information technology," is a broad concept that encompasses an array of technologies. Health IT is the use of computer hardware, software, or infrastructure to record, store, protect, and retrieve clinical, administrative, or financial information.

ELECTRONIC HEALTH RECORDS

An electronic health record (EHR) is a digital version of a patient's paper chart. EHRs are real time, patient-centered records that make information available instantly and securely to authorized users. While an EHR does contain the medical and treatment histories of patients, an EHR system is built to go beyond standard clinical data collected in a provider's office and can be inclusive of a broader view of a patient's care. EHRs are a vital part of health IT and can:

- Contain a patient's medical history, diagnoses, medications, treatment plans, immunization dates, allergies, radiology images, and laboratory and test results
- Allow access to evidence-based tools that providers can use to make decisions about a patient's care
- Automate and streamline provider workflow

One of the key features of an EHR is that health information can be created and managed by authorized providers in a digital format capable of being shared with other providers across more than one health-care organization. EHRs are built to share information with other health-care providers and organizations, such as laboratories, specialists, medical imaging facilities, pharmacies, emergency facilities, and school and workplace clinics, so they contain information from all clinicians involved in a patient's care.

PERSONAL HEALTH RECORDS

A personal health record (PHR) is an electronic application used by patients to maintain and manage their health information in a private, secure, and confidential environment. PHRs:

- Are managed by patients
- Can include information from a variety of sources, including health-care providers and patients themselves
- Can help patients securely and confidentially store and monitor health information, such as diet plans or data from home monitoring systems, as well as patient contact information, diagnosis lists, medication lists, allergy lists, immunization histories, and much more
- Are separate from, and do not replace, the legal record of any health-care provider
- Are distinct from portals that simply allow patients to view provider information or communicate with providers

ELECTRONIC MEDICAL RECORDS

Electronic health records and the ability to exchange health information electronically can help you provide higher quality and safer care for patients while creating tangible enhancements for your organization.

ELECTRONIC PRESCRIBING (E-PRESCRIBING)

With electronic prescribing, or "e-prescribing," health-care providers can enter prescription information into a computer device, such as a tablet, laptop, or desktop computer, and securely transmit the prescription to pharmacies using a special software program and connectivity to a transmission network. When a pharmacy receives a request, it can begin filling the medication right away.

The benefits of e-prescribing are to:

- Help improve health-care quality and patient safety by reducing medication errors and checking for drug interactions

- Make care more convenient by allowing providers to electronically request prescription refills

In short, e-prescribing is more convenient, cheaper, and safer for doctors, pharmacies, and patients.

PATIENT CONSENT DECISIONS

A number of different models for electronically capturing and managing patient consent exist, including:

- **Consent bundled with information.** Collecting patient consent at the place where healthcare is delivered and then transmitting the consent and corresponding health information when it is requested by others. For example, in some models, a consent document is sent along with the patient's health information.
- **Metadata tagging.** Adding a code to the health information to "tag" it with details related to the patient's consent choice. When this tagged information is sent from one health IT system to another, the sending and receiving organizations' health IT system needs to be able to read and understand what the tag means. The tag may also be a reference to a separate consent document that is stored locally or in a centralized database, showing the health IT system where to look for the most up-to-date consent choice for that piece of information.
- **Centralized approach.** Managing patient consent through a central database or repository that can be queried to decide how information may be accessed based on the patient's choice.

WHY IS TECHNOLOGY PARTICULARLY NEEDED FOR PROTECTING SENSITIVE HEALTH INFORMATION?

The following quick background on sensitive health information may be helpful in showing why technology is important in this

531

area. Sensitive health information is defined here as specific types of health information or health information generated by a specific type of provider.

Some of the categories of sensitive health information that may receive increased protection include:

- Subject of information (e.g., human immunodeficiency virus (HIV) related information, mental-health information)
- Provider type (e.g., substance abuse treatment provider)
- Type of information (e.g., psychotherapy notes)

Under the HIPAA Privacy Rule, patient consent is not required for the sharing of most health information for treatment, payment, and health-care operations. However, some federal and state laws require patient consent for the sharing of sensitive health information.

Some laws require that when sensitive health information is disclosed, the receiving organization be notified that it cannot further disclose the information without obtaining the patient's consent to do so. This restriction is often called a "prohibition on redisclosure." One federal law that has this requirement is 42 CFR Part 2, which protects the confidentiality of information related to substance abuse treatment received at federally-funded treatment centers.

In addition to these laws, some organizations have their own internal policies requiring patient consent in order to share particularly sensitive information.

Some providers or health information exchangers (HIEs) may be constrained by their technology's limitations. Some technologies offer patients only the choice to share all or none of their health information, including information that may be considered by many to be sensitive.

Section 41.2 | **Benefits of Health IT**

This section includes text excerpted from "Benefits of Health IT," HealthIT.gov, Office of the National Coordinator for Health Information Technology (ONC), September 15, 2017. Reviewed June 2021.

Over the past 20 years, our nation has undergone a major transformation due to information technology (IT). Today, we have at our fingertips access to a variety of information and services to help us manage our relationships with the organizations that are part of our lives: banks, utilities, government offices – even entertainment companies.

Until now, relatively few Americans have had the opportunity to use this kind of technology to enhance some of the most important relationships: those related to your health. Relationships with your doctors, your pharmacy, your hospital, and other organizations that make up your circle of care are now about to benefit from the next transformation in information technology: health IT.

For patients and consumers, this transformation will enhance both relationships with providers and providers' relationships with each other. This change will place you at the center of your care.

Although it will take years for healthcare to realize all these improvements and fully address any pitfalls, the first changes in this transformation are already underway. At the same time, numerous technology tools are becoming available to improve health for you, your family, and your community.

Most consumers will first encounter the benefits of health IT through an electronic health record, or EHR, at their doctor's office or at a hospital.

BENEFITS OF HEALTH IT FOR YOU AND YOUR FAMILY

On a basic level, an EHR provides a digitized version of the "paper chart" you often see doctors, nurses, and others using. But, when an EHR is connected to all of your health-care providers (and often, to you as a patient), it can offer so much more.

- **EHRs reduce your paperwork.** The clipboard and new patient questionnaire may remain a feature of your doctor's office for some time to come. But, as more information gets added to your EHR, your doctor and hospital will have more of that data available as soon as you arrive. This means fewer and shorter forms for you to complete, reducing the healthcare "hassle factor."

- **EHRs get your information accurately into the hands of people who need it.** Even if you have relatively simple health-care needs, coordinating information among care providers can be a daunting task and one that can lead to medical mistakes if done incorrectly. When all of your providers can share your health information via EHRs, each of them has access to more accurate and up-to-date information about your care. That enables your providers to make the best possible decisions, particularly in a crisis.

- **EHRs help your doctors coordinate your care and protect your safety.** Suppose you see three specialists in addition to your primary care physician. Each of them may prescribe different drugs, and sometimes, these drugs may interact in harmful ways. EHRs can warn your care providers if they try to prescribe a drug that could cause that kind of interaction. An EHR may also alert one of your doctors if another doctor has already prescribed a drug that did not work out for you, saving you from the risks and costs of taking ineffective medication.

- **EHRs reduce unnecessary tests and procedures.** Have you ever had to repeat medical tests ordered by one doctor because the results were not readily available to another doctor? Those tests may have been uncomfortable and inconvenient or have posed some risk, and they also cost money. Repeating tests – whether a $20 blood test or a $2,000 MRI results in higher costs to you in the form of bigger bills and increased insurance premiums. With EHRs, all of your care providers can have access to all your test results and records at once, reducing the potential for unnecessary repeat tests.

- **EHRs give you direct access to your health records.**
  In the United States, you already have a federally
  guaranteed right to see your health records, identify
  wrong and missing information, and make additions or
  corrections as needed. Some health-care providers with
  EHR systems give their patients direct access to their
  health information online in ways that help preserve
  privacy and security. This access enables you to keep
  better track of your care, and in some cases, answer
  your questions immediately rather than waiting hours
  or days for a returned phone call. This access may also
  allow you to communicate directly and securely with
  your health-care provider.

Section 41.3 | Consumer Health IT Applications

This section includes text excerpted from "Consumer Health IT Applications," Agency for Healthcare Research and Quality (AHRQ), U.S. Department of Health and Human Services (HHS), January 10, 2020.

As patients become more responsible for managing an increasing volume of health information, including their medical history, lab results, and medications, new consumer health information technology (health IT) applications are being developed that allow patients to manage, share, and control their health information electronically and to assume a more active role in the management of their health.

While the term "consumer health IT applications" is not yet well-defined, in general, it refers to a wide range of hardware, software, and web-based applications that allows patients to participate in their own healthcare via electronic means. The American Medical Informatics Association (AMIA) has developed a working definition for the field of consumer health informatics stating that it is "a subspecialty of medical informatics which studies from a patient/consumer perspective the use of electronic information and communication to improve medical outcomes and the healthcare decision-making process." In addition, as defined by Eysenbach, the study of consumer health informatics includes analyzing consumers' information needs, studying and implementing methods of making information accessible to consumers, and modeling and integrating consumers' preferences into medical information systems.

New consumer health IT applications are being developed to be used on a variety of different platforms, including via the web, messaging systems, and cell phones, and their use can benefit both patients and providers. These applications have various purposes including assisting with self-management through reminders and educational prompts, delivering real-time data on a patient's health condition to both patients and providers, facilitating web-based support groups, and compiling and storing personal health information in an easily accessible format. One example of the potential benefits of these kinds of applications is illustrated by the use of messaging capabilities available in certain consumer health IT applications that enable timely communication between patients and their providers. Moreover, consumer health IT applications that allow gathering and integrating data from various healthcare sources can serve as a comprehensive resource for patients and their providers. In addition to convenience, consumer health IT applications also can be important in emergency situations to provide critical health information to medical staff.

As described by Jimison et al., consumer health IT applications differ to the degree with which they integrate information about the patient in the application itself and the degree to which they provide patient-specific recommendations back to the user. Some examples of the range of applications are listed below.

SELF-MANAGEMENT SYSTEMS

This includes systems that are highly varied and include different combinations of functionality utilizing multiple platforms. The most effective systems provide a timely response to information about the current or evolving status of the user. Some of them allow for monitoring and transmission of information, such as blood pressure or blood glucose. Depending on system design, feedback to a patient regarding her or his health status can be received from the system directly or from the provider who receives information from the system.

ELECTRONIC PERSONAL HEALTH RECORDS AND PATIENT PORTALS

Electronic personal health records (PHRs) are defined as "an electronic record of health-related information on an individual that conforms to nationally recognized interoperability standards and that can be drawn from multiple sources while being managed, shared, and controlled by the individual." An electronic PHR can exist as a stand-alone application that allows information to be exported to or imported from other sources or applications or as a "tethered" application that is linked to a specific health-care organization's information system. Tethered PHRs, also referred to as "patient portals," typically allow patients to view, but not modify, data from the provider's electronic health record (EHR). Relevant information that is often retained in a PHR includes personal identifiers, contact information, health provider information, problem list, medication history, allergies, immunizations, lab, and test results, and other relevant medical histories. Some applications also allow patients to communicate electronically with their providers.

PEER INTERACTION SYSTEMS

Peer interaction can take the form of stand-alone applications or can sometimes be a part of multicomponent applications. These applications can increase perceived peer support and improve personal and social outcomes. Through online forums, discussion groups, and other peer communication features, patients can interact electronically with others who have similar conditions.

Section 41.4 | Trends in Use

This section includes text excerpted from "Trends in Individuals' Access, Viewing, and Use of Online Medical Records and Other Technology for Health Needs: 2017–2018," HealthIT.gov, Office of the National Coordinator for Health Information Technology (ONC), May 2019.

INDIVIDUALS WHO OFFERED ACCESS TO THEIR ONLINE MEDICAL RECORD

In 2018, three in 10 individuals were offered access to their online medical records and viewed their records at least once within the past year.

PERCENTAGE WHO VIEWED THEIR RECORD AT LEAST ONCE IN 2018

- Between 2017 and 2018, there were no differences in the frequency of viewing online medical records.
- In 2018, among individuals who were offered access to their online medical records, about three in 10 individuals viewed their data one to two times per year.
- In 2018, among individuals offered access to their online medical records, only about one in 10 viewed their data six or more times within the past year.

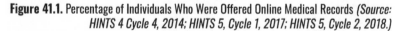

■ Offered access and viewed online medical record at least once within the past year

■ Offered access but did not view online medical record within the past year

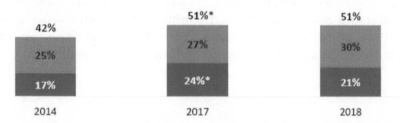

Figure 41.1. Percentage of Individuals Who Were Offered Online Medical Records *(Source: HINTS 4 Cycle 4, 2014; HINTS 5, Cycle 1, 2017; HINTS 5, Cycle 2, 2018.)*

*Note: *Significantly different from previous year (p<0.05). Denominator represents all individuals. Percentage reflects weighted national estimate.*

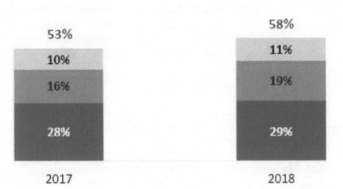

■ 1 to 2 times ■ 3 to 5 times ▨ 6 or more times

Figure 41.2. Percentage of Online Records Used *(Source: E: HINTS 5, Cycle 1, 2017; HINTS 5, Cycle 2, 2018.)*

Note: Numbers do not add up to 58 percent due to rounding. Denominator represents individuals who were offered access to their online medical record (52 percent of individuals nationwide in 2017; 51 percent of individuals nationwide in 2018).

INDIVIDUALS' VIEWING OF ONLINE MEDICAL RECORDS BY SELECTED CHARACTERISTICS

Table 41.1. Variation in Individuals Being Offered and Accessing Their Online Medical Records by Selected Characteristics, 2017–2018.

Characteristic		Percent of Individuals Who Were Offered Access to Online Medical Records by Characteristic (2017–2018)	Among Individuals Offered an Online Medical Record, Percent Who Viewed Their Record by Characteristic (2017–2018)
Gender	Male (reference)	45%	54%
	Female	57%*^	58%
Annual Household Income	$0 to $34,999	36%	*^ 41%*^

Table 41.1. Continued

Characteristic		Percent of Individuals Who Were Offered Access to Online Medical Records by Characteristic (2017–2018)	Among Individuals Offered an Online Medical Record, Percent Who Viewed Their Record by Characteristic (2017–2018)
	$35,000 to $74,999	49%*^	53%*^
	$75,000 or more (reference)	65%	66%
Education	College Degree or more	63%*	^ 68%*^
	Less than College (reference)	46%	48%
Internet access and use	Yes	57%*^	59%*^
	No (reference)	26%	24%
Geography	Urban	52%*	57%*^
	Rural (reference)	45%	45%
Doctor Visit in Past Year	Yes	57%*^	58%*^
	No (reference)	27%	38%
Health Insurance Coverage	Yes	54%*^	57%*
	No (reference)	25%	34%
Have a Chronic Condition	Yes	55%*^	57%^
	No (reference)	46%	54%

(Source: HINTS 5, Cycle 1, 2017; HINTS 5, Cycle 2, 2018.)
*Notes: Unadjusted weighted national estimate shown. *Unadjusted estimate significantly different from reference category (p<0.05). ^Adjusted estimate (not shown) significantly different from reference category (p<0.05). The adjusted estimates controlled for survey year (2017/2018), gender, age, race/ethnicity, income, education, geography, having seen a doctor in the past year, internet access, chronic condition, and health insurance. Chronic condition was defined as having at least one of the following conditions: diabetes, hypertension, chronic heart disease (CHD), chronic lung disease, arthritis, or a mental-health condition.*

- Access to online medical records varied by individuals' health-care use, socio-demographic characteristics, Internet access, and use, and whether they had a chronic health condition.
- Individuals with an annual household income of $75,000 were more likely to be offered access as well as view their online medical records compared to those with less income.
- Individuals who went to the doctor at least once within the past year were twice as likely to be offered access to their online medical record and were over 50 percent more likely to view their online medical record at least once compared to those who did not visit their doctor within the past year.
- Individuals with at least a college degree had higher rates of being offered access and subsequently viewing their online medical records compared to those with less than a college degree.
- Individuals with chronic health conditions were more likely to be offered access and view their online medical records compared to individuals without chronic health conditions.

PERCENTAGE WHO PREFERED TO SPEAK TO A PROVIDER DIRECTLY

- About three-quarters of individuals cited their preference to speak with their health-care provider directly as a reason for not using their online medical record within the past year.
- The percent of individuals who did not view their online medical records within the past year due to privacy and security concerns decreased by 11 percentage points between 2017 and 2018.
- Fewer individuals reported not having a way to access their online medical record's website as a reason for not viewing their record in 2018 compared to 2017.

Table 41.2. Reasons for Not Accessing Online Medical Record as Reported by Individuals Who Did Not View Their Online Medical Record within the Past Year, 2017–2018.

Reason for Not Using Online Record	2017	2018
Prefer to speak to health-care provider directly	76%	73%
Did not have a need to use your online medical record	59%	65%
Concerned about the privacy/security of online medical record	25%	14%*
No longer have an online medical record	19%	13%
Do not have a way to access the website	20%	10%*

(Source: HINTS 5, Cycle 1, 2017; HINTS 5, Cycle 2, 2018.)
*Notes: *Significantly different from previous year (p<0.05). Denominator represents individuals who were offered an online medical record but did not view their record within the past year.*

INDIVIDUALS WHO VIEWED AND DOWNLOADED THEIR MEDICAL RECORD DATA

Table 41.3. Those Who Viewed Their Record at Least Once within the Past Year, the Percentage That Used View, Download, or Transmit Functionalities 2017–2018.

View, Download, or Transmit	2017	2018
View test results	84%	–
Download online medical record data	17%	26%*
Transmitted data to at least one outside party listed below	14%	17%
Transmit to another health-care provider	10%	14%
Transmit to caregiver	4%	4%
Transmit to service or app	3%	3%

(Source: HINTS 5, Cycle 1, 2017; HINTS 5, Cycle 2, 2018.)
*Notes: *Significantly different from previous year (p<0.05). Denominator represents individuals who viewed their online medical records at least once within the last year (30 percent of respondents). Data for View Test Results were not collected in 2018.*

- One-quarter of individuals who viewed their online medical records also downloaded their data in 2018.
- In 2018, nearly one in five individuals who viewed their online medical records also transmitted their data to an

outside party (another health-care provider, caregiver, or app/service).

- In 2017 and 2018, only three percent of individuals who viewed their record within the past year transmitted their record data to a service or app.

INDIVIDUALS WHO USED ONLINE MEDICAL RECORDS TO SECURELY COMMUNICATE WITH THEIR HEALTH-CARE PROVIDERS

Table 41.4. Reported Online Medical Record Functionalities Used by Individuals amongst Those Who Were Offered and Viewed Their Record, 2017–2018.

Uses of Online Medical Record	2017	2018
Convenience Functions		
Request refill of medications	38%	39%
Fill out forms or paperwork related to your healthcare	38%	44%*
Updating Medical Record		
Request correction of inaccurate information	8%	7%
Add health information	19%	24%
Communicating with Health-Care Provider		
Securely message health-care provider and staff (e.g., e-mail)	48%	53%
Decision Making		
Help you make a decision about how to treat an illness or condition	19%	24%
Perceptions regarding Usefulness of Online Medical Record		
Consider online medical record useful for monitoring health	84%	83%

(Source: HINTS 5, Cycle 1, 2017; HINTS 5, Cycle 2, 2018.)
Notes: Denominator represents individuals who were offered access to the online medical record and viewed their online medical records at least once within the last year.

- Among those who viewed their online medical record, about four in 10 used it to request medical refills and fill out forms related to their healthcare in 2018.
- The percent of individuals who reported using their online medical records to fill out forms related to their healthcare increased by six percentage points between 2017 and 2018.

- Among individuals who viewed their online medical records, about 10 percent requested corrections to their online medical records in 2018.
- More than eight in 10 individuals who viewed their record reported that their online medical record was useful for monitoring their health in 2018.

INDIVIDUALS WHO USED A HEALTH OR WELLNESS APP

Table 41.5. Percent of Individuals Who Reported Having a Smartphone, Tablet, Electronic Monitoring Device, or Health and Wellness App, 2017–2018.

Type of Device	2017	2018
Electronic Monitoring Device (e.g., Fitbit, blood glucose meter, blood pressure device)	34%	35%
Tablet	62%	58%
Smartphone	79%	80%
Tablet or Smartphone	84%	84%
Health and Wellness App (among those with a tablet or smartphone)	44%	49%

(Source: HINTS 5, Cycle 1, 2017; HINTS 5, Cycle 2, 2018.)
Notes: Examples of an electronic monitoring device include Fitbit, blood glucose meter, and/or blood pressure monitor.

- The proportion of individuals who reported owning a tablet, smartphone, or other electronic monitoring device did not change between 2017 and 2018.
- Over eight in 10 individuals reported owning a tablet or smartphone in 2018.
- One-third of individuals owned an electronic monitoring device, such as a Fitbit, blood glucose meter, or blood pressure monitor in 2018.

HEALTH-RELATED GOAL PROGRESS TRACKING USING HEALTH AND WELLNESS APP

- The percentage of individuals who had a health and wellness app and used it to track progress on a

Table 41.6. Percent of Individuals Who Reported Using Their Health and Wellness App or Other Electronic Monitoring Device to Help Discuss, Track, and/or Make Decisions regarding Their Health, 2017–2018.

Use of Electronic Device	2017	2018
Individuals with a health & wellness app1		
Track progress on a health-related goal	69%	75%*
Make a decision about how to treat an illness or condition	45%	48%
Discuss your health with your health-care provider	43%	45%
Individuals with a health & wellness app or other electronic monitoring device2		
Shared information from a smartphone, tablet, or other electronic monitoring device with a health professional	26%	28%

(Source: HINTS 5, Cycle 1, 2017; HINTS 5, Cycle 2, 2018.)
*Notes: *Significantly different from previous year (p<0.05). Examples of an electronic monitoring device include Fitbit, blood glucose meter, and/or blood pressure monitor. [1]Denominator represents the sample of individuals that report having a health and wellness app; [2]Denominator represents the sample of individuals that report having a health and wellness app or electronic monitoring device.*

health-related goal increased by 6 percentage points between 2017 and 2018.

- In 2018, about half of individuals with a health and wellness app used it to make a decision about how to treat an illness or condition; a similar number used it to facilitate discussions with their health-care provider.
- More than a quarter of health and wellness app or other electronic monitoring device users shared information from their device with a health professional in 2018.

INDIVIDUALS WITH ACCESS TO SMARTPHONE OR TABLET BUT DID NOT VIEW THEIR ONLINE RECORD

- Almost three in 10 individuals owned a smartphone or tablet and viewed their online medical records at least once within the past year.
- Over one-third of individuals owned a smartphone or tablet and were not offered access to an online medical record.

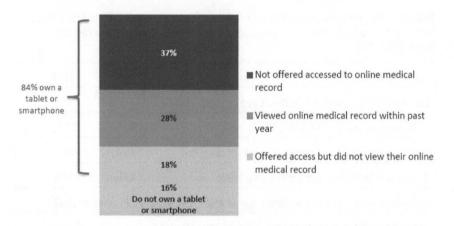

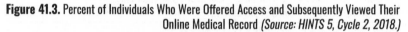

Figure 41.3. Percent of Individuals Who Were Offered Access and Subsequently Viewed Their Online Medical Record *(Source: HINTS 5, Cycle 2, 2018.)*

Notes: Denominator represents all individuals. Percentage reflects weighted national estimate. Percentages do not add up to 84 percent due to rounding.

Chapter 42 | Integrating Technology and Healthcare

Section 42.1 | **Health Information Technology Integration**

This section contains text excerpted from the following sources: Text in this section begins with excerpts from "Health Information Technology Integration," Agency for Healthcare Research and Quality (AHRQ), U.S. Department of Health and Human Services (HHS), August 2019; Text under the heading "Implementing Health IT" is excerpted from "Implementing Health IT," HealthIT.gov, Office of the National Coordinator for Health Information Technology (ONC), September 15, 2017. Reviewed June 2021.

The integration of health information technology (HIT) into primary care includes a variety of electronic methods that are used to manage information about people's health and healthcare, for both individual patients and groups of patients. The use of health IT can improve the quality of care, even as it makes healthcare more cost-effective.

The Agency for Healthcare Research and Quality's (AHRQ) health IT initiative is part of the Nation's strategy to put information technology to work in healthcare. The integration of health IT into primary care includes a variety of electronic methods that are used to manage information about people's health and healthcare, for both individual patients and groups of patients.

In primary care, examples of health IT include the following:
- Clinical decision support
- Computerized disease registries
- Computerized provider order entry
- Consumer health IT applications
- Electronic medical record systems (EMRs, EHRs, and PHRs)
- Electronic prescribing
- Telehealth

The AHRQ's National Resource Center for Health IT serves as the link between the health-care community and the researchers and experts who are on the front lines of health IT. The National Resource Center encourages adoption of health IT by providing the latest tools, best practices, and research results from this unique real-world laboratory. These health IT resources include:
- Workflow Assessment for Health IT Toolkit
- Health IT Tools and Resources
- Health IT Literacy Guide

WHY IS HEALTH IT IMPORTANT?

Health IT makes it possible for health-care providers to better manage patient care through the secure use and sharing of health information. By developing secure and private electronic health records for most Americans and making health information available electronically when and where it is needed, health IT can improve the quality of care, even as it makes healthcare more cost-effective.

With the help of health IT, health-care providers will have:

- Accurate and complete information about a patient's health. That way, providers can give the best possible care, whether during a routine visit or a medical emergency.
- The ability to better coordinate the care given. This is especially important if a patient has a serious medical condition.
- A way to securely share information with patients and their family caregivers over the Internet, for patients who opt for this convenience. This means patients and their families can more fully take part in decisions about their healthcare.
- Information to help diagnose health problems sooner, reduce medical errors, and provide safer care at lower costs.

IMPLEMENTING HEALTH IT

The successful implementation of a health IT system is essential to delivering safe care for patients and a more satisfying work experience for clinicians and staff.

The implementation process is complex, including components such as tailoring the system to support safe, high-quality patient care, and ensuring contingency plans are established to address system downtimes.

Health IT system implementation is a multi-stage process. When implementing a health IT system, it is critical to consider first what care processes it needs to support and how the hardware and software should be set up to support them in patient- and clinician-friendly ways. Configuring the system can be complex and requires a team that includes practicing clinicians to ensure the technology properly supports safe, effective clinical processes and complements efficient workflows.

Successful implementation involves assessing multiple aspects of communication within and outside the health IT system, the integration of its components with one another, and its interaction not only with other technology but also the people, processes, and culture of the organization. Early resolution of potential integration issues can reduce future patient safety risks.

Patient identification processes are also important to consider during implementation. A well-planned configuration alone does not ensure accurate patient identification. An organization implementing a health IT system should consider how its new technology will handle generating new patient records, patient registration, and retrieval of information. Defining and mapping these processes may detect, mitigate, and prevent problems caused by duplicate records, patient mix-ups, and comingled records.

In addition to resources relevant to other aspects of safety in a health IT enabled environment, ONC offers three SAFER Guides that may be particularly useful when implementing a health IT system.

- **System configuration.** It is a SAFER Guide that identifies recommended safety practices for EHR hardware and software set up. EHR safety and effectiveness can be improved by establishing proper configuration procedures, policies, and practices.
- **System interfaces.** It is a SAFER Guide that identifies recommended safety practices intended to optimize the safety and safe use of system-to-system interfaces between EHR-related software applications. Well-designed and well-developed system interfaces enable reliable connection of different systems.
- **Patient identification.** It is a SAFER Guide that recommends safety practices for reliable patient identification in the EHR. Accurate patient identification ensures that the information presented by and entered into the EHR is associated with the correct person.

Section 42.2 | **Information and Communication Technology**

This section includes text excerpted from "Health Communication and Health Information Technology," Office of Disease Prevention and Health Promotion (ODPHP), U.S. Department of Health and Human Services (HHS), June 11, 2021.

Ideas about health and behaviors are shaped by the communication, information, and technology that people interact with every day. Health communication and health information technology (HIT) are central to healthcare, public health, and the way our society views health. These processes make up the ways and the context in which professionals and the public search for, understand, and use health information, significantly impacting their health decisions and actions.

The objectives in this topic area describe many ways health communication and health IT can have a positive impact on health, healthcare, and health equity. They include:

- Supporting shared decision-making between patients and providers
- Providing personalized self-management tools and resources
- Building social support networks
- Delivering accurate, accessible, and actionable health information that is targeted or tailored
- Facilitating the meaningful use of health IT and the exchange of health information among health-care and public-health professionals
- Enabling quick and informed responses to health risks and public-health emergencies
- Increasing health literacy skills
- Providing new opportunities to connect with culturally diverse and hard-to-reach populations
- Providing sound principles in the design of programs and interventions that result in healthier behaviors
- Increasing Internet and mobile access

WHY ARE HEALTH COMMUNICATION AND HEALTH INFORMATION TECHNOLOGY IMPORTANT?

Effective use of communication and technology by health-care and public-health professionals can bring about an age of patient- and public-centered health information and services. By strategically combining health IT tools and effective health communication processes, there is the potential to:

- Improve health-care quality and safety
- Increase the efficiency of health-care and public-health service delivery
- Improve the public-health information infrastructure
- Support care in the community and at home
- Facilitate clinical and consumer decision-making
- Build health skills and knowledge

UNDERSTANDING HEALTH COMMUNICATION AND HEALTH INFORMATION TECHNOLOGY

All people have some ability to manage their health and the health of those they care for. However, with the increasing complexity of health information and health-care settings, most people need additional information, skills, and supportive relationships to meet their health needs.

Disparities in access to health information, services, and technology can result in lower usage rates of preventive services, less knowledge of chronic disease management, higher rates of hospitalization, and poorer reported health status.

Both public and private institutions are increasingly using the Internet and other technologies to streamline the delivery of health information and services. This results in an even greater need for health professionals to develop additional skills in the understanding and use of consumer health information.

The increase in online health information and services challenges users with limited literacy skills or limited experience using the Internet. For many of these users, the Internet is stressful and overwhelming – even inaccessible. Much of this stress can be reduced through the application of evidence-based best practices in user-centered design.

In addition, despite increased access to technology, other forms of communication are essential to ensuring that everyone, including nonweb users, is able to obtain, process, and understand health information to make good health decisions. These include printed materials, media campaigns, community outreach, and interpersonal communication.

EMERGING ISSUES IN HEALTH COMMUNICATION AND HEALTH INFORMATION TECHNOLOGY

During the coming decade, the speed, scope, and scale of adoption of health IT will only increase. Social media and emerging technologies promise to blur the line between expert and peer health information. Monitoring and assessing the impact of these new media, including mobile health, on public health will be challenging.

Equally challenging will be helping health professionals and the public adapt to the changes in health-care quality and efficiency due to the creative use of health communication and health IT. Continual feedback, productive interactions, and access to evidence on the effectiveness of treatments and interventions will likely transform the traditional patient-provider relationship. It will also change the way people receive, process, and evaluate health information. Capturing the scope and impact of these changes – and the role of health communication and health IT in facilitating them – will require multidisciplinary models and data systems.

Such systems will be critical to expanding the collection of data to better understand the effects of health communication and health IT on population health outcomes, health-care quality, and health disparities.

Chapter 43 | Digital-Health Records

Chapter Contents

Section 43.1 | Blue Button

This section contains text excerpted from the following sources: Text in this section begins with excerpts from "Blue Button® 2.0: Improving Medicare Beneficiary Access to Their Health Information," Centers for Medicare & Medicaid Services (CMS), December 27, 2019; Text beginning with the heading "About Blue Button" is excerpted from "Blue Button," HealthIT.gov, Office of the National Coordinator for Health Information Technology (ONC), April 8, 2019.

The Blue Button service was established in 2010 as a joint effort of the Centers for Medicare & Medicaid Services (CMS) and the U.S. Department of Veterans Affairs (VA). Since that time, Blue Button has been used by more than one million beneficiaries to download their CMS information via the MyMedicare.gov portal.

The current text and PDF downloadable files, while relatively easy to read, become challenging when handling large amounts of data, or converting the content into reusable data for further analysis.

As digital healthcare evolves, data becomes an important resource that patients can use to improve health outcomes for themselves, and as part of research groups. This drives the need for easier data interoperability.

ABOUT BLUE BUTTON

The Blue Button symbol signifies that a site has functionality for customers to download health records. You can use your health data to improve your health and to have more control over your personal health information and your family's healthcare.

- Do you want to feel more in control of your health and your personal health information?
- Do you have a health issue?
- Are you caring for an elderly parent?
- Are you changing doctors?
- Do you need to find the results of a medical test or a complete and current list of your medications?

Blue Button may be able to help.

Look for the Blue Button symbol and take action using your personal health information.

YOUR HEALTH RECORDS

Health information about you may be stored in many places, such as doctors' offices, hospitals, drug stores, and health insurance companies. The Blue Button symbol signifies that an organization has a way for you to access your health records electronically so you can:

- Share them with your doctor or trusted family members or caregivers.
- Check to make sure the information, such as your medication list, is accurate and complete.
- Keep track of when your child had his/her last vaccination.
- Have your medical history available in case of emergency, when traveling, seeking a second opinion, or switching health insurance companies.
- Plug your health information into apps and tools that help you set and reach personalized health goals.

You have a legal right to receive your personal-health information. Blue Button is one of the ways this information may be made available to you. Look for the Blue Button symbol, and ask your health-care providers or health insurance company if they offer you the ability to view online, download, and share your health records.

WHAT KIND OF INFORMATION IS AVAILABLE TO YOU?

It depends on whether you are getting information from your health-care provider (doctor, hospital, nursing home, etc.) your health insurance company, or another source such as a drug store or a lab since each has different kinds of information. In general, you may expect to be able to electronically access important information such as:

- Current medications you are taking
- Any allergies you have
- Medical treatment information from your doctor or hospital visits
- Your lab test results
- Your health insurance claims information (financial information, clinical information and more)

Until recently, many health records were stored in paper files, so it was not very easy for you to access or use this information. But, that is changing as more doctors and hospitals adopt electronic health records (EHRs) and other health information technologies, including mobile health apps.

Medicare beneficiaries can view and download their Medicare claims data in a more timely and user-friendly format than ever before. That information now covers three years of your health history, including claims information on services covered under Medicare Parts A and B, and a list of medications that were purchased under Part D. Look for the Blue Button symbol on the MyMedicare website.

Veterans can find the Blue Button symbol on the MyHealtheVet website (www.myhealth.va.gov/mhv-portal-web/home) and download demographic information (age, gender, ethnicity, and more), emergency contacts, a list of their prescription medications, clinical notes, and wellness reminders.

You may want to check back often as more and more organizations join the Blue Button movement. Online health records are not yet available to everyone, but access is rapidly growing, and if you ask for access you can help grow it faster.

YOUR RIGHTS

As Americans, you have the legal right to access your own health records held by doctors, hospitals and others who provide health-care services for you. And you have the option of getting your records on paper or electronically depending on how they are stored. You can exercise your rights by downloading your health records through an online portal, or by asking how to get a copy of your health records. Some doctors or hospitals may not be familiar with your rights to access your information about your own health. You can print out and share with them a letter that explains these rights.

Section 43.2 | E-prescription

This section includes text excerpted from "Electronic Prescribing," Digital Healthcare Research, Agency for Healthcare Research and Quality (AHRQ), U.S. Department of Health and Human Services (HHS), March 16, 2020.

Electronic prescription (e-prescribing) writing is defined by the eHealth Initiative as "the use of computing devices to enter, modify, review, and output or communicate drug prescriptions." Although the term e-prescribing implies the use of a computer for any type of prescribing action, a wide range of e-prescribing activities exist with varying levels of sophistication:

- Level 1: Electronic reference handbook
- Level 2: Stand alone prescription writer
- Level 3: Patient-specific prescription creation or refilling
- Level 4: Medication management (access to medication history, warnings, and alerts)
- Level 5: Connectivity to dispensing site
- Level 6: Integration with an electronic medical record

All levels of electronic prescription writing confer varying degrees of improvement in patient safety. Level 6, which is the most sophisticated, has been shown to confer the highest degree of patient safety and the largest return on investment. Over the last five years, national interest in e-prescribing has increased as the federal government has enacted legislation, including the Medicare Modernization Act of 2003 (MMA), aimed at increasing the adoption of e-prescribing.

The Centers for Medicare & Medicaid Services (CMS) released a report to Congress entitled Pilot Testing of Initial Electronic Prescribing Standards (digital.ahrq.gov/sites/default/files/docs/page/eRxReport_041607_1.pdf). This report was mandated by the MMA, and it details the rigorous pilot testing of information standards by five leading e-prescribing organizations. The Agency for Healthcare Research and Quality (AHRQ) and the National Resource Center's evaluation report recommended that the medication history, formulary and benefits, and prescription fill status indicator standards were ready for implementation under Part D. Prior authorization, structured and codified signature (sig), and the RxNorm standards were not ready for implementation in their current state.

In addition, the pilot projects evaluated key issues in e-prescribing such as reduction of adverse drug events, provider uptake, and potential gains in efficiency and effectiveness. The use of the proposed standards advances interoperability in the U.S. health-care system and greatly enhances the ability of health IT to improve safety and quality. Such efforts are integral to the AHRQ's mission to improve the quality, safety, efficiency, and effectiveness of health-care for all Americans.

AREAS OF CURRENT INVESTIGATION

Existing e-prescribing tools have begun to consider a variety of new uses for a medication history. Those uses include knowing what medications a patient has actually received from a pharmacist using data from pharmacy benefit managers (PBMs). Services such as SureScripts provide this information to electronic prescription writing systems, allowing providers to see a complete view of the patient's medication history. Another current trend is transmission of electronic prescriptions using a standard known as "NCPDP-SCRIPT." This standard supports interfaces to pharmacy information systems and is a foundation standard adopted by the U.S. Department of Health and Human Services (HHS) in 2005. A frequently used practice is to communicate via fax, which is often plagued by inaccurate fax numbers, poor management of faxes that are received by pharmacies, and poor systems to provide feedback about the status of fax delivery.

The MMA requires that Part D plans support an electronic prescription program, should any of their providers and pharmacies voluntarily choose to e-prescribe. This program is required to provide for the electronic transmittal of prescription orders themselves; plan eligibility queries and responses; plan benefit information; drug interactions, warnings or cautions, and any dosage adjustments related to the drug being prescribed or dispensed; appropriate lower-cost alternatives, if any, for a drug being prescribed;

and the patient's medical history related to a covered Part D drug being prescribed or dispensed. For each requirement, HHS released the final ruling on e-prescribing and the foundation standards in November 2005 in the federal Register. These standards are compatible with existing ones, especially the transactions specified in the administrative simplification provisions of the Health Insurance Portability and Accountability Act (HIPAA) of 1996.

The MMA also required pilot projects during 2006 to test any standards for which there is not adequate industry experience. The AHRQ and the Centers for Medicare & Medicaid Services (CMS) collaborated to issue grants and contracts for pilot testing e-prescribing standards. Results of these pilot projects were released in April 2007 in the form of an evaluation report from the AHRQ National Resource Center for Health Information Technology. Final e-prescribing standards were released in the federal Register on April 7, 2008, with implementation up to a year later. In the spring 2008 session of the U.S. Congress, the Medicare Improvements for Patients and Providers Act of 2008 was passed, offering physicians financial incentives for electronic prescribing. Under the new law, Medicare physicians who e-prescribe will receive a 2-percent payment bonus in 2009 and 2010, a 1-percent bonus in 2011 and 2012, and a 0.5-percent bonus in 2013. In addition, payments to Medicare physicians who do not e-prescribe will be reduced by 1 percent in 2012, 1.5 percent in 2013, and 2 percent in subsequent years.

In addition to the MMA, The Joint Commission for the Accreditation of Hospital Organizations (The Joint Commission) has recently endorsed medication reconciliation in 2006. Hospitals that are accredited by The Joint Commission need to demonstrate methods to verify that medication histories are reconciled and up-to-date with medication lists after each care transition (e.g., from outpatient to inpatient status; from inpatient ward to inpatient ICU; from outpatient hospital to nursing home facility). Medication reconciliation has been shown to be a time-intensive activity on the part of those people involved. E-prescribing tools may improve the process by providing more accurate and complete histories.

Chapter 44 | **Artificial Brains**

An artificial brain is a human-made machine with a set of software and hardware that mimic the cognitive abilities of the human or animal brain. The research to create an artificial brain is still a continuing discipline and is seeing significant advances in recent times. The approaches involved in creating artificial brains are of two types:

- Large-scale simulations are conducted that mirror the biological functions of the human brain with the current set of supercomputers.
- Constructing neuromorphic (like a neuron) computing devices that have an enormous storage capacity and are created to resemble neural tissues in the brain.

The initiative to create an artificial brain is driven by the need to study human consciousness and its mechanisms. The significance of research on artificial intelligence, constructing an artificial brain, and emulating the brain in science is seen in three primary roles:

- A continuing effort by neuroscientists to study cognitive neuroscience
- An experiment in artificial intelligence to test the theory whether a human-like machine can be created or simulated
- A long-term project based on artificial intelligence (AI) which encompasses technology and devices that are created to mirror human characteristics

"Artificial Brains," © 2021 Omnigraphics. Reviewed June 2021.

Studying and creating artificial brains can help improve neurological conditions in humans, such as Alzheimer and Parkinson diseases. Still, as many experts have pointed out, it can also lead to a machine- or simulation-dependent future.

MECHANISM OF AN ARTIFICIAL BRAIN

A brain model that resembles neuromolecular computing processes has three main components. The first component is the artificial neuron, whose input and output behavior is controlled by the internal dynamics of the artificial brain. For an artificial brain to function as expected, it must also possess simulated enzymatic neuron functions, which are controlled by cytoskeletal dynamics and reaction-diffusion neurons. The second component is the crucial learning algorithm. A significant reason for the artificial brain project is the learning capacity of the human brain. The learning algorithm will enable the artificial neurons to work in tandem to recognize patterns, seek targets, or any other specific function. The third component comprises the reference neuron scheme that is involved in memory manipulation. It is expected to direct the artificial brain to repeat neural networks for coherent behavior.

Much like how the neuron is the functional unit of the biological brain, an artificial neuron is the same for an artificial brain. A network of these neurons communicating together through artificial synapses is called an "artificial neural network" (ANN). An ANN helps create machines required to resemble human brains in terms of reasoning, imagination, and common sense, and is a simulation that helps to recreate the neural network in the human brain to help computers learn and make decisions similar to humans. ANNs are created by calibrating designated computers to interact with each other like interconnected neurons. ANNs use layers of mathematical processes to simplify ingoing data where the artificial neurons are arranged in layers. Input layers accept incoming data. The next layer consists of hidden units or layers that process the information into a usable form for the output units. The network learns about the data as it moves between layers.

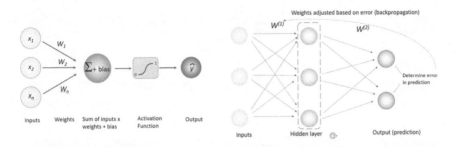

Figure 44.1. Artificial Neural Network (ANN) *(Source: U.S. Food and Drug Administration (FDA).)*

Artificial neural networks constantly try to replicate the hierarchy present in the human brain. Suppose the ANN makes an error in learning patterns or other information in the training process, it uses a technique called "back propagation" to adjust the learning and alter the mathematical equation accordingly. This determines the intelligence of the network. Various applications of ANN can be observed in Facebook's DeepFace technology, Google's Photos application, and in the watch next suggestions of YouTube.

Artificial brain models utilize parts and elements such as the most common metal-oxide-semiconductor-field-effect transistor (MOSFET). They are voltage-controlled similar to the neuron in the brain. Silicon is another element used in recreating the axon, dendrite, and soma regions of the neuron. A device known as the "single-transistor learning synapse" (STLS) is a kind of floating-gate transistor and is used to build synapses that help in machine learning and retrieval. The overall configuration of an artificial brain system consists of:

- An auditory module controlling sound localization, speech separation, speaker, and speech recognition. It uses a microphone as an input device.
- A vision module that controls object, expression, face recognition with a camera as an input device
- A service module that oversees dialogue, knowledge, content recognition management, and response management

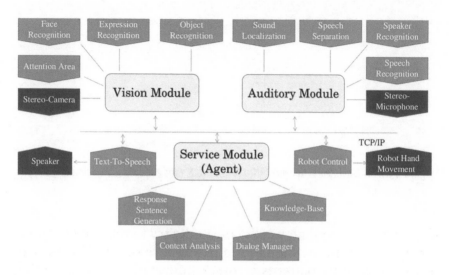

Figure 44.2. Artificial Brain System – Overall Configuration

Certain prominent projects involved in artificial brain technology include:

- The CAM-Brain Machine
- The Blue Brain Project
- Holographic Neural Technology (HNT)

Artificial brains can find purposes in different fields such as healthcare and employment. The recreation of the human brain can alter the dynamics of future civilizations where concepts such as physical death can have a different meaning. Certain artificial brain technologies are looking to reverse the deterioration of the brain cells affected by Alzheimer disease (AD), Parkinson disease (PD), or cerebral palsy (CP) and provide a cure for such conditions. There are ethical issues about creating artificial brains concerning human-machine interactions. Still, if these technologies are used for their intended purpose, artificial brains can become a boon for the future of medicine and other associated fields.

References

1. "Artificial Brain," Wikipedia, January 2, 2021.
2. "Artificial Brains," Artificial Brains, January 15, 2012.
3. Marr, Bernard. "What Are Artificial Neural Networks – a Simple Explanation for Absolutely Anyone," Bernard Marr and Co., September 24, 2018.
4. "A New Approach to Pharmacometrics: Recurrent Neural Networks for Modeling Drug Exposure and Drug Response," U.S. Food and Drug Administration (FDA), April 26, 2021.
5. Hasler, Jennifer. "We Could Build an Artificial Brain Right Now," IEEE Spectrum, June 1, 2017.
6. Zorpette, Glenn. "The Benefits of Building an Artificial Brain," IEEE Spectrum, May 31, 2017.

Chapter 45 | Artificial Intelligence: Improving Lives

Argonne implements laboratory-wide AI for Science initiative – leveraging world-class facilities, exploring new AI techniques, building collaboration, transforming traditional research methods, and driving discovery.

Commitment to developing artificial intelligence (AI) as a national research strategy in the United States may have unequivocally defined 2019 as the Year of AI – particularly at the federal level, more specifically throughout the U.S. Department of Energy (DOE) and its national laboratory complex.

In February, the White House established the Executive Order on Maintaining American Leadership in Artificial Intelligence (American AI Initiative) to expand the nation's leadership role in AI research. Its goals are to fuel economic growth, enhance national security and improve quality of life.

The initiative injects substantial and much-needed research dollars into federal facilities across the United States, promoting technology advances and innovation and enhancing collaboration with nongovernment partners and allies abroad.

In response, the DOE has made AI – along with exascale supercomputing and quantum computing – a major element of its $5.5 billion scientific research and development (R&D) budget and

This chapter includes text excerpted from "Artificial Intelligence: Transforming Science, Improving Lives," Argonne National Laboratory (ANL), U.S. Department of Energy (DOE), September 30, 2019.

established the Artificial Intelligence and Technology Office, which will serve to coordinate AI work being done across the DOE.

Engaging nearly 350 members of the AI community, the town hall served to stimulate conversation around expanding the development and use of AI, while addressing critical challenges by using the initiative framework called "AI for Science."

"AI for Science requires new research and infrastructure, and we have to move a lot of data around and keep track of thousands of models," says Rick Stevens, Associate Laboratory Director for Argonne's Computing, Environment and Life Sciences (CELS) Directorate and a professor of computer science at the University of Chicago.

"How do we distribute this production capability to thousands of people? We need to have system software with different capabilities for AI than for simulation software to optimize workflows. And these are just a few of the issues we have to begin to consider."

The conversation has just begun and continues through laboratory-wide talks and events, such as a recent AI for Science workshop aimed at growing interest in AI capabilities through technical hands-on sessions.

Argonne also will host DOE's Innovation XLab Artificial Intelligence Summit in Chicago, meant to showcase the assets and capabilities of the national laboratories and facilitate an exchange of information and ideas between industry, universities, investors, and end-use customers with Lab innovators and experts.

WHAT EXACTLY IS ARTIFICIAL INTELLIGENCE?

Ask any number of researchers to define AI and you are bound to get – well, first, a long pause and perhaps a chuckle – a range of answers from the more conventional "utilizing computing to mimic the way we interpret data but at a scale not possible by human capability" to "a technology that augments the human brain."

Taken together, AI might well be viewed as a multicomponent toolbox that enables computers to learn, recognize patterns, solve problems, explore complex datasets and adapt to changing conditions – much like humans, but one day, maybe better.

While the definitions and the tools may vary, the goals remain the same: utilize or develop the most advanced AI technologies to more effectively address the most pressing issues in science, medicine, and technology, and accelerate discovery in those areas.

At Argonne, AI has become a critical tool for modeling and prediction across almost all areas where the Laboratory has significant domain expertise: chemistry, materials, photon science, environmental and manufacturing sciences, biomedicine, genomics, and cosmology.

A key component of Argonne's AI toolbox is a technique called "machine learning" and its derivatives, such as deep learning. The latter is built on neural networks comprising many layers of artificial neurons that learn internal representations of data, mimicking human information-gathering-processing systems such as the brain.

"Deep learning is the use of multi-layered neural networks to do machine learning, a program that gets smarter or more accurate as it gets more data to learn from. It is very successful at learning to solve problems," says Stevens.

A staunch supporter of AI, particularly deep learning, Stevens is principal investigator on a multi-institutional effort that is developing the deep neural network application CANDLE (CANcer Distributed Learning Environment), that integrates deep learning with novel data, modeling, and simulation techniques to accelerate cancer research.

Coupled with the power of Argonne's forthcoming exascale computer Aurora – which has the capacity to deliver a billion-billion calculations per second – the CANDLE environment will enable a more personalized and effective approach to cancer treatment.

And that is just a small sample of AI's potential in science. Currently, all across Argonne, researchers are involved in more than 60 AI-related investigations, many of them driven by machine learning.

Argonne Distinguished Fellow Valerie Taylor's work looks at how applications execute on computers and large-scale, high-performance computing systems. Using machine learning, she and her colleagues model an execution's behavior and then use that model to provide feedback on how to best modify the application for better performance.

"Better performance may be shorter execution time or, using generated metrics such as energy, it may be reducing the average power," says Taylor, director of Argonne's Mathematics and Computer Science (MCS) division. "We use statistical analysis to develop the models and identify hints on how to modify the application."

Material scientists are exploring the use of machine learning to optimize models of complex material properties in the discovery and design of new materials that could benefit energy storage, electronics, renewable energy resources, and additive manufacturing, to name just a few areas.

And still more projects address complex transportation and vehicle efficiency issues by enhancing engine design, minimizing road congestion, increasing energy efficiency, and improving safety.

BEYOND THE DEEP

Beyond deep learning, there are many subranges of AI that people have been working on for years, notes Stevens. "And while machine learning now dominates, something else might emerge as a strength."

Natural language processing, for example, is commercially recognizable as voice-activated technologies – think Siri – and on-the-fly language translators. Exceeding those capabilities is its ability to review, analyze and summarize information about a given topic from journal articles, reports, and other publications, and extract and coalesce select information from massive and disparate datasets.

Immersive visualization can place us into 3D worlds of our own making, interject objects or data into our current reality or improve upon human pattern recognition. Argonne researchers have found applications for virtual and augmented reality in the 3D visualization of complicated data sets and the detection of flaws or instabilities in mechanical systems.

And of course, there is robotics – a program started at Argonne in the late 1940s and rebooted in 1999 – that is just beginning to take advantage of Argonne's expanding AI toolkit, whether to conduct research in a specific domain or improve upon its more utilitarian use in decommissioning nuclear power plants.

Until recently, according to Stevens, AI has been a loose collection of methods using very different underlying mechanisms, and the people using them were not necessarily communicating their progress or potentials with one another.

But, with a federal initiative in hand and a laboratory-wide vision, that is beginning to change.

Among those trying to find new ways to collaborate and combine these different AI methods is Marius Stan, a computational scientist in Argonne's Applied Materials division (AMD) and a senior fellow at both the University of Chicago's Consortium for Advanced Science and Engineering and the Northwestern-Argonne Institute for Science and Engineering.

Stan leads a research area called "intelligent materials design" that focuses on combining different elements of AI to discover and design new materials and to optimize and control complex synthesis and manufacturing processes.

Work on the latter has created a collaboration between Stan and colleagues in the Applied Materials and Energy Systems divisions, and the Argonne Leadership Computing Facility (ALCF), a DOE Office of Science User Facility.

Merging machine learning and computer vision with the Flame Spray Pyrolysis technology at Argonne's Materials Engineering Research Facility, the team has developed an AI "intelligent software" that can optimize, in real time, the manufacturing process.

"Our idea was to use the AI to better understand and control in real time – first in a virtual, experimental setup, then in reality – a complex synthesis process," says Stan.

Automating the process leads to a safer and much faster process compared to those led by humans. But, even more, intriguing is the potential that the AI process might observe materials with better properties than did the researchers.

WHAT DROVE US TO ARTIFICIAL INTELLIGENCE

Whether or not they concur on a definition, most researchers will agree that the impetus for the escalation of AI in scientific research was the influx of massive data sets and the computing power to sift, sort, and analyze it.

Not only was the push coming from big corporations brimming with user data, but the tools that drive science were getting more expansive – bigger and better telescopes and accelerators and of course supercomputers, on which they could run larger, multiscale simulations.

"The size of the simulations we are running is so big, the problems that we are trying to solve are getting bigger so that these AI methods can no longer be seen as a luxury, but as a must-have technology," notes Prasanna Balaprakash, a computer scientist in MCS and ALCF.

Data and compute size also drove the convergence of more traditional techniques, such as simulation and data analysis, with machine and deep learning. Where analysis of data generated by simulation would eventually lead to changes in an underlying model, that data is now being fed back into machine learning models and used to guide more precise simulations.

"More or less anybody who is doing large-scale computation is adopting an approach that puts machine learning in the middle of this complex computing process and AI will continue to integrate with simulation in new ways," says Stevens.

"And where the majority of users are in theory-modeling-simulation, they will be integrated with experimentalists on data-intense efforts. So the population of people who will be part of this initiative will be more diverse."

But, while AI is leading to faster time-to-solution and more precise results, the number of data points, parameters, and iterations required to get to those results can still prove monumental.

Focused on the automated design and development of scalable algorithms, Balaprakash and his Argonne colleagues are developing new types of AI algorithms and methods to more efficiently solve large-scale problems that deal with different ranges of data. These additions are intended to make existing systems scale better on supercomputers, such as those housed at the ALCF; a necessity in the light of exascale computing.

"We are developing an automated machine learning system for a wide range of scientific applications, from analyzing cancer drug data to climate modeling," says Balaprakash. "One way to speed up a simulation is to replace the computationally expensive part with an AI-based predictive model that can make the simulation faster."

INDUSTRY SUPPORT

The AI techniques that are expected to drive discovery are only as good as the tech that drives them, making collaboration between industry and the national labs essential.

"Industry is investing a tremendous amount in building up AI tools," says Taylor. "Their efforts should not be duplicated, but they should be leveraged. Also, industry comes in with a different perspective, so by working together, the solutions become more robust."

Argonne has long had relationships with computing manufacturers to deliver a succession of ever-more-powerful machines to handle the exponential growth in data size and simulation scale. Its most recent partnership is that with semiconductor chip manufacturer Intel and supercomputer manufacturer Cray to develop the exascale machine Aurora.

But, the Laboratory is also collaborating with a host of other industrial partners in the development or provision of everything from chip design to deep learning-enabled video cameras.

One of these, Cerebras, is working with Argonne to test a first-of-its-kind AI accelerator that provides a 100–500 times improvement over existing AI accelerators. As its first U.S. customer, Argonne will deploy the Cerebras CS-1 to enhance scientific AI models for cancer, cosmology, brain imaging, and materials science, among others.

The National Science Foundation-funded Array of Things, a partnership between Argonne, the University of Chicago, and the City of Chicago, actively seeks commercial vendors to supply technologies for its edge computing network of programmable, multisensor devices.

But, Argonne and the other national labs are not the only ones to benefit from these collaborations. Companies understand the value in working with such organizations, recognizing that the AI tools developed by the labs, combined with the kinds of large-scale problems they seek to solve, offer industry unique benefits in terms of business transformation and economic growth, explains Balaprakash.

"Companies are interested in working with us because of the type of scientific applications that we have for machine learning," he adds "What we have is so diverse, it makes them think a lot harder about how to architect a chip or design software for these types of workloads and science applications. It's a win-win for both of us."

ARTIFICIAL INTELLIGENCE'S FUTURE, OUR FUTURE

"There is one area where I do not see AI surpassing humans any time soon, and that is hypotheses formulation," says Stan, "because that requires creativity. Humans propose interesting projects and for that, you need to be creative, make correlations, propose something out of the ordinary. It is still human territory but machines may soon take the lead.

"It may happen," he says and adds that he is working on it.

In the meantime, Argonne researchers continue to push the boundaries of existing AI methods and forge new components for the AI toolbox. Deep learning techniques such as neuromorphic algorithms that exhibit the adaptive nature of insects in an equally small computational space can be used at the "edge" – where there are few computing resources; as in cell phones or urban sensors.

An optimizing neural network called a "neural architecture search," where one neural network system improves another, is helping to automate deep-learning-based predictive model development in several scientific and engineering domains, such as cancer drug discovery and weather forecasting using supercomputers.

Just as big data and better computational tools drove the convergence of simulation, data analysis, and visualization, the introduction of the exascale computer Aurora into the Argonne complex of leadership-class tools and experts will only serve to accelerate the evolution of AI and witness its full assimilation into traditional techniques.

The tools may change, the definitions may change, but AI is here to stay as an integral part of the scientific method and our lives.

Chapter 46 | **Augmented Reality**

The COVID-19 pandemic has highlighted the need for transformation of remote learning to not only survive a wave of crisis but to potentially fit the new normal. A trend among governments across the world has been emerging to emphasize the potential for new technologies such as artificial intelligence and virtual/augmented reality to mitigate the problems remote learning has compared to on-site learning, such as academic dishonesty, decreased social aspects of studying, lack of practical kinesthetic interactions, problems keeping students' attention, the practice of technological boundaries, etc. As these are complex and expensive technologies, a decision for their use must be based not on technological hype but scientifically validated outcomes. When it became clear that remote learning will have to be extended after the first wave, the government of The Republic of Latvia initiated a research program in technological transformation of remote education.

A six month long research program providing a 500,000 EUR grant to an interdisciplinary team of researchers from multiple research institutions to evaluate how the Latvian society dealt with the coronavirus crisis and to provide recommendations for societal resilience in the future. The project has several work packages including study of societal dynamics in Latvia during this crisis, evaluation of labor market and employment structures, psychological effects of COVID-19 on individuals and families, evaluation of media and health communication, strategic communication, and

This chapter includes text excerpted from "Use of Augmented and Virtual Reality in Remote Higher Education: A Systematic Umbrella Review," Education Resources Information Center (ERIC), U.S. Department of Education (ED), December 31, 2020.

governance, and finally education transformation. This work is part of this project, specifically the last work package, and is aimed at finding evidence of the impact of virtual reality (VR) and augmented reality (AR) technologies on remote learning in higher education-specifically impact on performance and engagement. This is done through a systematic umbrella literature review-a review of literature reviews. The review conforms to PRISMA guidelines.

In order to determine if AR/VR technologies might be beneficial to technological transformation of remote learning, in this chapter an umbrella review of related literature is described. The results show that most of the current experiments pertain to organizing laboratory or practical exercises within virtual or augmented reality in cases when physical presence is not feasible. This overall seems to provide positive results, except for a few cases. In cases where practical, spatial, or kinesthetic skills have required the results were very encouraging, especially in medicine-related education. In addition to the specific results extracted, the literature also suggests that virtual/augmented reality is not capable of completely replacing on-site studies, because whenever it was tried, the student grades suffered.

This could be explained by multiple mechanisms, the three more plausible ones are (a) either the AR/VR technologies actually impact the learning process directly, or (b) they impact the outcomes indirectly for example, these technologies might improve social contact, which in turn improves overall outcomes or (c) the result might be due to a novelty and thus diminish in time as well as stop functioning if new novelty technique is introduced. The latter can only be distinguished if the same group of students is followed through several semesters. The fact that in all interventions where engagement was measured, the engagement increased, leads to speculate that the novelty of technology used has a direct positive impact on engagement. If this is the case, it means that novelty itself is a potential intervention, and any newly hyped technology could provide similar results. If this is true then another question should be researched – whether there exists a cumulative novelty resistance and whether it accumulates for a person in general with any novelty, or just a subset. Does "acumulative novelty resistance"-the effect when introducing next new technology to study process with purpose of increasing the engagement and/or performance of students have any effect due to satiation. The possibility of such novelty requirements could lead to future experiments to determine the best way to keep the engagement and performance of students until the end of the study year. In every study that showed an increase in performance or engagement, the course was well designed and teachers had good qualifications to use the benefits of AR/VR for learning purposes, however, AR/VR is not a panacea. In cases when students or teachers were not familiar with AR/VR technologies or when courses were not adapted well for AR/VR usage or when teacher of the course was not prepared enough to work with AR/VR, a notable decrease in performance was noted in the articles explored. This leads to a highly vital conclusion-an unprepared teacher cannot prepare a student well. The potential solution is 1. create courses for teachers and lecturers on how to prepare/adapt courses for AR/VR; 2. create a framework that would allow teachers easily prepare/adopt their material for AR/VR; 3. Do not overload students with need to get familiar with AR/VR in a short time. there should be a possibility to use classical methods to get through the course; At the same time, AR/VR proved that it could help to understand abstract and complex content more easily due to good visualization capabilities and interactivity. In multiple of the reviewed articles, it was shown that kinesthetic learning, when instead of a classic lecture, students are working in 3-D world, performing experiments alone or together with a teacher, is much more efficient than, previously mentioned, classic method.

The creation of AR/VR adopted courses could have a great effect on knowledge availability. An opinion in the educational community and society at large that has been reinforced by the 2020 lockdown, is that online learning currently could be the future of education. If this is the case, then based on the fact that multiple papers show that AR/VR labs are of similar benefits as traditional "offline" labs with real equipment, it could be argued that properly adopted AR/VR based courses could, potentially, raise good, qualified specialists all around the globe, not only in local regions, democratizing education in hands-on skills. Performance is not the only factor that needs to be taken into account, emotional wellness is at least as important, as performance in terms of grades. Scientific groups that were researching Virtual Worlds as a substitution for university environment showed that students feel much better if they could see their avatar in some virtual world, they could associate with, walk around virtual campus and explore it, like it would be real university. It also must be noted that VR is still relatively complex and expensive technology and even though the prices are going down, still outfitting each student with VR/AR systems for remote learning is a complex and expensive task, which suggests that some of the future remote learning could happen from semi-centralized labs outfitted with VR/AR technologies, where students could arrive at work, but educators would connect remotely.

Chapter 47 | **Virtual Reality**

Research has shown that virtual reality (VR) can be put to medical use to help distract patients during painful procedures, such as changing the bandages on severe burn victims. For example, some people with severe burns who used VR during wound care reported not noticing what is normally an excruciating process.

Brennan Spiegel, M.D., sees technology as far more powerful than a short-term distraction. "The question now is, can it really help not just with acute pain, but with chronic pain," asks Spiegel, Cedars-Sinai Medical Center in Los Angeles, California.

Spiegel personally tested VR after a colleague recommended that he check it out.

"First he had me jump off a building, and I realized my brain had been hijacked, completely commandeered by this headset," Spiegel, said of his first VR experience. "That is when I realized the power of this and how it could change our perception of the world."

Spiegel is investigating the use of VR to help ease chronic pain. His research is part of the Back Pain Consortium (BACPAC), a patient-centered effort to address the need for effective and personalized therapies for chronic low back pain. BACPAC is an innovative, integrative approach looking at biological and psychological contributors to pain within the Helping to End Addiction LongtermSM Initiative, or the National Institutes of Health (NIH) HEAL InitiativeSM's clinical research in the pain management focus area.

In this work, VR involves the use of a headset over the eyes to allow people to experience three-dimensional immersive environments. The simulated sights, sounds, and engaging experiences, such as swimming with dolphins or walking up waterfalls, transport users to a different world far from their pain.

This chapter includes text excerpted from "Using Virtual Reality to Treat Real Pain," National Institutes of Health (NIH), December 22, 2020.

Spiegel and his colleagues hope VR can provide immersive experiences that absorb more of the brain's attention. With fewer mental resources left to process pain signals, people perceive less pain. Usually, he explains, less pain means less dependence on pain medication and a lower risk of opioid addiction.

Spiegel describes chronic low back pain as "one of the most common forms of chronic pain in America, and one that frequently leads to opioid use."

He hopes to integrate VR into the management of chronic lower back pain "not just for a few minutes, but to actually teach people something about their body and their mind – their consciousness even."

As part of this effort, Spiegel and his team are engaged in a three-part research study to determine the effectiveness of different VR approaches. The first, educational part of the study examines whether VR can be used to effectively teach techniques, such as mental imagery and biofeedback to slow heart rate, reduce anxiety, and manage pain, which is essentially the same techniques used for centuries to alleviate pain during childbirth.

In one example, VR users see a computer image of a tree. Changing how a person breathes alters the tree in a game-like scenario. Spiegel describes breathing life into the tree as a way to learn ways to cope with pain later without the aid of VR.

The second, part immerses participants in a virtual world to distract them from real-world sensations. It is the same approach used to help burn patients better endure bandage changes.

The final part looks at whether the act of putting on a VR headset, regardless of the content being shown, affects the perception of pain. In this scenario, study participants wear VR headsets, but their experience is more like watching a nature show on a widescreen television, rather than being fully immersed in a three-dimensional environment.

Despite the on-going COVID-19 pandemic, Spiegel's team has been able to continue moving forward since the entire study is being carried out remotely. Participants receive a VR headset and other equipment by mail and interact with researchers over the Internet.

Spiegel likens the VR process to home delivery of "a pain psychologist that can be experienced in three-dimensional fantastical worlds at a time and place of [participants'] choosing."

This model for VR therapy could be especially helpful in isolated, rural areas with limited access to specialty care. These same areas tend to be hard-hit by opioid misuse.

WHAT THE FUTURE HOLDS

A growing number of researchers are optimizing VR for medical use. If the trend continues, Spiegel hopes that in the future, VR technology could be used routinely to augment existing pain management techniques.

In line with this trend, the U.S. Department of Food and Drug Administration (FDA) is looking to create frameworks for how to manage future VR products as they are developed. Current chronic low back pain treatment options are not very effective, which has led to increased use of opioids. As the VR medical research field grows, Spiegel predicts that it has the potential to be a useful medical tool to augment existing pain management techniques.

Chapter 48 | **Computational Modeling**

WHAT IS COMPUTATIONAL MODELING?

Computational modeling is the use of computers to simulate and study complex systems using mathematics, physics, and computer science. A computational model contains numerous variables that characterize the system being studied. Simulation is done by adjusting the variables alone or in combination and observing the outcomes. Computer modeling allows scientists to conduct thousands of simulated experiments by computer. The thousands of computer experiments identify the handful of laboratory experiments that are most likely to solve the problem being studied.

Today's computational models can study a biological system at multiple levels. Models of how the disease develops include molecular processes, cell to cell interactions, and how those changes affect tissues and organs. Studying systems at multiple levels is known as "multiscale modeling" (MSM).

HOW IS COMPUTATIONAL MODELING USED TO STUDY COMPLEX SYSTEMS?

Weather forecasting models make predictions based on numerous atmospheric factors. Accurate weather predictions can protect life and property and help utility companies plan for power increases that occur with extreme climate shifts.

Flight simulators use complex equations that govern how aircraft fly and react to factors, such as turbulence, air density, and

This chapter includes text excerpted from "Computational Modeling," National Institute of Biomedical Imaging and Bioengineering (NIBIB), May 2020.

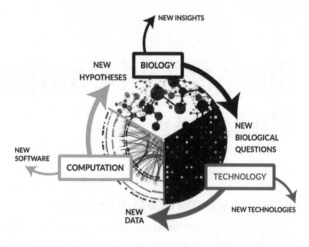

Figure 48.1. Computational Modeling

precipitation. Simulators are used to train pilots, design aircraft, and study how aircraft are affected as conditions change.

Earthquake simulations aim to save lives, buildings, and infrastructure. Computational models predict how the composition, and motion of structures interact with the underlying surfaces to affect what happens during an earthquake.

HOW CAN COMPUTATIONAL MODELING IMPROVE MEDICAL CARE AND RESEARCH?
Tracking Infectious Diseases

Computational models are being used to track infectious diseases in populations, identify the most effective interventions, and monitor and adjust interventions to reduce the spread of disease. Identifying and implementing interventions that curb the spread of disease is critical for saving lives and reducing stress on the health-care system during infectious disease pandemics.

Clinical Decision Support

Computational models intelligently gather, filter, analyze and present health information to provide guidance to doctors for disease treatment based on detailed characteristics of each patient. The systems help to provide informed and consistent care of a patient as they transfer to appropriate hospital facilities and departments and receive various tests during their course of treatment.

Predicting Drug Side Effects
Researchers use computational modeling to help design drugs that will be the safest for patients and least likely to have side effects. The approach can reduce the many years needed to develop a safe and effective medication.

HOW ARE NIBIB-FUNDED RESEARCHERS USING COMPUTATIONAL MODELING TO IMPROVE HEALTH?
Modeling Infectious Disease Spread to Identify Effective Interventions
Modeling infectious diseases accurately rely on numerous large sets of data. For example, evaluation of the efficacy of social distancing on the spread of flu-like illness must include information on friendships and interactions of individuals, as well as standard biometric and demographic data. The National Institute of Biomedical Imaging and Bioengineering (NIBIB)-funded researchers are developing new computational tools that can incorporate newly available data sets into models designed to identify the best courses of action and the most effective interventions during the pandemic spread of infectious disease and other public-health emergencies.

Tracking Viral Evolution during the Spread of Infectious Disease
Ribonucleic acid (RNA) viruses, such as HIV, hepatitis B, and coronavirus continually mutate to develop drug resistance, escape immune response, and establish new infections. Samples of sequenced pathogens from thousands of infected individuals can be used to identify millions of evolving viral variants. The NIBIB-funded researchers are creating computational tools to incorporate this important data into infectious disease analysis by health-care professionals. The new tools will be created in partnership with the Centers for Disease Control (CDC) and made available online

to researchers and health-care workers. The project will enhance worldwide disease surveillance and treatment and enable the development of more effective disease eradication strategies.

Transforming Wireless Health Data into Improved Health and Healthcare

Health monitoring devices at hospitals and wearable sensors, such as smartwatches generate vast amounts of health data in real time. Data-driven medical care promises to be fast, accurate, and less expensive, but the continual data streams currently overwhelm the ability to use the information. NIBIB-funded researchers are developing computational models that convert streaming health data into a useful form. The new models will provide real-time physiological monitoring for clinical decision-making at the Nationwide Children's Hospital. A team of mathematicians, biomedical informaticians, and hospital staff will generate publicly shared data and software. The project will leverage the $11 billion wireless health market to significantly improve healthcare.

Human and Machine Learning for Customized Control of Assistive Robots

The more severe a person's motor impairment, the more challenging it is to operate assistive machines, such as powered wheelchairs and robotic arms. Available controls, such as sip-and-puff devices are not adequate for persons with severe paralysis. NIBIB-funded researchers are engineering a system to enable people with tetraplegia to control a robotic arm while promoting exercise and maintenance of residual motor skills. The technology uses body-machine interfaces that respond to minimal movement in limbs, head, tongue, shoulders, and eyes. Initially, when the user moves, machine learning augments the signal to perform a task with a robotic arm. Help is scaled back as the machine transfers control to the progressively skilled user. The approach aims to empower people with severe paralysis and provide an interface to safely learn to control robotic assistants.

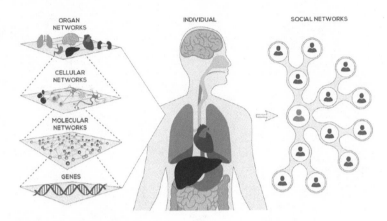

Figure 48.2. Multiscale Modeling

Chapter 49 | **Stem Cell Research**

WHAT ARE STEM CELLS, AND WHY ARE THEY IMPORTANT?

Stem cells have the remarkable potential to renew themselves. They can develop into many different cell types in the body during early life and growth. Researchers study many different types of stem cells. There are several main categories: the "pluripotent stem cells" (embryonic stem cells and induced pluripotent stem cells) and "nonembryonic" or "somatic" stem cells (commonly called "adult stem cells"). Pluripotent stem cells have the ability to differentiate into all of the cells of the adult body. Adult stem cells are found in a tissue or organ and can differentiate to yield the specialized cell types of that tissue or organ.

Pluripotent Stem Cells

Early mammalian embryos at the blastocyst stage contain two types of cells – cells of the inner cell mass, and cells of the trophectoderm. The trophectodermal cells contribute to the placenta. The inner cell mass will ultimately develop into the specialized cell types, tissues, and organs of the entire body of the organism. Previous work with mouse embryos led to the development of a method in 1998 to derive stem cells from the inner cell mass of preimplantation human embryos and to grow human embryonic stem cells (hESCs) in the laboratory. In 2006, researchers identified conditions that would allow some mature human adult cells to be reprogrammed

This chapter contains text excerpted from the following sources: Text beginning with the heading "Pluripotent Stem Cells" is excerpted from "Stem Cell Basics," National Institute on Aging (NIA), National Institutes of Health (NIH), March 13, 2020; Text under the heading "Engineering New Tissues and Organs" is excerpted from "Fixing Flawed Body Parts," *NIH News in Health*, National Institutes of Health (NIH), February 2015. Reviewed June 2021.

into an embryonic stem cell-like state. Those reprogramed stem cells are called "induced pluripotent stem cells" (iPSCs).

Adult Stem Cells

Throughout the life of the organism, populations of adult stem cells serve as an internal repair system that generates replacements for cells that are lost through normal wear and tear, injury, or disease. Adult stem cells have been identified in many organs and tissues and are generally associated with specific anatomical locations. These stem cells may remain quiescent (nondividing) for long periods of time until they are activated by a normal need for more cells to maintain and repair tissues.

WHAT ARE THE UNIQUE PROPERTIES OF ALL STEM CELLS?

Stem cells have unique abilities to self-renew and to recreate functional tissues.

Stem Cells Have the Ability to Self-Renew

Unlike muscle cells, blood cells, or nerve cells – which do not normally replicate – stem cells may replicate many times. When a stem cell divides, the resulting two daughter cells may be: 1) both stem cells, 2) a stem cell and a one more differentiated cell, or 3) both more differentiated cells. What controls the balance between these types of divisions to maintain stem cells at an appropriate level within a given tissue is not yet well-known.

Discovering the mechanism behind self-renewal may make it possible to understand how cell fate (stem versus nonstem) is regulated during normal embryonic development and postnatally, or misregulated as during aging, or even in the development of cancer. Such information may also enable scientists to grow stem cells more efficiently in the laboratory. The specific factors and conditions that allow pluripotent stem cells to remain undifferentiated are of great interest to scientists. It has taken many years of trial and error to learn to derive and maintain pluripotent stem cells in the laboratory without the cells spontaneously differentiating into specific cell types.

Stem Cells Have the Ability to Recreate Functional Tissues

Pluripotent stem cells are undifferentiated; they do not have any tissue-specific characteristics (such as morphology or gene expression pattern) that allow them to perform specialized functions. Yet they can give rise to all of the differentiated cells in the body, such as heart muscle cells, blood cells, and nerve cells. On the other hand, adult stem cells differentiate to yield the specialized cell types of the tissue or organ in which they reside, and may have defining morphological features and patterns of gene expression reflective of that tissue.

Different types of stems cells have varying degrees of potency; that is, the number of different cell types that they can form. While differentiating, the cell usually goes through several stages, becoming more specialized at each step. Scientists are beginning to understand the signals that trigger each step of the differentiation process. Signals for cell differentiation include factors secreted by other cells, physical contact with neighboring cells, and certain molecules in the microenvironment.

HOW DO YOU CULTURE STEM CELLS IN THE LABORATORY?

How Are Stem Cells Grown in the Laboratory?

Growing cells in the laboratory is known as "cell culture." Stem cells can proliferate in laboratory environments in a culture dish that contains a nutrient broth known as "culture medium" (which is optimized for growing different types of stem cells). Most stem cells attach, divide, and spread over the surface of the dish.

The culture dish becomes crowded as the cells divide, so they need to be replated in the process of subculturing, which is repeated periodically many times over many months. Each cycle of subculturing is referred to as a "passage." The original cells can yield millions of stem cells. At any stage in the process, batches of cells can be frozen and shipped to other laboratories for further culture and experimentation.

How Do You "Reprogram" Regular Cells to Make iPSCs?

Differentiated cells, such as skin cells, can be reprogrammed back into a pluripotent state. Reprogramming is achieved over several weeks by forced expression of genes that are known to be master regulators of pluripotency. At the end of this process, these master regulators will remodel the expression of an entire network of genes. Features of differentiated cells will be replaced by those associated with the pluripotent state, essentially reversing the developmental process.

How Are Stem Cells Stimulated to Differentiate?

As long as the pluripotent stem cells are grown in culture under appropriate conditions, they can remain undifferentiated. To generate cultures of specific types of differentiated cells, scientists may change the chemical composition of the culture medium, alter the surface of the culture dish, or modify the cells by forcing the expression of specific genes. Through years of experimentation, scientists have established some basic protocols, or "recipes," for the differentiation of pluripotent stem cells into some specific cell types.

What Laboratory Tests Are Used to Identify Stem Cells?

At various points during the process of generating stem cell lines, scientists test the cells to see whether they exhibit the fundamental properties that make them stem cells. These tests may include:

- Verifying expression of multiple genes that have been shown to be important for the function of stem cells
- Checking the rate of proliferation
- Checking the integrity of the genome by examining the chromosomes of selected cells
- Demonstrating the differentiation potential of the cells by removing signals that maintain the cells in their undifferentiated state, which will cause pluripotent stem cells to spontaneously differentiate, or by adding signals that induce adult stem cells to differentiate into appropriate cell phenotypes

HOW ARE STEM CELLS USED IN BIOMEDICAL RESEARCH AND THERAPIES?

Given their unique regenerative abilities, there are many ways in which human stem cells are being used in biomedical research and therapeutics development.

Understanding the Biology of Disease and Testing Drugs

Scientists can use stem cells to learn about human biology and for the development of therapeutics. A better understanding of the genetic and molecular signals that regulate cell division, specialization, and differentiation in stem cells can yield information about how diseases arise and suggest new strategies for therapy. Scientists can use iPSCs made from a patient and differentiate those iPSCs to create "organoids" (small models of organs) or tissue chips for studying diseased cells and testing drugs, with personalized results.

Cell-Based Therapies

An important potential application is the generation of cells and tissues for cell-based therapies, also called "tissue engineering." The current need for transplantable tissues and organs far outweighs the available supply. Stem cells offer the possibility of a renewable source. There is typically a very small number of adult stem cells in each tissue, and once removed from the body, their capacity to divide is limited, making generation of large quantities of adult stem cells for therapies difficult. In contrast, pluripotent stem cells are less limited by starting material and renewal potential.

To realize the promise of stem cell therapies in diseases, scientists must be able to manipulate stem cells so that they possess the necessary characteristics for successful differentiation, transplantation, and engraftment. Scientists must also develop procedures for the administration of stem cell populations, along with the induction of vascularization (supplying blood vessels), for the regeneration and repair of three-dimensional solid tissues.

To be useful for transplant purposes, stem cells must be reproducibly made to:
- Proliferate extensively and generate sufficient quantities of cells for replacing lost or damaged tissues.
- Differentiate into the desired cell type(s).
- Survive in the recipient after transplant.
- Integrate into the surrounding tissue after transplant.
- Avoid rejection by the recipient's immune system.
- Function appropriately for the duration of the recipient's life. While stem cells offer exciting promise

for future therapies, significant technical hurdles remain that will likely only be overcome through years of intensive research.

ENGINEERING NEW TISSUES AND ORGANS

How can you mend a broken heart? Or repair a damaged liver, kidney, or knee? NIH-funded scientists are exploring innovative ways to fix faulty organs and tissues or even grow new ones. This type of research is called "tissue engineering." Exciting advances continue to emerge in this fast-moving field.

Tissue engineering could allow doctors to repair or replace worn-out tissues and organs with living, working parts. Most important, tissue engineering might help some of the 120,000 people on the waitlist to receive donated kidneys, livers, or other organs.

Doctors have long used tissue-engineered skin to heal severe burns or other injuries. But, most tissue engineering methods are still experimental. They have been tested only in laboratory dishes and sometimes in animals, but only a few new approaches have been tested in people. Several clinical studies (involving human volunteers) are in the early stages of testing newly developed tissues.

"With this approach, scientists are combining engineering and biology to restore a damaged organ or tissue, whether it is been damaged by disease or injury or something else," says Dr. Martha Lundberg, an NIH expert in heart-related tissue engineering.

Some scientists are creating special net-like structures, or scaffolds, in desired shapes and then coaxing cells to grow within them. Some use a mixture of natural substances called "growth factors," which direct cells to grow and develop in certain ways.

"Other scientists are using different 3-D bioprinting technologies – some are like fancy inkjet printers – to create new tissues or organs," Lundberg says. They've printed 3-D kidneys and other organs that look like the real thing. But, while most of these printed body parts have the right shape, they're not fully functional.

"Scientists have not yet figured out how to print an organ that includes the correct blood vessel patterns, nerve connections, and other components that come together in a mature organ," Lundberg says. "When creating a new organ, if it can perform the right job and functions, it may not need to look like the real thing."

Many tissue engineering methods use stem cells, which can be nudged to turn into different cell types. One research team guided human stem cells to become a 3-D structure that can respond to light. The method might one day lead to new therapies for eye disorders. Other stem cell approaches may lead to improved treatment for spinal cord injuries, diabetes, and more.

Another approach, called "decellularization," involves removing all the cells from an organ. What's left behind is a thin, pale framework that contains the organ's natural structural proteins, including the pathways for tiny blood vessels and nerves. By infusing new cells into this mesh-like matrix, some researchers have successfully created working animal kidneys, livers, hearts, lungs, and other organs.

The decellularization technique was used by Dr. Martin Yarmush and his colleagues to create a functional rat liver that included a network of working blood vessels. Yarmush is a biomedical engineer at Rutgers University and the Massachusetts General Hospital. The engineered livers his team created were kept alive in the laboratory for days and functioned for several hours after transplantation into rats. The researchers are now working to help those transplanted livers survive even longer. They're also scaling up the methods to create a decellularized human liver that can be repopulated with functional cells.

"A parallel effort we are pursuing involves taking a donated organ that is not considered transplantable for a particular reason, and then using a reconditioning solution and perhaps even stem cells to revitalize the organ so it becomes transplantable," Yarmush says.

Other researchers are working to repair damaged body parts that are still in the body. At the University of Washington in Seattle, Dr. Charles Murry and colleagues are searching for ways to fix injured hearts. One of their latest studies used human stem cells to repair damaged hearts in monkeys. The stem cells were coaxed to become early-stage heart cells, which were then infused near the heart injury.

The new cells made their way into the damaged heart muscle and organized into muscle fibers in all of the treated monkeys. The infused stem cells replaced nearly half of the damaged heart tissue and began beating in sync with the heart. Still, the scientists note they need years of research before this type of therapy might be tried in people.

Some methods are already being tested in humans. Dr. Martha Murray, a surgeon at Boston Children's Hospital, is exploring new ways to heal a common knee injury known as a "torn anterior cruciate ligament" (ACL). Athletes who do a lot of twisting and turning, as in basketball or soccer, are at risk for damaging the ACL.

"Typical treatment today, called "ACL reconstruction," works well, and it gets patients back to the playing field at a relatively high rate," Murray says. But, the surgery involves removing a piece of tendon from elsewhere in the body and using that to replace the ACL. "So it involves making 2 injuries that the body has to heal from. And even with this treatment, patients still develop arthritis in the knee 15 to 20 years later," Murray adds. "We wanted to find a better therapy – something less invasive."

After testing several biomaterials, Murray's team found that stitching a bioengineered sponge between the torn ends of an injured ACL allows blood to clot and collect around the damaged ligament. Because blood naturally contains stem cells and growth factors, the blood-soaked sponge acts as a "bridge" that encourages ACL healing. The sponge is made of some of the same proteins normally found in ligaments, and it dissolves after a few weeks.

Studies in large animals showed that the bioengineered sponge was much less likely to lead to arthritis, and it healed ACL injuries as well as standard reconstruction surgery. The U.S. Food and Drug Administration (FDA) recently approved human safety testing of the sponge in 10 people with ACL injuries.

Metal, plastic, and other nonbiological devices can also replace or enhance malfunctioning body parts. One promising possibility still in development is an artificial kidney that could be implanted in the body and used in place of dialysis to treat end-stage kidney disease. Scientists are also studying a synthetic glue modeled after a natural adhesive that might help to repair tissues in the body. You can learn more about these and other cutting-edge studies at www.nibib.nih.gov/science-education/bionic-man.

Chapter 50 | Genome Sequencing

WHAT IS DNA SEQUENCING?

Sequencing deoxyribonucleic acid (DNA) means determining the order of the four chemical building blocks – called "bases" – that make up the DNA molecule. The sequence tells scientists the kind of genetic information that is carried in a particular DNA segment. For example, scientists can use sequence information to determine which stretches of DNA contain genes and which stretches carry regulatory instructions, turning genes on or off. In addition, and importantly, sequence data can highlight changes in a gene that may cause disease.

In the DNA double helix, the four chemical bases always bond with the same partner to form "base pairs." Adenine (A) always pairs with thymine (T); cytosine (C) always pairs with guanine (G). This pairing is the basis for the mechanism by which DNA molecules are copied when cells divide, and the pairing also underlies the methods by which most DNA sequencing experiments are done. The human genome contains about 3 billion base pairs that spell out the instructions for making and maintaining a human being.

HOW NEW IS DNA SEQUENCING?

Since the completion of the Human Genome Project, technological improvements and automation have increased speed and lowered costs to the point where individual genes can be sequenced

This chapter includes text excerpted from "DNA Sequencing Fact Sheet," National Human Genome Research Institute (NHGRI), August 16, 2020.

routinely, and some labs can sequence well over 100,000 billion bases per year, and an entire genome can be sequenced for just a few thousand dollars.

Many of these new technologies were developed with support from the National Human Genome Research Institute (NHGRI) Genome Technology Program and its Advanced DNA Sequencing Technology awards. One of NHGRI's goals is to promote new technologies that could eventually reduce the cost of sequencing a human genome of even higher quality than is possible today and for less than $1,000.

ARE NEWER SEQUENCING TECHNOLOGIES UNDER DEVELOPMENT?

One new sequencing technology involves watching DNA polymerase molecules as they copy DNA – the same molecules that make new copies of DNA in our cells – with a very fast movie camera and microscope, and incorporating different colors of bright dyes, one each for the letters A, T, C, and G. This method provides different and very valuable information than what is provided by the instrument systems that are in most common use.

Another new technology in development entails the use of nanopores to sequence DNA. Nanopore-based DNA sequencing involves threading single DNA strands through extremely tiny pores in a membrane. DNA bases are read one at a time as they squeeze through the nanopore. The bases are identified by measuring differences in their effect on ions and electrical current flowing through the pore. Using nanopores to sequence DNA offers many potential advantages over current methods. The goal is for sequencing to cost less and be done faster. Unlike sequencing methods currently in use, nanopore DNA sequencing means researchers can study the same molecule over and over again.

WHAT DO IMPROVEMENTS IN DNA SEQUENCING MEAN FOR HUMAN HEALTH?

Researchers now are able to compare large stretches of DNA – 1 million bases or more – from different individuals quickly and cheaply. Such comparisons can yield an enormous amount of information about the role of inheritance in susceptibility to disease and in response to environmental influences. In addition, the ability to sequence the genome more rapidly and cost-effectively creates vast potential for diagnostics and therapies.

Although routine DNA sequencing in the doctor's office is still many years away, some large medical centers have begun to use sequencing to detect and treat some diseases. In cancer, for example, physicians are increasingly able to use sequence data to identify the particular type of cancer a patient has. This enables the physician to make better choices for treatments.

Researchers in the NHGRI-supported Undiagnosed Diseases Program use DNA sequencing to try to identify the genetic causes of rare diseases. Other researchers are studying its use in screening newborns for disease and disease risk.

Moreover, The Cancer Genome Atlas project, which is supported by NHGRI and the National Cancer Institute, is using DNA sequencing to unravel the genomic details of some 30 cancer types. Another National Institutes of Health program examines how gene activity is controlled in different tissues and the role of gene regulation in disease. Ongoing and planned large-scale projects use DNA sequencing to examine the development of common and complex diseases, such as heart disease and diabetes, and in inherited diseases that cause physical malformations, developmental delay, and metabolic diseases.

Comparing the genome sequences of different types of animals and organisms, such as chimpanzees and yeast, can also provide insights into the biology of development and evolution.

Chapter 51 | Medical Applications of 3D Printing

Three-dimensional (3D) printers are used to manufacture a variety of medical devices, including those with complex geometry or features that match a patient's unique anatomy.

Some devices are printed from a standard design to make multiple identical copies of the same device. Other devices, called "patient-matched" or "patient-specific devices," are created from a specific patient's imaging data.

Commercially available 3D printed medical devices include:
- Instrumentation (e.g., guides to assist with the proper surgical placement of a device),
- Implants (e.g., cranial plates or hip joints), and
- External prostheses (e.g., hands).

Scientists are researching how to use the 3D printing process to manufacture living organs, such as a heart or liver, but this research is in the early stages of development.

The 3D printing process can be accomplished using any of several different technologies. The choice of technology can depend on many factors including how the final product will be used and how easy the printer is to use. The most common technology used for

This chapter contains text excerpted from the following sources: Text in this chapter begins with excerpts from "Medical Applications of 3D Printing," U.S. Food and Drug Administration (FDA), December 4, 2017. Reviewed June 2021; Text beginning with the heading "Medical Devices, Accessories, Components, and Parts during the COVID-19 Pandemic" is excerpted from "3D Printing Medical Equipment in Response to the COVID-19 Pandemic," National Institutes of Health (NIH), August 7, 2020.

3D printing medical devices is called "powder bed fusion." Powder bed fusion is commonly used because it works with a variety of materials used in medical devices, such as titanium and nylon.

The powder bed fusion process builds a three-dimensional product from very fine metal or plastic powder, which is poured onto a platform and leveled carefully. A laser or electron beam then moves across the powder layer and melts the material it touches. Melted material fuses to the layer below it and to the powder around it to create a solid. Once a layer is completed, the platform moves down and one more layer of carefully leveled powder is placed on top.

The U.S. Food and Drug Administration (FDA) has several 3D printers that help us better understand the capabilities of 3D printing of medical devices and the public-health benefit of this technology. For example, the FDA has printers that use different printing technologies, including powder bed fusion, to evaluate what parts of the printing processes and workflows are critical to ensure the quality of the finished medical device.

PATIENT-MATCHED DEVICES

While 3D printers are often used to create identical copies of the same device, they can also be used to create devices unique to a specific patient. Patient-matched (or patient-specific) devices are created specifically for the patient based on individual features, such as anatomy. They can be based on a template model that is matched to a patient using medical imaging. Patient-matching can be accomplished by techniques, such as scaling of the device using one or more anatomic features from patient data.

The FDA regulates 3D printed medical devices through the same pathways as traditional medical devices; therefore they are evaluated according to the safety and effectiveness information submitted to us by the manufacturer. While traditionally manufactured medical devices come in discrete sizes, patient-matched devices can be made in a continuous range of shapes with predefined minimum and maximum specifications that we can use to review the devices in the same way as standard-sized devices. For instance, the specification may define a minimum and maximum wall thickness or how sharp a curve can be to maintain device performance for its intended use.

There is a provision in federal law that exempts "custom" medical devices from the FDA review, but patient-matched devices do not automatically meet all the requirements.

OTHER USES OF 3D PRINTING

The use of 3D printing is not limited to medical devices. Other industries and government departments are also interested in its use. For instance, the U.S. Department of Energy (DOE) is investing resources to study 3D printing, and how it can be used to reduce waste by using fewer raw materials and require fewer manufacturing steps. The DOE has compiled information on how 3D printing works, the different types of printers, and for what they are used.

MEDICAL DEVICES, ACCESSORIES, COMPONENTS, AND PARTS DURING THE COVID-19 PANDEMIC

Personal protective equipment (PPE) includes protective clothing, gowns, gloves, face shields, goggles, face masks, and respirators, or other equipment designed to protect the wearer from injury or the spread of infection or illness. While it is possible to use 3D printing to make certain PPE, there are technical challenges that have to be overcome to be effective enough. 3D-printed PPE can be used to provide a physical barrier to the environment. However, 3D-printed PPE are unlikely to provide the same fluid barrier and air filtration protection as U.S. Food and Drug Administration (FDA)-cleared surgical masks and N95 respirators.

PUBLIC–PRIVATE PARTNERSHIP TO COORDINATE ON OPEN-SOURCE MEDICAL PRODUCTS FOR THE COVID-19 RESPONSE

The U.S. Food and Drug Administration (FDA), the U.S. Veterans Health Administration (VHA), the National Institutes of Health (NIH), and America Makes are partnering to coordinate the additive manufacturing response to coronavirus.

The FDA is striving to facilitate the use of 3D printing and other advanced manufacturing technology to bring PPE and other needed medical device parts to health-care organizations through emergency use authorization.

The NIH 3D Print Exchange is providing access to a collection of design files for sharing with the community.

The Veterans Health Administration is leading a process to review protective equipment and other devices in demand for the COVID-19 crisis. Prototypes that meet applicable standards will be designated as "Clinically Reviewed."

America Makes is a large public-private partnership with members that span many different 3D printing industries. They have created an online repository to connect the capabilities of the additive manufacturing industry with specific needs of health-care providers.

Members of the collaboration will work continuously to evaluate 3D printable parts and other improvised designs for their effectiveness and identify several designs that are likely to be the most useful for health-care providers and patients in shortage situations.

CURRENT INITIATIVES

- The Biomedical Library at the University of Pennsylvania is working with the Penn Health Tech Rapid Response Team to create face shields, masks, and ventilators.
- Stony Brook University is producing face shields with partners on Long Island.
- Do-It-Yourself Medical Devices and Protective Gear Fuel Battle Against COVID-19 at Georgia Tech
- Maker Mask
- 3D for COVID
- MatterHackers COVID-19 Maker Response Hub
- COVID-19 Response Projects from the Stanford BioEngineering Prakash Lab
- Make4Covid
- Formlabs 3D Printed Test Swabs for COVID-19 Testing and COVID-19 Community Part Library
- How Academic Medical Centers and the 3D Printing Industry Teamed Up to Respond to COVID-19

Chapter 52 | Microneedle Patch for Flu Vaccination

A National Institutes of Health (NIH) funded study led by a team at the Georgia Institute of Technology and Emory University has shown that an influenza vaccine can produce robust immune responses and be administered safely with an experimental patch of dissolving microneedles. The method is an alternative to needle-and-syringe immunization; with further development, it could eliminate the discomfort of an injection as well as the inconvenience and expense of visiting a flu clinic.

"This bandage-strip sized patch of painless and dissolvable needles can transform how we get vaccinated," said Roderic I. Pettigrew, Ph.D., M.D., director of the National Institute of Biomedical Imaging and Bioengineering (NIBIB), which funded the study. "A particularly attractive feature is that this vaccination patch could be delivered in the mail and self-administered. In addition, this technology holds promise for delivering other vaccines in the future."

The researchers received funding through an NIBIB Quantum Grant and from the National Institute of Allergy and Infectious Diseases.

The study, published online June 27, 2017, in *The Lancet*, was led by Nadine Rouphael, M.D., associate professor of medicine, and Mark J. Mulligan, M.D., distinguished professor of medicine, Emory University School of Medicine, in collaboration with Mark

This chapter contains text excerpted from the following sources: Text in this chapter begins with excerpts from "Researchers Develop Microneedle Patch for Flu Vaccination," National Institute of Biomedical Imaging and Bioengineering (NIBIB), June 27, 2017. Reviewed June 2021; Text under the heading "Microneedle Patch for COVID-19 Vaccine" is excerpted from "Prickly Patch Delivery of Experimental COVID-19 Vaccine Shows Promise in Animal Study," National Institute of Allergy and Infectious Diseases (NIAID), April 3, 2020.

R. Prausnitz, Ph.D., Regents Professor, and J. Erskine Love Chair in Chemical and Biomolecular Engineering, Georgia Institute of Technology. A team led by Prausnitz designed the dime-sized patch of microneedles used in the study.

The vaccine patch consists of 100 solid, water-soluble needles that are just long enough to penetrate the skin. "The skin is an immune surveillance organ," Prausnitz said. "It is our interface with the outside world, so it is very well equipped to detect a pathogen and mount an immune response against it."

Adhesive helps the patch grip the skin during the administration of the vaccine, which is encapsulated in the needles and is released as the needle tips dissolves, within minutes. The patch is peeled away and discarded such as a used bandage strip.

The researchers enrolled 100 adult participants, dividing them into four random groups: vaccination with microneedle patch given by a health-care provider; vaccination with microneedle patch self-administered by the study participant; vaccination with intramuscular injection given by a health-care provider; and placebo microneedle patch given by a health-care provider. The researchers used an inactivated influenza vaccine formulated for the 2014–2015 flu season to inoculate participants other than those in the placebo group.

The researchers found that vaccination with the microneedle patches was safe, with no serious related adverse events reported. Some participants developed local skin reactions to the patches, described as faint redness and mild itching that lasted two to three days.

The results also showed that antibody responses generated by the vaccine, as measured through analysis of blood samples, were similar in the groups vaccinated using patches and those receiving intramuscular injection, and these immune responses were still present after six months. More than 70 percent of patch recipients reported they would prefer patch vaccination over injection or intranasal vaccination for future vaccinations.

No significant difference was seen between the doses of vaccine delivered by the health-care workers and the volunteers who self-administered the patches, showing that participants were able to correctly self-administer the patch. After vaccination, imaging of the used patches found that the microneedles had dissolved in the skin, suggesting that the used patches could be safely discarded as nonsharps waste. The vaccines remained potent in the patches without refrigeration for at least one year.

The prospective vaccine technology could offer economic and manufacturing advantages. The manufacturing cost for the patch is expected to be competitive with prefilled syringe costs. The patch, however, can dramatically reduce the cost of vaccination, since self-administration can eliminate the need to have health workers oversee the process. It can be easily packaged for transportation, requires no refrigeration, and is stable.

MICRONEEDLE PATCH FOR COVID-19 VACCINE

A candidate vaccine delivered through a thumbnail-sized patch studded with microneedles could help address the coronavirus disease 2019 (COVID-19) pandemic. The National Institute of Allergy and Infectious Diseases (NIAID) funded scientists at the University of Pittsburgh School of Medicine tested the vaccine delivery device in mice and published the results on April 2, 2020 in *The Lancet* journal *EBioMedicine*.

Previous research on the coronaviruses that cause severe acute respiratory syndrome (SARS) and the Middle East respiratory syndrome (MERS) by co-lead investigator Andrea Gambotto, M.D., and his colleagues laid the groundwork for the current investigation of the spike (S) protein of the novel coronavirus, SARS-CoV-2, which causes COVID-19. The virus uses the S protein to enter cells and initiate infection. In response, the body eventually develops antibodies directed against SARS-CoV-2, and they help control and end the infection. Vaccination gives the immune system a "preview" of a virus or other disease-causing pathogen so that protective antibodies can be rapidly produced if a vaccinated person later encounters that pathogen. If vaccine-generated antibodies and other immune responses are sufficiently robust, infection is prevented.

The experimental Pittsburgh coronavirus vaccine, PittCoVacc, is made from parts of the virus S protein impregnated into 400 tiny needles on a small adhesive patch. Once attached, the microneedles, which are made of sugar, dissolve and deliver the viral protein directly to immune cells in the skin that are especially responsive to viral invaders.

When tested in mice, PittCoVacc generated a surge of antibodies against SARS-CoV-2 within two weeks of the microneedle prick. The vaccinated animals have not yet been tracked longterm, but the researchers note that mice vaccinated with a microneedle patch against MERS-CoV produced sufficient antibody levels to neutralize the virus for at least a year. The antibody levels of the SARS-CoV-2-vaccinated animals are following a similar trend, the team reports.

The SARS-CoV-2 microneedle vaccine maintains its potency after gamma radiation sterilization – a useful feature for the eventual manufacture of products suitable for human use. Additionally, the components of the experimental vaccine can be made rapidly and at large-scale, say the investigators, and the final product does not require refrigeration, which means that vaccine patches could be produced and placed in storage until needed.

Chapter 53 | **Photonic Dosimetry**

As part of the National Institute of Standards and Technology (NIST) on a Chip program, the Photonic Dosimetry project is developing in-situ submicrometer ionizing-radiation dosimetry and calorimetry leading to new chip-based metrology for industrial and medical applications. Deployed as standalone chips, such devices may provide dosimetry alternatives for radiation processing of bulk materials and radiotherapy treatment planning. If fabricated or embedded into materials, arrays of such devices could enable highly resolved dose imaging for applications such as x-ray scanning of semiconductor devices and surface sterilization processes for medical equipment.

With this effort, NIST is responding to industry needs for traceable, measurement solutions that can resolve spatial variations of absorbed dose at the level of individual components on a silicon wafer or bacteria on surgical instruments.

Presently, there is only limited traceability to national standards for measuring radiation dose at the very small length scales where industry is pushing, and NIST is investing in new technology to meet this need. Now is a critical time for U.S. manufacturing in the large and growing markets for precise delivery of radiation for uses such as:

- Medical device sterilization by radiation, including low-energy electron and x-ray beams

This chapter contains text excerpted from the following sources: Text in this chapter begins with excerpts from "Photonic Dosimetry," National Institute of Standards and Technology (NIST), May 4, 2021; Text beginning with the heading "What Does a Photonic Dosimeter Do?" is excerpted from "Photonic Dosimeter and Process for Performing Dosimetry," National Institute of Standards and Technology (NIST), February 11, 2021.

- Food irradiation for safety and quality, including low-energy electron and x-ray beams
- Ionizing radiation medical therapy, including proton and ion therapy

To remain competitive in these fields, U.S. manufacturers are expanding capabilities in machine-based electron and ion beams, which are effective, efficient, and secure. However, the newer techniques such as low-energy electron irradiation deliver dose gradients over very short distances (microns) and therefore require high-resolution absorbed-dose sensors for irradiation planning, validation, and quality assurance.

No sensors are currently able to meet all industrial and medical needs for these new techniques, but the NIST on a Chip program is working to harness commercial silicon chip fabrication and telecommunications photonics technology to create a new sensor that is accurate enough for NIST calibrations, but small enough to be field-deployable or embeddable within semiconductor microcircuits.

To this end, NIST is studying the impact of ionizing radiation on the performance of silicon photonic devices. In the first round of testing, the team irradiated chips with up to 1 MGy dose – well beyond the dose required for many industrial applications, and several thousand times higher than most medical radiation treatment levels – with little to no damage to the photonic devices. Studies are ongoing of in-beam irradiation effects on patented photonic calorimeter and dosimeter prototypes and material and device designs for ionizing radiation applications.

WHAT DOES A PHOTONIC DOSIMETER DO?

A photonic dosimeter accrues cumulative dose and includes: a substrate; a waveguide disposed on the substrate and that: receives a primary input light; transmits secondary input light from the primary input light to a dosimatrix; receives a secondary output light from the dosimatrix and produces primary output light from the secondary output light; the dosimatrix disposed on the substrate and in optical communication with the waveguide and that:

receives the secondary input light from the waveguide; produces the secondary output light that is communicated to the waveguide; and includes an active element that undergoes conversion from a prime state to a dosed state in response to receipt, by the active element, of a dose of radiation; and a cover layer disposed on waveguide and the dosimatrix.

PROCESS FOR PERFORMING DOSIMETRY

Radiation-induced materials modification is ubiquitous. These applications rely on dosimetry to reliably deliver the desired amount of radiation to the right place. Currently, the dosimetry standard is based on calorimetry of a large water phantom irradiated exclusively by Co-60 gamma rays. The thermistor used is large – half of a millimeter. The current dosimetry standards permit traceable dosimetry that is limited by the size of the probes used in primary standard calorimeters and the requirement of field uniformity over the probe (thus, field ~ 10x probe diameter). This works for bulk sterilization but for surfaces or small dimensions, this existing dose standard is too crude by several orders of magnitude. While higher-energy electron beams can penetrate matter, beams of low-energy electrons have the opposite characteristic: they penetrate no more than 100 microns or so into most materials. This makes them valuable for industrial processes such as surface sterilization of medical instruments and bandages or curing of inks used on labels for food items – wherever the benefits of radiation dose are confined to the outside of something (and could harm what's inside). Lack of traceability thus leaves huge industries without the support needed to meet regulatory requirements. Thus, NIST has developed a chip-scale calorimeter for radiation dosimetry that could serve as a new standard to extend traceability and allow quantitative dosimetry on micron dimension.

FEATURES OF A PHOTONIC DOSIMETER

This invention is technically superior by enabling absolute dosimetry at an unprecedented physical scale due to micron-scale spatial resolution across six orders-of-magnitude of absorbed dose, from medical diagnostic and therapeutic procedures up through industrial materials processing, sterilization, and applications lead I ng to commercialization of space.

Part 7 | Medical Technology – Legal and Ethical Concerns

Chapter 54 | Health Information Privacy Law and Policy

WHAT TYPE OF PATIENT CHOICE EXISTS UNDER HEALTH INFORMATION PRIVACY LAW AND POLICY?

Most health-care providers must follow the Health Insurance Portability and Accountability Act (HIPAA) Privacy Rule (Privacy Rule), a federal privacy law that sets a baseline of protection for certain individually identifiable health information ("health information").

The Privacy Rule generally permits but does not require, covered health-care providers to give patients the choice as to whether their health information may be disclosed to others for certain key purposes. These key purposes include treatment, payment, and health-care operations.

HOW CAN PATIENT CHOICE BE IMPLEMENTED IN ELECTRONIC HEALTH INFORMATION EXCHANGE (eHIE)?

While it is not required, health-care providers may decide to offer patients a choice as to whether their health information may be exchanged electronically, either directly or through a Health Information Exchange (HIE) Organization. That is, they may offer an "opt-in" or "opt-out" policy or a combination.

This chapter includes text excerpted from "Health Information Privacy Law and Policy," HealthIT.gov, Office of the National Coordinator for Health Information Technology (ONC), September 19, 2018.

ARE THERE SPECIFIC LEGAL REQUIREMENTS FOR OPT-IN OR OPT-OUT POLICIES?

The U.S. Department of Health and Human Services (HHS) does not set out specific steps or requirements for obtaining a patient's choice of whether to participate in eHIE. However, adequately informing patients of these new models for exchange and giving them the choice of whether to participate is one means of ensuring that patients trust these systems. Providers are therefore encouraged to enable patients to make a "meaningful" consent choice rather than an uninformed one.

ARE THERE PRIVACY LAWS THAT REQUIRE PATIENT CONSENT?

Yes. There are some federal and state privacy laws (e.g., 42 CFR Part 2, Title 10) that require health-care providers to obtain patients' written consent before they disclose their health information to other people and organizations, even for treatment. Many of these privacy laws protect information that is related to health conditions considered "sensitive" by most people.

HOW DOES HIPAA AFFECT THESE OTHER PRIVACY LAWS?

HIPAA created a baseline of privacy protection. It overrides (or "preempts") other privacy laws that are less protective. But, HIPAA leaves in effect other laws that are more privacy-protective. Under this legal framework, health-care providers and other implementers must continue to follow other applicable federal and state laws that require obtaining patients' consent before disclosing their health information.

Chapter 55 | Health Information Technology Legislation and Regulations

21st CENTURY CURES ACT

There are many provisions of the 21st Century Cures Act (Cures Act) that will improve the flow and exchange of electronic health information. The Office of the National Coordinator for Health Information Technology (ONC) is responsible for implementing those parts of Title IV, delivery, related to advancing interoperability, prohibiting information blocking, and enhancing the usability, accessibility, privacy, and security of health IT. ONC works to ensure that all individuals, their families, and their health-care providers have appropriate access to electronic health information to help improve the overall health of the nation's population.

In addition to supporting medical research, advancing interoperability, clarifying HIPAA privacy rules, and supporting substance abuse and mental-health services, the Cures Act defines interoperability as the ability to exchange and use electronic health information without special effort on the part of the user and as not constituting information blocking.

This chapter includes text excerpted from "Health IT Legislation," HealthIT.gov, Office of the National Coordinator for Health Information Technology (ONC), June 8, 2021.

The ONC focuses on the following provisions:

- Section 4001: Health IT Usability
- Section 4002(a): Conditions of Certification
- Section 4003(b): Trusted Exchange Framework and Common Agreement
- Section 4003(c): Health Information Technology Advisory Committee
- Section 4004: Identifying reasonable and necessary activities that do not constitute information blocking

The ONC is also supporting and collaborating with the federal partners, such as the Centers for Medicare and Medicaid Services, the HHS Office of Civil Rights, the HHS Inspector General, the Agency for Healthcare Research and Quality, and the National Institute for Standards and Technology.

THE MEDICARE ACCESS AND CHIP REAUTHORIZATION ACT

The Medicare Access and CHIP Reauthorization Act of 2015 (MACRA) ended the Sustainable Growth Rate formula and established the Quality Payment Program (QPP). The QPP rewards high-value, high-quality Medicare clinicians with payment increases, while reducing payments to clinicians who do not meet performance standards. The Quality Eligible clinicians have two tracks to choose from in the Quality Payment Program based on their practice size, specialty, location, or patient population:

- Advanced Alternative Payment Models (APMs)
- The Merit-based Incentive Payment System (MIPS)

Under MACRA, the Medicare EHR Incentive Program, commonly referred to as "meaningful use," was transitioned to become one of the four components of MIPS, which consolidated multiple, quality programs into a single program to improve care. Clinicians participating in MIPS earn a performance-based payment adjustment while clinicians participating in an Advanced APM may earn an incentive payment for participating in an innovative payment model.

THE HEALTH INFORMATION TECHNOLOGY FOR ECONOMIC AND CLINICAL HEALTH ACT

The Health Information Technology for Economic and Clinical Health (HITECH) Act of 2009 provides HHS with the authority to establish programs to improve health-care quality, safety, and efficiency through the promotion of health IT, including electronic health records and private and secure electronic health information exchange.

THE FOOD AND DRUG ADMINISTRATION SAFETY AND INNOVATION ACT

Section 618 of the Food and Drug Administration Safety and Innovation Act (FDASIA) of 2012 directed the Secretary of Health and Human Services, acting through the Commissioner of the U.S. Food and Drug Administration (FDA), and in consultation with ONC and the Chairman of the Federal Communications Commission, to develop a report that contains a proposed strategy and recommendations on an appropriate, risk-based regulatory framework for health IT, including medical mobile applications, that promotes innovation, protects patient safety, and avoids regulatory duplication. The Health IT Policy Committee formed an FDASIA workgroup and issued recommendations to ONC, FDA, and FCC as of the September 4th, 2013 HIT Policy Committee meeting.

THE HEALTH INSURANCE PORTABILITY AND ACCOUNTABILITY ACT

The Health Insurance Portability and Accountability Act (HIPAA) of 1996 protects health insurance coverage for workers and their families when they change or lose their jobs, requires the establishment of national standards for electronic health-care transactions, and requires establishment of national identifiers for providers, health insurance plans, and employers.

The HHS Office for Civil Rights administers the HIPAA Privacy and Security Rules. The HIPAA Privacy Rule describes what information is protected and how protected information can be used and disclosed. The HIPAA Security Rule describes who is covered by the HIPAA privacy protections and what safeguards must be in place to ensure appropriate protection of electronically protected health information.

The Centers for Medicare and Medicaid Services administer and enforce the HIPAA Administrative Simplification Rules, including the Transactions and Code Set Standards, Employer Identifier Standard, and National Provider Identifier Standard. The HIPAA Enforcement Rule provides standards for the enforcement of all the Administrative Simplification Rules.

AFFORDABLE CARE ACT

The Affordable Care Act of 2010 establishes comprehensive healthcare insurance reforms that aim to increase access to healthcare, improve quality and lower healthcare costs, and provide new consumer protections.

Chapter 56 | **HIPAA Privacy Rule's Right of Access and Health Information Technology**

Twenty-two years ago this month, the U.S. Congress enacted the Health Insurance Portability and Accountability Act of 1996 (HIPAA). The federal Privacy, Security, and Breach Notification Rules implemented under HIPAA, and administered and enforced by the HHS Office for Civil Rights (OCR), continue to serve as the national foundation of protections for individually identifiable health information, and of individuals' rights with respect to their information, including the right to see and obtain copies of their health information from their health-care providers and health plans. In addition, HIPAA covered entities and their business associates continue to use the required HIPAA electronic transactions and code set standards to exchange health information for essential administrative purposes, such as submitting insurance claims.

HIPAA SUPPORTS DATA PORTABILITY

HIPAA recognizes the importance of providing individuals with portability of their data. With limited exceptions, the HIPAA Privacy Rule provides individuals with a right, upon request, to see and receive copies of information in their medical and other health

This chapter includes text excerpted from "HIPAA & Health Information Portability: A Foundation for Interoperability," HealthIT.gov, Office of the National Coordinator for Health Information Technology (ONC), August 30, 2018.

records (a designated record set) maintained by a HIPAA covered entity, such as an individual's health-care provider or health plan. At the direction of an individual or personal representative, a covered entity must transmit health information about the individual directly to any person or designated entity within 30 days (with the possibility of one 30-day extension). Covered entities are strongly encouraged to provide individuals with access to their health information much sooner, and to take advantage of technologies that enable individuals to have faster or even immediate access to the information.

ONC and OCR recently began a campaign encouraging individuals to get, check, and use copies of their health information and the two offices offer training for health-care providers about the HIPAA right of access. OCR and ONC have developed guidance to empower individuals to take more control of decisions regarding their health and well-being through easy access to their health information. These guidelines include access guidance for professionals, HIPAA right of access training for health-care providers, and Get It. Check It. Use It. resources for individuals.

HIPAA also supports the sharing of health information among health-care providers, health plans, and those operating on their behalf, for treatment, payment, and healthcare operations (TPO) purposes, and provides avenues for transmitting health information to loved ones involved in an individual's care as well as for research, public health, and other important activities.

TECHNOLOGY FACILITATES PORTABILITY – PAST, PRESENT, AND FUTURE

To further promote the portability of health information, the development, refinement, and use of health information technology (health IT) is encouraged to provide health-care providers, health plans, and individuals and their personal representatives the ability to more rapidly access, exchange, and use health information electronically

Now, more health-care providers and health plans are offering individuals electronic access to their health information. In addition, the Cures Act directs HHS to address information blocking and promote the trusted exchange of health information, which will further promote the portability of this information.

HHS and its components such as the Centers for Medicare & Medicaid Services (CMS) and the National Institutes for Health (NIH), along with the White House Office of American Innovation, are working to support the portability of health information and encourage the growth of a health ecosystem that encourages health-care providers, health plans, and individuals to share health information electronically.

The CMS is calling on health-care providers and health plans (HIPAA covered entities) to share health information directly with patients, upon their request.

NIH has established a research program to help improve health-care for all individuals that will require the portability of health information.

The White House Office of American Innovation also has an initiative, MyHealthEData, that aims to break down the barriers preventing patients from having electronic access to their own health records; this initiative also facilitates individuals of their HIPAA Privacy Rule right of access to obtain their health information and direct copies to share with third parties.

Health IT can improve the portability of digital-health information and facilitate the HIPAA individual right of access. For example, health-care providers using Certified Electronic Health Record Technology (CEHRT) certified to the 2015 Edition of standards, implementation specifications and certification criteria (2015 Edition) adopted by HHS for ONC's Health IT Certification Program have view, download, and transmit (VDT) technical capabilities. These capabilities support individuals' ability to use Internet-based technology to transmit their health information to a third-party, directly from the provider's technology (such as through a patient portal or personal health record) to any email address, as requested by the patient. In the 2015 Edition, the "application access" certification criteria requires health IT developers to demonstrate that the health IT can provide application access to a common set of patient clinical data via an application programming interface (API). An API is technology that allows one software application to programmatically access the services another software application provides, including supporting the sharing of electronic health information.

The OCR's health app developer portal offers resources for health IT developers and others interested in the intersection of health IT and HIPAA privacy and security protections, including those wanting to build privacy and security protections into technology to enable individual choices for secure health information access and sharing. Assistance is also available at www.HHS.gov/hipaa.

The Cures Act builds on the capabilities of the 2015 Edition by calling for the development of APIs that enable the user to access and use health information "without special effort." As researchers focus on accelerating individuals' ability to access, share, and use their health information on their smartphones or other mobile devices, APIs should increase data portability and serve as a technology to further implement the health information portability concept. For example, researchers are currently looking at how developers and users of health IT enable individuals to use an API to make a request to exercise their HIPAA right of access and to request that their health information be transmitted to a designated third-party, such as the All of Us Research Program.

LOOKING AHEAD

The HHS' guiding principle is to make policy choices that will give consumers, health-care professionals, and innovators more options for getting and using health information. Our interoperability efforts focus on improving individuals' ability to access and share their health information to better enable them to shop for and coordinate their own care. Researchers are dedicated to putting patients first, allowing them to be empowered consumers of healthcare by making the information they need to be engaged and active decision-makers in their care available on their smartphones or other mobile devices.

As the HHS continues working toward achieving the interoperability priorities of the 21st Century Cures Act, HIPAA puts researchers one step closer to doing so. Now, twenty-two years after it was enacted, and at a time when the European Union's General Data Protection Regulation (GDPR) includes data portability as a fundamental right of individuals, HIPAA still serves as a nationwide foundation for portability of electronic health information as well as its privacy and security.

Chapter 57 | **Personal Health Records and the HIPAA Privacy Rule**

A personal health record (PHR) is an emerging health information technology that individuals can use to engage in their own healthcare to improve the quality and efficiency of that care. In this rapidly developing market, there are several types of PHRs available to individuals with varying functionalities. Some PHRs are offered by health-care providers and health plans covered by the Health Insurance Portability and Accountability Act of 1996 (HIPAA) Privacy Rule, known as "HIPAA covered entities." The HIPAA Privacy Rule applies to these PHRs and protects the privacy of the information in them. Alternatively, some PHRs are not offered by HIPAA-covered entities, and, in these cases, it is the privacy policies of the PHR vendor as well as any other applicable laws, which will govern how information in the PHR is protected. This chapter describes how the Privacy Rule may apply to and supports the use of PHRs.

WHAT IS A PHR?

There is currently no universal definition of a PHR, although several relatively similar definitions exist within the industry. In general, a PHR is an electronic record of an individual's health information by which the individual controls access to the information and

This chapter includes text excerpted from "Personal Health Records and the HIPAA Privacy Rule," U.S. Department of Health and Human Services (HHS), December 15, 2008. Reviewed June 2021.

may have the ability to manage, track, and participate in her or his own healthcare. A PHR should not be confused with an electronic health record (EHR). An EHR is held and maintained by a health-care provider and may contain all the information that once existed in a patient's paper medical record, but in electronic form.

The PHRs universally focus on providing individuals with the ability to manage their health information and to control, to vary-ing extents, who can access that health information. A PHR has the potential to provide individuals with a way to create a longitu-dinal health history and may include common information such as medical diagnoses, medications, and test results. Most PHRs also provide individuals with the capability to control who can access the health information in the PHR, and because PHRs are electronic and generally accessible over the Internet, individuals have the flexibility to view their health information at any time and from any computer at any location. The accessibility of health information in a PHR may facilitate appropriate and improved treatment for conditions or emergencies that occur away from an individual's usual health-care provider. Additionally, the ability to access one's own health information in a PHR may assist individu-als in identifying potential errors or mistakes in their information.

Depending on the type of PHR, individuals also may be able to input family histories and emergency contact information, to track and chart their own health information and the health information of their children or others whose care they manage, to schedule and receive reminders about upcoming appointments or proce-dures, to research medical conditions, to renew prescriptions, and to communicate directly with their health-care providers through secure messaging systems. The PHR also may function as a way for both individuals and health-care providers to streamline the administrative processes involved in transferring patient records or for coordinating patient care.

TYPES OF PHRS

The PHR market continues to evolve at a rapid pace, with new types of PHRs continually emerging. However, the universe of PHRs can be broken down into two categories: those subject to the Privacy

Rule and those that fall outside of its scope. PHRs that are subject to the Privacy Rule are those that a covered health-care provider or health plan offers. Examples of PHRs that fall outside the scope of the Privacy Rule are those offered by an employer (separate from the employer's group health plan) or those made available directly to an individual by a PHR vendor that is not a HIPAA covered entity. Some stand-alone software packages or portable devices also may be available for use by individuals as PHRs.

THE HIPAA PRIVACY RULE'S APPLICATION TO PHRS OFFERED BY COVERED ENTITIES

The Privacy Rule protects the privacy of certain individually iden-tifiable health information, known as "protected health formation" (PHI), created or maintained by covered entities. Covered entities include health plans and those health-care providers that transmit any health information in electronic form in connection with cer-tain standard transactions, such as health-care claims. The Privacy Rule governs how these covered entities may use and disclose an individual's PHI and grants individuals certain rights regarding their health information. PHRs that are offered by a covered entity will contain PHI and thus, the covered entity must appropriately safeguard this information as required by the Privacy Rule.

Business Associates

Covered entities offering a PHR may hire another entity as a busi-ness associate to administer the PHR or perform other PHR-related services or functions. The Privacy Rule allows a covered entity to use a business associate to perform functions or activities on behalf of, or provide services to, the covered entity that involve the use or disclosure of PHI, provided the covered entity obtains satisfactory assurances, through a contract or agreement, that the business associate will appropriately safeguard the information. A business associate agreement must specify, among other things, the business associate's permitted uses and disclosures of PHI and that the business associate will appropriately safeguard the information. The business associate may not use or disclose the information for any purpose that would violate the Privacy Rule. The agreement may specify the manner in which the individual will control access to the information in the PHR, including whether, and the circumstances under which, the business associate is to allow third parties and even the covered entity access to the information.

The Use and Disclosure of Protected Health Information

Covered entities may not use or disclose an individual's PHI except as the Privacy Rule expressly permits or requires, or with an individual's written authorization. The Privacy Rule's use and disclosure provisions were designed with the typical business or clinical health-care record in mind, whether paper or electronic, and the uses and disclosures covered entities would need to make of this information for their core health-care functions. Thus, the Privacy Rule generally allows covered entities to use and disclose an individual's PHI for treatment, payment of healthcare, and health-care operations (certain functions that support treatment and payment). Also, in recognition that there are certain legitimate and important additional uses of an individual's health information, the Privacy Rule allows a covered entity to disclose, subject to conditions, an individual's PHI for certain other purposes, such as research and public health.

With respect to offering and maintaining a PHR, a covered entity is generally permitted by the Privacy Rule to use and disclose an individual's PHI for purposes of providing this service to the individual, as well as communicating with the individual through the use of a PHR. With respect to PHI within the PHR, a covered entity offering a PHR may establish privacy policies that restrict its uses and disclosures of such information beyond what is required by the Privacy Rule. Because the fundamental purpose of a PHR is to give individuals more control over, and access to, their health information, covered entities are encouraged to reassess what uses and disclosures of individuals' information in the PHR may be appropriate, and to give individual greater control over the information in their PHRs. This may include, for example, allowing an individual to control not only access to the information in the PHR by third parties, but even by the covered entity itself.

However, covered entities should be aware of the circumstances in which they may need to access or disclose information within an individual's PHR to comply with other legal obligations, and should make these circumstances clear to the individual.

Individual Rights

The Privacy Rule grants individuals several rights with respect to their own health information, such as the right to view and obtain a copy of much of their health information and to have corrections made to such information. Because PHRs provide individuals with access to their health information and can facilitate communication between individuals and their health-care providers or health plans, PHRs may be useful mechanisms for covered entities to facilitate providing individuals with their HIPAA rights.

ACCESS

The Privacy Rule gives individuals a right of access to inspect and obtain a copy of their PHI in a designated record set held by a covered entity. A designated record set is the medical records, billing records, enrollment and claims records, and other information used by the covered entity to make decisions about the individual. A PHR offered by a HIPAA covered entity may allow individuals to view all or part of their PHI held by a covered entity and to download and print this information. Thus, depending on the breadth and usefulness of the information to which the individual has access, a PHR could eliminate or reduce the need for individuals to otherwise request access to their complete designated record set held by the HIPAA covered entity.

However, access to health information through a PHR would not replace an individual's right to obtain access to health information in her or his designated record set that is not available through the PHR and to which she or he is entitled under the Privacy Rule. Thus, covered entities providing the individual with access to only a portion of the individual's health information in a designated record set through a PHR should make clear the individual's right to obtain access to the information in the designated record set that is not available through the PHR. Also, individuals always retain the right to a paper copy of the individual's health information in the designated record set held by the covered entity. In addition, the Privacy Rule requires a covered entity to have a mechanism to provide an individual's personal representatives with access to the individual's PHI and, as with access provided to the individual, a PHR may be a way to eliminate or reduce the need for personal representatives to otherwise request access to the complete designated record set about the individual.

Additionally, covered entities are not precluded from setting up a PHR system that allows individuals to designate family members or other persons to have access to the information in their PHRs.

AMENDMENT

The Privacy Rule gives individuals the right to have amendments or corrections made to the PHI in their health records or other designated record set held by a covered entity. PHRs that replicate some or all of the information in the health record may be helpful mechanisms for individuals to identify potential errors in their health information and to request that the covered entity correct the information. If there is a mistake, the covered entity can correct or append additional information to the individual's health information held in the covered entity's health records system and can update the PHR with the corrected information. The individual control inherent in PHRs also may allow individuals to revise and update some information, such as that information they themselves have entered in their PHRs.

NOTICE OF PRIVACY PRACTICES

The Privacy Rule requires covered entities to provide individuals with a notice of privacy practices (NPPs) outlining individuals' rights with respect to their health information and how the covered entity may use and disclose this information. The PHR may be a useful mechanism for a covered entity to distribute its HIPAA NPP, in addition to the other distribution methods required by the Privacy Rule. Also, a covered entity that offers a PHR to individuals is encouraged to consider highlighting its privacy practices with respect to the PHR explicitly in its HIPAA NPP, particularly to the extent such practices provide greater restrictions on the use and disclosure of health information compared to the covered entity's policies generally with respect to PHI. Alternatively, covered entities may consider creating a separate and more detailed NPP specific to PHRs that outlines the privacy practices and highlights the extent to which individuals can control information in their PHRs. Making available to individuals specific information about the privacy protections and controls over information in a PHR may build trust in, and help promote use of, PHRs by individuals.

ACCOUNTING OF DISCLOSURES

The Privacy Rule gives individuals the right to receive an accounting of certain disclosures of their PHI made by a covered entity for the six years prior to the request for the accounting, so that individuals are aware of how their information has been shared. However, because disclosures from the PHR will generally be to the individual or for limited other purposes, such as for administering the PHR, disclosures of information from a PHR generally would not be subject to the HIPAA accounting requirement. However, consistent with the intent of the accounting for disclosures, covered entities may want to consider setting up a functionality within a PHR that provides individuals with the ability to view a log of who accessed their PHR.

PHRS NOT OFFERED BY HIPAA-COVERED ENTITIES

In contrast to the PHRs discussed earlier, some PHRs fall outside the scope of the Privacy Rule because they are not offered by covered entities. For example, PHRs may be offered by employers (separate from the employer's group health plan) or by PHR vendors directly to individuals. Although some of these PHRs may advertise that they are "HIPAA-compliant," the Privacy Rule does not apply to or protect the health information within these PHRs. These PHRs are governed by the privacy policies and practices of the entities offering or administering the PHRs, as well as by any other applicable laws. When selecting a PHR, individuals should evaluate these privacy policies to decide if they are comfortable with the protections and rights offered, such as how their information will be safeguarded, for what purposes their information will be used and disclosed, and the extent to which the individual will control access to information in the PHR. Additionally, in some cases, an entity offering a PHR may share an individual's health information with contractors or other business partners.

Individuals may wish to evaluate whether these contractors or business partners also will be limited in how they can use or disclose the individual's health information.

Although the information in these PHRs is not covered by the Privacy Rule, the Privacy Rule does govern how PHI held by a covered entity enters a PHR. There are a number of ways in which a covered entity may disclose PHI about an individual for purposes of populating a third party PHR consistent with the Privacy Rule.

Authorization

The Privacy Rule permits a covered entity to disclose an individual's PHI to a third party with the individual's written authorization. Thus, in cases where the entity offering the PHR is able to or has agreed to input information directly into the PHR for the individual, a covered entity is permitted to disclose PHI about the individual directly to the entity administering the PHR if the covered entity has a written authorization from the individual for the disclosure.

The Privacy Rule specifies the required elements of the authorization, including that it describe the information to be disclosed, identify the recipients of the information, be signed by the individual, and include an expiration date or expiration event.

However, the Privacy Rule does not require that a HIPAA authorization be drafted or distributed by the covered entity, and a PHR vendor, for example, could create a HIPAA compliant authorization form that the individual could use to authorize her or his healthcare providers or health plans to disclose PHI directly to the PHR vendor. HIPAA authorizations also may be executed on paper or electronically, provided any electronic signature obtained from the individual complies with applicable law.

Disclosure to the Individual

The Privacy Rule also permits a covered entity to disclose PHI about an individual to the individual. The individual may grant the covered entity authority to upload information about the individual directly into the individual's PHR. Alternatively, a covered entity may provide this information directly to the individual for the individual to enter into the PHR.

Individual's Right of Access

In addition to covered entities being permitted to disclose an individual's PHI to the individual, individuals also have a right under the Privacy Rule to obtain a copy of their PHI in a designated record set, such as a medical or billing record, maintained by the covered entity. A covered entity generally must provide the individual with access to the information to which the individual is entitled within 30 days of the request. In addition, the covered entity must provide the individual with access to the PHI in the form or format requested by the individual, if it is readily producible in such form or format. Thus, covered entities are required to provide the individual with a copy of the PHI in the electronic form requested by the individual if such form is readily producible by the covered entity. Here, as above, a covered entity may provide the PHI directly to the individual for the individual to enter into the PHR or, if the functionality exists, and where the individual has granted the covered entity authority to upload information directly to the PHR, the covered entity can comply with the access request by entering the information directly into the PHR rather than giving the individual a separate paper or electronic copy.

Chapter 58 | **Privacy, Security, and Electronic Health Records**

The Office of the National Coordinator for Health Information Technology (ONC), in coordination with the U.S. Department of Health and Human Services (HHS) Office for Civil Rights (OCR), created the Guide to help you integrate privacy and security into your practice. The Guide covers a variety of topics highlighted below.

HIPAA BASICS

The HIPAA Rules provide federal protections for patient health information held by Covered Entities (CEs) and Business Associates (BAs). HIPAA gives patients many rights with respect to their health information.

The Guide provides details on the HIPAA Privacy, Security, and Breach Notification Rules, such as:
- What types of information HIPAA protects
- Who must comply with HIPAA
- How patient information can be used and disclosed under the HIPAA Privacy Rule

This chapter includes text excerpted from "Guide to Privacy & Security of Electronic Health Information," HealthIT. gov, Office of the National Coordinator for Health Information Technology (ONC), April 9, 2019.

PATIENT HEALTH INFORMATION RIGHTS

Under the HIPAA Privacy Rule, you have responsibilities to patients, which include:

- Providing a Notice of Privacy Practices (NPP)
- Responding to patients' requests for:
  - Access to their Protected Health Information (PHI)
  - Amendments to their PHI
  - Accounting of disclosures
  - Restrictions on uses and disclosures of their health information
  - Confidential communications

ELECTRONIC HEALTH RECORDS (EHRs) AND CYBERSECURITY

Electronic PHI (ePHI) may exist in your practice in a variety of systems, including electronic health records (EHRs). Because all electronic systems are vulnerable to cyber-attacks, you must consider all of your practice's systems and technologies when conducting security efforts.

An Internet connection is a necessity to conduct the many online activities that can be part of EHR and ePHI use. Exchanging patient information electronically, submitting claims electronically, generating electronic records for patients' requests, and e-prescribing are all examples of online activities that rely on cybersecurity practices to safeguard systems and information.

Cybersecurity refers to ways to prevent, detect, and respond to attacks against or unauthorized access against a computer system and its information. Cybersecurity protects your information or any form of digital asset stored in your computer or in any digital memory device.

It is important to have strong cybersecurity practices in place to protect patient information, organizational assets, your practice operations, and your personnel, and of course to comply with the HIPAA Security Rule. Cybersecurity is needed whether you have your EHR locally installed in your office or access it over the Internet from a cloud service provider.

The Office of the National Coordinator for Health Information Technology (ONC) offers online Cybersecurity information, including the Top 10 Tips for Cybersecurity in healthcare, to help you reduce your risk. For a full overview of security standards and required protections for ePHI under the HIPAA Security Rule, visit OCR's HIPAA Security Rule webpage.

PRIVACY AND SECURITY IN MEANINGFUL USE

You may be familiar with the Medicare and Medicaid EHR Incentive Programs (also called "Meaningful Use Programs"). The Meaningful Use Programs set staged requirements for providers. Providers receive incentive payments as they demonstrate progressively integrated EHR use.

Some of the Meaningful Use requirements relate to your practice's obligations under the HIPAA Privacy and Security Rules.

Meaningful Use must be demonstrated by:

- Using the capabilities of Certified EHR Technology (CEHRT) adopted by the U.S. Department of Health and Human Services (HHS) as standards, implementation specifications, and certification criteria (in the Office of the National Coordinator for Health Information Technology's Standards and Certification Criteria regulations),
- Meeting CMS-defined criteria through a phased approach based on anticipated technology and capabilities development. To define meaningful use, CMS sought to balance the sometimes competing considerations of improving health-care quality, encouraging widespread EHR adoption, promoting innovation, and avoiding imposing excessive or unnecessary burdens on health-care providers.

The Stage 1 Meaningful Use criteria, consistent with other provisions of Medicare and Medicaid law, focuses on:

- Electronically capturing health information in a structured format;
- Using that information to track key clinical conditions and communicating that information for care coordination purposes (whether that information is

641

structured or unstructured, but in structured format whenever feasible);

- Implementing clinical decision support tools to facilitate disease and medication management;
- Using EHRs to engage patients and families; and
- Reporting clinical quality measures and public-health information.

The Stage 2 Meaningful Use criteria, consistent with other provisions of Medicare and Medicaid law, expanded upon the Stage 1 criteria to encourage the use of health information technology (health IT) for continuous quality improvement at the point of care and the exchange of information in the most structured format possible. Examples of such use include the electronic transmission of orders entered using Computerized Provider Order Entry (CPOE) and the electronic transmission of diagnostic test results (such as blood tests, microbiology, urinalysis, pathology tests, radiology, cardiac imaging, nuclear medicine tests, pulmonary function tests, genetic tests, genomic tests and other such data needed to diagnose and treat disease).

SAMPLE SEVEN-STEP APPROACH FOR IMPLEMENTING A SECURITY MANAGEMENT PROCESS

Before you start, ask your local Regional Extension Center (REC) where you can get help. In addition:

- Check the Office of the National Coordinator for Health Information Technology (ONC) Health IT Privacy and Security Resources webpage.
- Review the Office for Civil Rights (OCR) Security Rule Guidance Material.
- Look at the OCR audit protocols.
- Let your EHR developer(s) know that health information security is one of your major goals in adopting an EHR.
- Check with your membership associations to see if they have training resource lists or suggestions.

The sample seven steps which will be discussed here are:

- Step 1: Lead Your Culture, Select Your Team, and Learn
  - Step 1A: Designate a Security Officer(s)
  - Step 1B: Discuss HIPAA Security Requirements with Your EHR Developer
  - Step 1C: Consider Using a Qualified Professional to Assist with Your Security Risk Analysis
  - Step 1D: Use Tools to Preview Your Security Risk Analysis
  - Step 1E: Refresh Your Knowledge Base of the HIPAA Rules
  - Step 1F: Promote a Culture of Protecting Patient Privacy and Securing Patient Information
- Step 2: Document Your Process, Findings, and Actions
- Step 3: Review Existing Security of ePHI (Perform Security Risk Analysis)
- Step 4: Develop an Action Plan
- Step 5: Manage and Mitigate Risks
  - Step 5A: Implement Your Action Plan
  - Step 5B: Prevent Breaches by Educating and Training Your Workforce
  - Step 5C: Communicate with Patients
  - Step 5D: Update Your BA Contracts
- Step 6: Attest for Meaningful Use Security-Related Objective
- Step 7: Monitor, Audit, and Update Security on an Ongoing Basis

BREACH NOTIFICATION AND HIPAA ENFORCEMENT

A breach is, generally, an impermissible use or disclosure under the Privacy Rule that compromises the security or privacy of PHI. An impermissible use or disclosure of unsecured PHI is presumed to be a breach unless the CE or BA demonstrates (based on a risk assessment) that there is a low probability that the PHI has been compromised. When a breach of unsecured PHI occurs, the Rules require your practice to notify affected individuals, the Secretary of HHS, and, in some cases, the media.

The Breach Notification Rule requires HIPAA CEs to notify individuals and the Secretary of HHS of the loss, theft, or certain other impermissible uses or disclosures of unsecured PHI. In particular, health-care providers must promptly notify the Secretary of HHS if there is any breach of unsecured PHI that affects 500 or more individuals, and they must notify the media if the breach affects more than 500 residents of a state or jurisdiction. If a breach affects fewer than 500 individuals, the CE must notify the Secretary and affected individuals. Reports of breaches affecting fewer than 500 individuals are due to the Secretary no later than 60 days after the end of the calendar year in which the breaches occurred.

- Significant breaches are investigated by OCR, and penalties may be imposed for failure to comply with the HIPAA Rules. Breaches that affect 500 or more patients are publicly reported on the OCR website.
- Similar breach notification provisions implemented and enforced by the Federal Trade Commission apply to Personal Health Record (PHR) developers and their third-party service providers.

If you can demonstrate through a risk assessment that there is a low probability that the use or disclosure compromised unsecured PHI, then breach notification is not necessary. (Please note that this breach-related risk assessment is different from the periodic security risk analysis required by the Security Rule.)

And, if you encrypt your data in accordance with the OCR guidance regarding rendering data unusable, unreadable, or indecipherable, you may avoid reporting what would otherwise have been a reportable breach. Remember, encryption depends on the encryption key being kept highly confidential, so do not store it with the data or in a location that would compromise it.

REPORTING BREACHES

If you choose not to conduct the risk assessment, or if, after performing the risk assessment outlined above, you determine that breach notification is required, there are three types of notification to be made to individuals, to the Secretary of HHS, and, in some cases, to the media. The number of individuals that are affected by the breach of unsecured PHI determines your notification requirements. Visit the OCR Breach Notification Rule webpage for more information on notifying individuals, the Secretary, and the media. If you determine that breach notification is required, you should also visit the OCR website for instructions on how to submit the breach notification form to the Secretary of HHS. Once notified, HHS publicly reports, on the OCR website, breaches that affect 500 or more individuals. OCR opens a compliance review of all reported breaches that affect 500 or more individuals and many breaches affecting fewer than 500. (Note that similar breach notification provisions, which are implemented and enforced by the Federal Trade Commission, apply to developers of PHRs that are not providing this service for a CE.)

OTHER LAWS AND REQUIREMENTS

Besides HIPAA Rules, HITECH, and Meaningful Use privacy- and security-related requirements, your medical practice may also need to comply with additional privacy and security laws and requirements. Your state, state board of medicine, state associations, Regional Extension Center (REC), and HIE initiatives also may have guidance.

A good place to start privacy- and security-related compliance implementation within your practice is to:

- Stay abreast of privacy and security updates. Sign up for OCR's privacy and security listservs to receive updates, and contact your local association to learn about available assistance sources.
- Integrate privacy and security updates into your policies and procedures.
- Identify and monitor violations and demonstrate good faith efforts to promptly cure any violation that may occur. Keep your workforce training materials up-to-date and conduct regular training sessions.
- Continually raise your practice's level of awareness about how to minimize the likelihood of privacy and security breaches.

Chapter 59 | **Cloning and Law**

The term cloning describes a number of different processes that can be used to produce genetically identical copies of a biological entity. The copied material, which has the same genetic makeup as the original, is referred to as a "clone." Researchers have cloned a wide range of biological materials, including genes, cells, tissues, and even entire organisms, such as sheep.

DO CLONES EVER OCCUR NATURALLY?

Yes. In nature, some plants and single-celled organisms, such as bacteria, produce genetically identical offspring through a process called "asexual reproduction." In asexual reproduction, a new individual is generated from a copy of a single cell from the parent organism.

Natural clones, also known as "identical twins," occur in humans and other mammals. These twins are produced when a fertilized egg splits, creating two or more embryos that carry almost identical deoxyribonucleic acid (DNA). Identical twins have nearly the same genetic makeup as each other, but they are genetically different from either parent.

WHAT ARE THE TYPES OF ARTIFICIAL CLONING?

There are three different types of artificial cloning: gene cloning, reproductive cloning and therapeutic cloning.

This chapter includes text excerpted from "Cloning Fact Sheet," National Human Genome Research Institute (NHGRI), August 15, 2020.

Gene cloning produces copies of genes or segments of DNA. Reproductive cloning produces copies of whole animals. Therapeutic cloning produces embryonic stem cells for experiments aimed at creating tissues to replace injured or diseased tissues.

Gene cloning, also known as "DNA cloning," is a very different process from reproductive and therapeutic cloning. Reproductive and therapeutic cloning share many of the same techniques, but are done for different purposes.

WHAT SORT OF CLONING RESEARCH IS GOING ON AT NHGRI?

Gene cloning is the most common type of cloning done by researchers at National Human Genome Research Institute (NHGRI). NHGRI researchers have not cloned any mammals and NHGRI does not clone humans.

HOW ARE GENES CLONED?

Researchers routinely use cloning techniques to make copies of genes that they wish to study. The procedure consists of inserting a gene from one organism, often referred to as "foreign DNA," into the genetic material of a carrier called a "vector." Examples of vectors include bacteria, yeast cells, viruses or plasmids, which are small DNA circles carried by bacteria. After the gene is inserted, the vector is placed in laboratory conditions that prompt it to multiply, resulting in the gene being copied many times over.

HOW ARE ANIMALS CLONED?

In reproductive cloning, researchers remove a mature somatic cell, such as a skin cell, from an animal that they wish to copy. They then transfer the DNA of the donor animal's somatic cell into an egg cell, or oocyte, that has had its own DNA-containing nucleus removed.

Researchers can add the DNA from the somatic cell to the empty egg in two different ways. In the first method, they remove the DNA-containing nucleus of the somatic cell with a needle and inject it into the empty egg. In the second approach, they use an electrical current to fuse the entire somatic cell with the empty egg.

In both processes, the egg is allowed to develop into an early-stage embryo in the test-tube and then is implanted into the womb of an adult female animal.

Ultimately, the adult female gives birth to an animal that has the same genetic make up as the animal that donated the somatic cell. This young animal is referred to as a "clone." Reproductive cloning may require the use of a surrogate mother to allow development of the cloned embryo, as was the case for the most famous cloned organism, Dolly the sheep.

WHAT ANIMALS HAVE BEEN CLONED?

Over the last 50 years, scientists have conducted cloning experiments in a wide range of animals using a variety of techniques. In 1979, researchers produced the first genetically identical mice by splitting mouse embryos in the test tube and then implanting the resulting embryos into the wombs of adult female mice. Shortly after that, researchers produced the first genetically identical cows, sheep and chickens by transferring the nucleus of a cell taken from an early embryo into an egg that had been emptied of its nucleus.

It was not until 1996, however, that researchers succeeded in cloning the first mammal from a mature (somatic) cell taken from an adult animal. After 276 attempts, Scottish researchers finally produced Dolly, the lamb from the udder cell of a 6-year-old sheep. Two years later, researchers in Japan cloned eight calves from a single cow, but only four survived.

Besides cattle and sheep, other mammals that have been cloned from somatic cells include: cat, deer, dog, horse, mule, ox, rabbit and rat. In addition, a rhesus monkey has been cloned by embryo splitting.

HAVE HUMANS BEEN CLONED?

Despite several highly publicized claims, human cloning still appears to be fiction. There currently is no solid scientific evidence that anyone has cloned human embryos.

In 1998, scientists in South Korea claimed to have successfully cloned a human embryo, but said the experiment was interrupted very early when the clone was just a group of four cells. In 2002, Clonaid, part of a religious group that believes humans were created by extraterrestrials, held a news conference to announce the birth of what it claimed to be the first cloned human, a girl named Eve. However, despite repeated requests by the research community and the news media, Clonaid never provided any evidence to confirm the existence of this clone or the other 12 human clones it purportedly created.

In 2004, a group led by Woo-Suk Hwang of Seoul National University in South Korea published a paper in the journal *Science* in which it claimed to have created a cloned human embryo in a test tube. However, an independent scientific committee later found no proof to support the claim and, in January 2006, *Science* announced that Hwang's paper had been retracted.

From a technical perspective, cloning humans and other primates are more difficult than in other mammals. One reason is that two proteins essential to cell division, known as "spindle proteins," are located very close to the chromosomes in primate eggs. Consequently, removal of the egg's nucleus to make room for the donor nucleus also removes the spindle proteins, interfering with cell division. In other mammals, such as cats, rabbits, and mice, the two spindle proteins are spread throughout the egg. So, removal of the egg's nucleus does not result in loss of spindle proteins. In addition, some dyes and the ultraviolet light used to remove the egg's nucleus can damage the primate cell and prevent it from growing.

DO CLONED ANIMALS ALWAYS LOOK IDENTICAL?

No. Clones do not always look identical. Although clones share the same genetic material, the environment also plays a big role in how an organism turns out.

For example, the first cat to be cloned, named Cc, is a female calico cat that looks very different from her mother. The explanation for the difference is that the color and pattern of the coats of cats cannot be attributed exclusively to genes. A biological phenomenon involving inactivation of the X chromosome in every cell of the female cat (which has two X chromosomes) determines which coat color genes are switched off and which are switched on. The distribution of X inactivation, which seems to occur randomly, determines the appearance of the cat's coat.

WHAT ARE THE POTENTIAL APPLICATIONS OF CLONED ANIMALS?

Reproductive cloning may enable researchers to make copies of animals with the potential benefits for the fields of medicine and agriculture.

For instance, the same Scottish researchers who cloned Dolly have cloned other sheep that have been genetically modified to produce milk that contains a human protein essential for blood clotting. The hope is that someday this protein can be purified from the milk and given to humans whose blood does not clot properly. Another possible use of cloned animals is for testing new drugs and treatment strategies. The great advantage of using cloned animals for drug testing is that they are all genetically identical, which means their responses to the drugs should be uniform rather than variable as seen in animals with different genetic makeups.

After consulting with many independent scientists and experts in cloning, the U.S. Food and Drug Administration (FDA) decided in January 2008 that meat and milk from cloned animals, such as cattle, pigs, and goats, are as safe as those from noncloned animals. The FDA action means that researchers are now free to using cloning methods to make copies of animals with desirable agricultural traits, such as high milk production or lean meat. However, because cloning is still very expensive, it will likely take many years until food products from cloned animals actually appear in supermarkets.

Another application is to create clones to build populations of endangered, or possibly even extinct, species of animals. In 2001, researchers produced the first clone of an endangered species: a type of Asian ox known as a "guar." Sadly, the baby guar, which had developed inside a surrogate cow mother, died just a few days after its birth. In 2003, another endangered type of ox, called the "Banteg," was successfully cloned. Soon after, three African wildcats were cloned using frozen embryos as a source of DNA. Although some experts think cloning can save many species that would otherwise disappear, others argue that cloning produces a population of genetically identical individuals that lack the genetic variability necessary for species survival.

Some people also have expressed interest in having their deceased pets cloned in the hope of getting a similar animal to replace the dead one. But, as shown by Cc the cloned cat, a clone may not turn out exactly like the original pet whose DNA was used to make the clone.

WHAT ARE THE POTENTIAL DRAWBACKS OF CLONING ANIMALS?

Reproductive cloning is a very inefficient technique and most cloned animal embryos cannot develop into healthy individuals. For instance, Dolly was the only clone to be born live out of a total of 277 cloned embryos. This very low efficiency, combined with safety concerns, presents a serious obstacle to the application of reproductive cloning.

Researchers have observed some adverse health effects in sheep and other mammals that have been cloned. These include an increase in birth size and a variety of defects in vital organs, such as the liver, brain, and heart. Other consequences include premature aging and problems with the immune system. Another potential problem centers on the relative age of the cloned cell's chromosomes. As cells go through their normal rounds of division, the tips of the chromosomes, called "telomeres," shrink. Over time, the telomeres become so short that the cell can no longer divide and, consequently, the cell dies. This is part of the natural aging process that seems to happen in all cell types. As a consequence, clones created from a cell taken from an adult might have chromosomes that are already shorter than normal, which may condemn the clones' cells to a shorter life span. Indeed, Dolly, who was cloned from the cell of a 6-year-old sheep, had chromosomes that were shorter than those of other sheep her age. Dolly died when she was six years old, about half the average sheep's 12-year lifespan.

WHAT IS THERAPEUTIC CLONING?

Therapeutic cloning involves creating a cloned embryo for the sole purpose of producing embryonic stem cells with the same DNA as the donor cell. These stem cells can be used in experiments aimed at understanding disease and developing new treatments for disease. To date, there is no evidence that human embryos have been produced for therapeutic cloning.

The richest source of embryonic stem cells is tissue formed during the first five days after the egg has started to divide. At this stage of development, called the "blastocyst," the embryo consists of a cluster of about 100 cells that can become any cell type. Stem cells are harvested from cloned embryos at this stage of development, resulting in the destruction of the embryo while it is still in the test tube.

WHAT ARE THE POTENTIAL APPLICATIONS OF THERAPEUTIC CLONING?

Researchers hope to use embryonic stem cells, which have the unique ability to generate virtually all types of cells in an organism, to grow healthy tissues in the laboratory that can be used replace injured or diseased tissues. In addition, it may be possible to learn more about the molecular causes of disease by studying embryonic stem cell lines from cloned embryos derived from the cells of animals or humans with different diseases. Finally, differentiated tissues derived from ES cells are excellent tools to test new therapeutic drugs.

WHAT ARE THE POTENTIAL DRAWBACKS OF THERAPEUTIC CLONING?

Many researchers think it is worthwhile to explore the use of embryonic stem cells as a path for treating human diseases. However, some experts are concerned about the striking similarities between stem cells and cancer cells. Both cell types have the ability to proliferate indefinitely and some studies show that after 60 cycles of cell division, stem cells can accumulate mutations that could lead to cancer. Therefore, the relationship between stem cells and cancer cells needs to be more clearly understood if stem cells are to be used to treat human disease.

WHAT ARE SOME OF THE ETHICAL ISSUES RELATED TO CLONING?

Gene cloning is a carefully regulated technique that is largely accepted today and used routinely in many labs worldwide. However, both reproductive and therapeutic cloning raise important ethical issues, especially as related to the potential use of these techniques in humans.

Reproductive cloning would present the potential of creating a human that is genetically identical to another person who has previously existed or who still exists. This may conflict with long-standing religious and societal values about human dignity, possibly infringing upon principles of individual freedom, identity and autonomy. However, some argue that reproductive cloning could help sterile couples fulfill their dream of parenthood. Others see human cloning as a way to avoid passing on a deleterious gene that runs in the family without having to undergo embryo screening or embryo selection.

Therapeutic cloning, while offering the potential for treating humans suffering from disease or injury, would require the destruction of human embryos in the test tube. Consequently, opponents argue that using this technique to collect embryonic stem cells is wrong, regardless of whether such cells are used to benefit sick or injured people.

Part 8 | Additional Help and Information

Chapter 60 | **Glossary of Terms Related to Health Technology**

angiography: A diagnostic x-ray imaging procedure used to see how blood flows through the blood vessels and organs of the body. This is done by injecting special dyes, known as "contrast agents," into the blood vessel and using x-ray techniques such as fluoroscopy to monitor blood flow.

biocompatibility: A measure of how a biomaterial interacts in the body with the surrounding cells, tissues, and other factors.

bioengineering: The application of concepts and methods of engineering, biology, medicine, physiology, physics, materials science, chemistry, mathematics, and computer sciences to develop methods and technologies to solve health problems in humans.

bioinformatics: The branch of biology that is concerned with the acquisition, storage, display, and analysis of biological information.

biomaterial: Any matter, surface, or construct that interacts with biological systems. Biomaterials can be derived from nature or synthesized in the laboratory using metallic components, polymers, ceramics, or composite materials. Medical devices made of biomaterials are often used to replace or augment a natural function.

biomedical imaging: The science and the branch of medicine concerned with the development and use of imaging devices and techniques, to obtain internal anatomic images, and to provide biochemical and physiological analysis of tissues and organs.

This glossary contains terms excerpted from documents produced by several sources deemed reliable.

biomimetics: Using biological form and function seen in nature, to inspire the design of solutions to engineering problems.

biosensors: A device that uses biological material, such as deoxyribonucleic acid (DNA), enzymes, and antibodies, to detect specific biological, chemical, or physical processes and then transmits or reports this data.

blood-brain barrier (BBB): A highly selective, semi-impermeable boundary that divides the brain from the rest of the body. It allows the passage of vital molecules through specialized transport proteins and diffusion mechanisms.

brain-computer interface (BCI): A system that uses the brain's electrical signals to allow individuals with limited mobility to learn to use their thoughts to move a computer cursor or other devices such as a robotic arm or a wheelchair.

cardiovascular disease (CVD): Also called "heart disease" it is a class of diseases that involve the heart, the blood vessels (arteries, capillaries, and veins,) or both.

clinical decision support (CDS): An interactive software-based system designed to assist physicians and other health professionals as well as patients with diagnostic and treatment decisions and reminders.

computational modeling: The use of mathematics, statistics, physics and computer science to study the mechanism and behavior of complex systems by computer simulation.

computed tomography (CT): A computerized x-ray imaging procedure in which a narrow beam of x-rays is aimed at a patient and quickly rotated around the body, producing signals that are processed by the machine's computer, to generate cross-sectional images – or "slices" – of the body.

computerized provider order entry (CPOE): A computer application that allows a physician's orders for diagnostic and treatment services (such as medications, laboratory, and other tests) to be entered electronically instead of being recorded on order sheets or prescription pads. The computer compares the order against standards for dosing, checks for allergies or interactions with other medications, and warns the physician about potential problems.

contrast agent: A substance used to enhance the imaged appearance of structures, processes or fluids within the body in biomedical imaging.

control group: The group of participants in a trial that receives standard treatment or a placebo. The control group may also be made up of healthy volunteers. Researchers compare results from the control group with results from the experimental group to find and learn from any differences.

deep brain stimulation: A neurosurgical treatment utilizing a neurostimulator placed in the brain to deliver electrical signals to specific parts of the brain to help control unwanted movements such as in Parkinson disease (PD) or regulate the firing of neurons in the brain to help control the symptoms of disorders such as epilepsy or depression.

drug delivery systems: Engineered technologies for the targeted delivery and/or controlled release of therapeutic agents.

elastography: A medical imaging technique that measures the elasticity or stiffness of a tissue. The technique captures snapshots of shear waves, a special type of sound wave, as they move through the tissue.

electroencephalography (EEG): The recording of electrical activity along the scalp resulting from current flowing within the neurons of the brain. EEG can be used to diagnose epilepsy and other disorders associated with altered brain electrical activity.

electromagnetic radiation (EMR): Radiation that has both electric and magnetic fields and travels in waves. It comes from natural and human-made sources. Electromagnetic radiation can vary in strength from low energy to high energy. It includes radio waves, microwaves, infrared light, visible light, ultraviolet light, x-rays, and gamma rays. Also called "EMR."

electronic health record (EHR): A real-time patient health record with access to evidence-based decision support tools that can be used to aid clinicians in decision-making. The EHR can automate and streamline a clinician's workflow, ensuring that all clinical information is communicated.

electronic health record system (EHRS): An information technology (IT) system designed to store and manage electronic health records (EHRs).

electronic medical record (EMR): An electronic record of health-related information on an individual that can be created, gathered, managed, and consulted by authorized clinicians and staff within one health-care organization.

electronic prescribing (e-prescribing): A technology where health-care providers can enter prescription information into a computer device – such as a tablet, laptop, or desktop computer – and securely transmit the prescription to pharmacies using a special software program and connectivity to a transmission network. When a pharmacy receives a request, it can begin filling the medication right away.

endoscope: A thin illuminated flexible or rigid tube-like optical system used to examine the interior of a hollow organ or body cavity by direct insertion.

exoskeleton: The external skeleton that supports and protects an animal's body in contrast to the bones of an internal skeleton. Rehabilitation engineers have used this design in nature to develop exoskeletons that attach to the outside of the body and assist individuals with functions such as arm and leg movement.

extracellular matrix (ECM): The ECM is a collection of extracellular molecules secreted by support cells that provides structural and biochemical support to the surrounding cells.

fluorescence: The emission of light by a substance that has absorbed light or other electromagnetic radiation. The absorbed and emitted light are usually different wavelengths and therefore produce different colors.

functional magnetic resonance imaging (fMRI): An MRI-based technique for measuring brain activity. It works by detecting the changes in blood oxygenation and flow that occur in response to neural activity – when a brain area is more active it consumes more oxygen and to meet this increased demand blood flow increases to the active area. fMRI can be used to produce activation maps showing which parts of the brain are involved in a particular mental process.

gamma ray: Electromagnetic radiation of the shortest wavelength and the highest energy.

health information exchange (HIE): The electronic movement of health-related information across organizations within a region, community or hospital system and according to nationally recognized standards.

health information technology (HIT): The application of information processing involving both computer hardware and software that deals with the storage, retrieval, sharing, and use of health-care information, data, and knowledge for communication and decision-making.

image-guided robotic interventions: Medical procedures, primarily minimally invasive surgery, performed through a small incision or natural orifice using robotic tools operated remotely by a surgeon with visualization by devices such as cameras small enough to fit into a minimal incision.

implantable device: Human-made medical devices implanted in the body to replace or augment biological functions. Such devices range from those that provide structural support, such as a hip replacement to those that contain electronics, such as pacemakers. Some implants are bioactive such as a drug-eluting stent used to open a blocked artery.

in vitro: A laboratory experiment or process performed in a test tube, culture dish, or elsewhere outside a living animal.

induced pluripotent stem cell (iPSC): A stem cell that is formed by the introduction of stem-cell inducing factors into a differentiated cell of the body, typically a skin cell.

interoperability: It refers to the ability of health information systems to work together within and across organizational boundaries in order to advance the effective delivery of healthcare for individuals and communities.

ionizing radiation: A type of electromagnetic radiation (EMR) that can strip electrons from an atom or molecule – a process called "ionization." Ionizing radiation has a relatively short wavelength on the electromagnetic spectrum (EMS). Examples of ionizing radiation include gamma rays, and x-rays. Lower energy ultraviolet, visible light, infrared, microwaves, and radio waves are considered nonionizing radiation.

magnetic resonance elastography (MRE): A special MRI technique to capture snapshots of shear waves that move through the tissue and create "elastograms" or images that show tissue stiffness. MRE is used to non-invasively detect hardening of the liver caused by chronic liver disease (CLD). MRE also has the potential to diagnose diseases in other parts of the body.

magnetic resonance imaging (MRI): A noninvasive imaging technology used to investigate anatomy and function of the body without the use of damaging ionizing radiation. It is often used for disease detection, diagnosis, and treatment monitoring. It is based on sophisticated technology that excites and detects changes in protons found in the water that makes up living tissues.

mammography: An x-ray imaging method used to image the breast for the early detection of cancer and other breast diseases. It is used as both a diagnostic and screening tool.

mesenchymal stem cells: A term used to define nonblood adult stem cells from a variety of tissues.

mHealth: An abbreviation for mobile health, which is the practice of medicine and public health supported with mobile devices such as mobile phones for health services and information.

microfluidics: A multidisciplinary field including engineering, physics, chemistry and biotechnology involving the design of systems for the precise control and manipulation of fluids on a small, submillimeter scale. Typically fluids are moved, mixed, separated or processed in various ways.

microscopy: Using microscopes to view samples and objects that cannot be seen with the unaided eye.

minimally invasive surgery: A surgical procedure typically utilizing one or more small incisions through which laparoscopic surgical tools are inserted and manipulated by a surgeon. Minimally invasive surgery can reduce damage to surrounding healthy tissue, decrease the need for pain medication, and reduce patient recovery time.

molecular imaging: A discipline that involves the visualization of molecular processes and cellular functions in living organisms. With the inclusion of a biomarker, which interacts chemically with tissues and structures of interest, many imaging techniques can be used for molecular imaging including ultrasound, x-rays, magnetic resonance imaging (MRI), optical imaging, positron emission tomography (PET), and single photon emission computed tomography (SPECT).

multiscale modeling: It uses mathematics and computation to quantitatively represent and simulate a system at more than one scale while functionally linking the mathematical models across these scales. Biological and behavioral scales include atomic, molecular, molecular complexes, subcellular, cellular, multicell systems, tissue, organ, multi-organ systems, organism/individual, group, organization, market, environment, and populations.

nanoparticle: Ultrafine particles between 1 and 100 nanometers in size. The size is similar to that of most biological molecules and structures. Nanoparticles can be engineered for a wide variety of biomedical uses including diagnostic devices, contrast agents, physical therapy applications, and drug delivery vehicles. A nanoparticle is approximately 1/10,000 the width of a human hair. Nanoparticles are generally 1000 times smaller than microparticles.

nanotechnology: Nanotechnology is science, engineering, and technology conducted at the nanoscale, which is about 1 to 100 nanometers. Nanoscience and nanotechnology are the study and application of extremely small things and can be used across all the other science fields, such as chemistry, biology, physics, materials science, and engineering.

Glossary of Terms Related to Health Technology

neuroimaging: Includes the use of a number of techniques to image the structure and function of the brain, spinal cord, and associated structures.

nuclear medicine: A medical specialty that uses radioactive tracers (radiopharmaceuticals) to assess bodily functions and to diagnose and treat disease. Diagnostic nuclear medicine relies heavily on imaging techniques that measure cellular function and physiology.

optical coherence tomography (OCT): A technique for obtaining subsurface images such as diseased tissue just below the skin. For example, ophthalmologists use OCT to obtain detailed images from within the retina. Cardiologists also use it to help diagnose coronary artery disease (CAD).

optical imaging: A technique for noninvasively looking inside the body, as is done with x-rays. Unlike x-rays, which use ionizing radiation, optical imaging uses visible light and the special properties of photons to obtain detailed images of organs and tissues as well as smaller structures including cells and molecules.

personal health record (PHR): An electronic application through which individuals can maintain and manage their health information (and that of others for whom they are authorized) in a private, secure, and confidential environment.

photon: A particle of light or electromagnetic radiation. The energies of photons range from high-energy gamma rays and x-rays to low-energy radio waves.

point of care (POC): Testing and treating of patients at sites close to where they live. Rapid diagnostic tests are used to obtain immediate, on-site results.

polymer: A large molecule composed of many repeating subunits. Polymers range from familiar synthetic plastics such as polystyrene to natural biopolymers such as deoxyribonucleic acid (DNA). Polymers have unique physical properties, including strength, flexibility and elasticity.

positron emission tomography (PET): These scans use radiopharmaceuticals to create three-dimensional (3-D) images. The decay of the radiotracers used with PET scans produce small particles called "positrons." When positrons react with electrons in the body they annihilate each other. This annihilation produces two photons that shoot off in opposite directions. The detectors in the PET scanner measure these photons and use this information to create images of internal organs.

progenitor cells: They are cells that are similar to stem cells but instead of the ability to become any type of cell, they are already predisposed to develop into a particular type of cell.

prosthetics: The design, fabrication, and fitting of artificial body parts.

radiation: The emission of energy as electromagnetic waves or as moving subatomic particles, especially high-energy particles that cause ionization.

radiopharmaceuticals/radioactive tracers: They are made up of carrier molecules that are bonded tightly to a radioactive atom. The carrier molecule is designed to bind to the tissue being examined so that the radioactive atom can be scanned to produce an image from inside the body.

Raman spectroscopy: This technique relies on inelastic scattering of visible, near-infrared, or near-ultraviolet light that is delivered by a laser. The laser light interacts with molecular vibrations in the material being examined, and shifts in energy are measured that reveal information about the properties of the material. The technique has a wide variety of applications including identifying chemical compounds and characterizing the structure of materials and crystals. In medicine, Raman gas analyzers are used to monitor anesthetic gas mixtures during surgery.

regenerative medicine: A broad field that includes tissue engineering but also incorporates research on self-healing – where the body uses its own systems, sometimes with the help of foreign biological material to rebuild tissues and organs.

rehabilitation engineering: The use of engineering science and principles to develop technological solutions and devices to assist individuals with disabilities, and aid the recovery of physical and cognitive functions lost because of disease or injury.

robotic surgery: Surgery performed through very small incisions or natural orifices using thin finger-like robotic tools controlled remotely by the surgeon through a telemanipulator or computer interface.

scaffold: A structure of artificial or natural materials on which tissue is grown to mimic a biological process outside the body or to replace a disease or damaged tissue inside the body.

sensors: In medicine and biotechnology, sensors are tools that detect specific biological, chemical, or physical processes and then transmit or report this data. Some sensors work outside the body while others are designed to be implanted within the body. Sensors help health-care providers and patients monitor health conditions. Sensors are also used to monitor the safety of medicines, foods and other environmental substances that may be encountered.

single photon emission computed tomography (SPECT): A nuclear medicine imaging technique using gamma rays. SPECT imaging instruments provide three-dimensional (3-D) images of the distribution of radioactive tracer molecules that have been introduced into the patient's body. The 3-D images are computer generated from a large number of images of the body recorded at different angles by cameras that rotate around the patient.

spectroscopy: The branch of science concerned with the investigation and measurement of spectra produced when matter interacts with or emits electromagnetic radiation.

stem cell: An undifferentiated cell of a multicellular organism that is capable of giving rise to more of the same cell type indefinitely, and has the ability to differentiate into many other types of cells that form the structures of the body.

telehealth: The use of communication technologies to provide and support healthcare at a distance.

theranostics: The relatively experimental science of combining therapy and diagnosis into a single procedure or molecule. Towards this end, bioengineers are building multifunctional nanoparticles that can be introduced into a patient, find the site of disease, diagnose the condition, and deliver the appropriate, personalized therapy.

tissue engineering: An interdisciplinary and multidisciplinary field that aims at the development of biological substitutes that restore, maintain, or improve tissue function.

ultrasound: A form of acoustic energy, or sound, that has a frequency that is higher than the level of human hearing. As a medical diagnostic technique, high-frequency sound waves are used to provide real-time medical imaging image inside the body without exposure to ionizing radiation. As a therapeutic technique, high-frequency sound waves interact with tissues to destroy diseased tissue such as tumors, or to modify tissues, or target drugs to specific locations in the body.

x-ray: A form of high-energy electromagnetic radiation (EMR) that can pass through most objects, including the body. X-rays travel through the body and strike an x-ray detector (such as radiographic film, or a digital x-ray detector) on the other side of the patient, forming an image that represents the "shadows" of objects inside the body.

Chapter 61 | Directory of Agencies That Provide Information about Health Technology

GOVERNMENT AGENCIES THAT PROVIDE INFORMATION ABOUT HEALTH TECHNOLOGY

Agency for Healthcare Research and Quality (AHRQ)
5600 Fishers Ln.
Rockville, MD 20857
Phone: 301-427-1364
Fax: 301-427-1873
Website: www.ahrq.gov

Centers for Disease Control and Prevention (CDC)
1600 Clifton Rd.
Atlanta, GA 30333
Toll-Free: 800-CDC-INFO
(800-232-4636)
Phone: 404-639-3311
Toll-Free TTY: 888-232-6348
Website: www.cdc.gov
E-mail: cdcinfo@cdc.gov

Eunice Kennedy Shriver National Institute on Child Health and Human Development (NICHD)
P.O. Box 3006
Rockville, MD 20847
Toll-Free: 800-370-2943
Phone: 301-496-5133
Toll-Free TTY: 888-320-6942
Toll-Free Fax: 866-760-5947
Website: www.nichd.nih.gov
E-mail: nichdinformationresource-center@mail.nih.gov

Federal Trade Commission (FTC)
600 Pennsylvania Ave., N.W.
Washington, DC 20580
Phone: 202-326-2222
Website: www.ftc.gov

Resources in this chapter were compiled from several sources deemed reliable; all contact information was verified and updated in June 2021.

Health Resources and Services Administration (HRSA)

5600 Fishers Ln.
Rockville, MD 20857
Toll-Free: 800-221-9393
Phone: 301-443-3376
Toll-Free TTY: 877-897-9910
Website: www.hrsa.gov

Healthfinder®

P.O. Box 1133
Washington, DC 20013-1133
Toll-Free: 800-336-4797
Phone: 301-565-4167
Fax: 301-984-4256
Website: www.healthfinder.gov
E-mail: healthfinder@nhic.org

MedlinePlus

8600 Rockville Pike
Bethesda, MD 20894
Toll-Free: 888-FIND-NLM
(888-346-3656)
Phone: 301-594-5983
Website: www.medlineplus.gov

National Aeronautics and Space Administration (NASA)

300 E. St., S.W., Ste. 5R30
Washington, DC 20546
Phone: 202-358-0001
Fax: 202-358-4338
Website: www.nasa.gov

National Cancer Institute (NCI)

9609 Medical Center Dr.
Bethesda, MD 20892-9760
Toll-Free: 800-4-CANCER
(800-422-6237)
Phone: 240-276-6600
Toll-Free TTY: 800-332-8615
Website: www.cancer.gov
E-mail: cancergovstaff@mail.nih.gov

National Human Genome Research Institute (NHGRI)

31 Center Dr., MSC 2152
Bldg. 31, Rm. 4B09
Bethesda, MD 20892-2152
Phone: 301-402-0911
Fax: 301-402-2218
Website: www.genome.gov

National Institute of Arthritis and Musculoskeletal and Skin Diseases (NIAMS)

One AMS Cir.
Bethesda, MD 20892-3675
Toll-Free: 877-226-4267
Phone: 301-495-4484
TTY: 301-565-2966
Fax: 301-718-6366
Website: www.niams.nih.gov
E-mail: niamsinfo@mail.nih.gov

National Institute of Biomedical Imaging and Bioengineering (NIBIB)

6707 Democracy Blvd., Ste. 202
Bethesda, MD 20892-5469
Phone: 301-496-8859
Website: www.nibib.nih.gov
E-mail: info@nibib.nih.gov

National Institute of Diabetes, Digestive and Kidney Diseases (NIDDK)
31 Center Dr., MSC 2560
Bldg. 31, Rm. 9A06
Bethesda, MD 20892-2560
Toll-Free: 800-472-0424
Phone: 301-496-3583
Website: www.niddk.nih.gov
E-mail: niddkinquiries@nih.gov

National Institute of Standards and Technology (NIST)
100 Bureau Dr.
Gaithersburg, MD 20899
Phone: 301-975-2000
Website: www.nist.gov

National Institute on Deafness and Other Communication Disorders (NIDCD)
31 Center Dr., MSC 2320
Bethesda, MD 20892-2320
Website: www.nidcd.nih.gov
E-mail: nidcdinfo@nidcd.nih.gov

National Institute on Mental Health (NIMH)
6001 Executive Blvd., MSC 9663
Rm. 6200
Bethesda, MD 20892-9663
Toll-Free: 866-615-6464
Phone: 301-443-4513
TTY: 301-443-8431
Toll-Free TTY: 866-415-8051
Fax: 301-443-4279
Website: www.nimh.nih.gov
E-mail: nimhinfo@nih.gov

National Institutes of Health (NIH)
9000 Rockville Pike
Bethesda, MD 20892
Phone: 301-496-4000
TTY: 301-402-9612
Website: www.nih.gov
E-mail: nihinfo@od.nih.gov

National Science Foundation (NSF)
2415 Eisenhower Ave.
Alexandria, VA 22314
Toll-Free: 800-877-8339
Phone: 703-292-5111
Toll-Free TDD: 800-281-8749
Website: www.nsf.gov

The Networking and Information Technology Research and Development Program (NITRD)
2415 Eisenhower Ave.
Alexandria, VA 22314
Phone: 202-459-9674
Fax: 202-459-9673
Website: www.nitrd.gov

NIH News in Health
Bldg. 31, Rm. 5B52
Bethesda, MD 20892-2094
Phone: 301-451-8224
Website: newsinhealth.nih.gov
E-mail: nihnewsinhealth@od.nih.gov

Office of the National Coordinator for Health Information Technology (ONC)

330 C St., S.W.
7th Fl.
Washington, DC 20201
Phone: 202-690-7151
Fax: 202-690-6079
Website: www.healthit.gov
E-mail: onc.request@hhs.gov

Office on Women's Health (OWH)

200 Independence Ave., S.W.
Rm. 712E
Washington, DC 20201
Toll-Free: 800-994-9662
Phone: 202-690-7650
Fax: 202-205-2631
Website: www.womenshealth.gov

Substance Abuse and Mental Health Services Administration (SAMHSA)

5600 Fishers Ln.
Rockville, MD 20857
Toll-Free: 877-726-4727
Toll-Free TTY: 800-487-4889
Fax: 240-221-4292
Website: www.samhsa.gov

U.S. Congressional Budget Office (CBO)

Ford House Office Bldg.
4th Fl., 2nd D St., S.W.
Washington, DC 20515-6925
Website: www.cbo.gov
E-mail: communications@cbo.gov

U.S. Consumer Product Safety Commission (CPSC)

4330 E.W., Hwy.
Bethesda, MD 20814
Toll-Free: 800-638-2772
Toll-Free TTY: 800-638-8270
Fax: 301-504-0124
Website: www.cpsc.gov

U.S. Department of Energy (DOE)

1000 Independence Ave., S.W.
Washington, DC 20585
Phone: 202-586-5000
Website: www.energy.gov
E-mail: LM@hq.doe.gov

U.S. Department of Health and Human Services (HHS)

200 Independent Ave., S.W.
Washington, DC 20201
Toll-Free: 877-696-6775
Website: www.hhs.gov

U.S. Department of Justice (DOJ)

950 Pennsylvania Ave., N.W.
Washington, DC 20530-0001
Phone: 202-514-2000
Toll-Free TTY: 800-877-8339
Website: www.justice.gov

U.S. Department of Labor (DOL)

200 Constitution Ave., N.W.
Washington, DC 20210
Toll-Free: 866-4-USA-DOL
(866-4487-2365)
Toll-Free TTY: 877-889-5627
Website: www.dol.gov

U.S. Department of Veterans Affairs (VA)
50 Irving St., N.W.
Washington, DC 20422-0001
Toll-Free: 800-698-2411
Phone: 202-745-8000
Website: www.va.gov

U.S. Food and Drug Administration (FDA)
10903 New Hampshire Ave.
Silver Spring, MD 20993
Toll-Free: 888-INFO-FDA
(888-463-6332)
Website: www.fda.gov

U.S. Library of Congress (LOC)
101 Independence Ave., S.E.
Washington, DC 20540
Phone: 202-707-5000
Website: www.loc.gov

U.S. National Library of Medicine (NLM)
8600 Rockville Pike
Bethesda, MD 20894
Toll-Free: 888-FIND-NLM
(888-346-3656)
Phone: 301-594-5983
Website: www.nlm.nih.gov
E-mail: custserv@nlm.nih.gov

U.S. Senate Special Committee on Aging
G41 Dirksen Senate Office Bldg.
Washington, DC 20510
Phone: 202-224-5364
Fax: 202-224-8660
Website: www.aging.senate.gov

PRIVATE AGENCIES THAT PROVIDE INFORMATION ABOUT HEALTH TECHNOLOGY

AdvaMed
701 Pennsylvania Ave., N.W.
Ste. 800
Washington, DC 20004-2654
Phone: 202-783-8700
Fax: 202-783-8750
Website: www.advamed.org
E-mail: info@advamed.org

American Academy of Family Physicians (AAFP)
11400 Tomahawk Creek Pkwy.
Leawood, KS 66211-2680
Toll-Free: 800-274-2237
Phone: 913-906-6000
Fax: 913-906-6075
Website: www.aafp.org
E-mail: aafp@aafp.org

American Academy of Pediatrics (AAP)

141 N.W., Pt., Blvd.
Elk Grove Village, IL 60007-1098
Toll-Free: 800-433-9016
Fax: 847-434-8000
Website: www.aap.org
E-mail: international@aap.org

American Association for the Advancement of Science (AAAS)

1200 New York Ave., N.W.
Washington, DC 20005
Phone: 202-326-6400
Website: www.aaas.org

American Federation for Medical Research (AFMR)

500 Cummings Ctr., Ste. 4400
Beverly, MA 01915
Phone: 978-927-8330
Fax: 978-524-0461
Website: afmr.org

American Heart Association (AHA)

7272 Greenville Ave.
Dallas, TX 75231
Toll-Free: 800-AHA-USA-1
(800-242-8721)
Website: www.heart.org

American Medical Association (AMA)

AMA Plaza 330 N. Wabash Ave.
Ste. 39300
Chicago, IL 60611-5885
Toll-Free: 800-621-8335
Website: www.ama-assn.org

American Optometric Association (AOA)

243 N. Lindbergh Blvd.
St. Louis, MO 63141
Toll-Free: 800-365-2219
Phone: 314-991-4100
Fax: 314-991-4101
Website: www.aoa.org

American Society of Health-System Pharmacists (ASHP)

4500 East-West Hwy., Ste. 900
Bethesda, MD 20814
Toll-Free: 866-279-0681
Website: www.ashp.org

American Society of Ophthalmic Plastic and Reconstructive Surgery (ASOPRS)

1043 Grand Ave., Ste. 132
St Paul, MN 55105
Phone: 612-601-3168
Website: www.asoprs.org/i4a/
pages/index.cfm?pageid=3504
E-mail: info@asoprs.org

Americans for Medical Progress (AMP)

444 N. Capitol St., N.W., Ste. 417
Washington, DC 20001
Phone: 202-624-8810
Website: www.amprogress.org/
about/contact-us
E-mail: outreach@amprogress.org

Biotechnology Innovation Organization (BIO)

1201 Maryland Ave., S.W., Ste. 900
Washington, DC 20024
Phone: 202-962-9200
Fax: 202-488-6301
Website: www.bio.org/contact-bio
E-mail: info@bio.org

Cincinnati Children's Hospital Medical Center

3333 Burnet Ave.
Cincinnati, OH 45229-3026
Toll-Free: 800-344-2462
Phone: 513-636-4200
TTY: 513-636-4900
Website: www.cincinnatichildrens.org

Cleveland Clinic

9500 Euclid Ave.
Cleveland, OH 44195
Toll-Free: 800-223-2273
Website: www.my.clevelandclinic.org

Drug, Chemical & Associated Technologies Association (DCAT)

One Union St., Ste. 207
Robbinsville, NJ 08691
Toll-Free: 800-640-DCAT
(800-640-3228)
Phone: 609-208-1888
Fax: 609-208-0599
Website: www.dcat.org/Contact
E-mail: info@dcat.org

Health Volunteers Overseas (HVO)

1900 L St., N.W., Ste. 310
Washington, DC 20036
Phone: 202-296-0928
Fax: 202-296-8018
Website: www.hvousa.org
E-mail: info@hvousa.org

The Healthcare Association of New York State (HANYS)

499 S. Capitol St., S.W., Ste. 410
Washington, DC 20003
Website: www.hanys.org

Healthcare Information and Management Systems Society (HIMSS)

33 W. Monroe St., Ste. 1700
Chicago, IL 60603-5616
Phone: 312-664-HIMSS
(312-664-4467)
Fax: 312-664-6143
Website: www.himss.org

Immunization Action Coalition (IAC)

2550 University Ave., W., Ste. 415 N.
St. Paul, MN 55114
Phone: 651-647-9009
Fax: 651-647-9131
Website: www.immunize.org
E-mail: admin@immunize.org

Materials Research Society (MRS)
506 Keystone Dr.
Warrendale, PA 15086-7537
Phone: 724-779-3003
Fax: 724-779-8313
Website: www.mrs.org
E-mail: info@mrs.org

Mental Health America
500 Montgomery St., Ste. 820
Alexandria, VA 22314
Toll-Free: 800-969-6642
Phone: 703-684-7722
Fax: 703-684-5968
Website: www.mhanational.org
E-mail: info@mhanational.org

National Alliance on Mental Illness (NAMI)
3803 N. Fairfax Dr., Ste. 100
Arlington, VA 22203
Toll-Free: 800-950-6264
Phone: 703-524-7600
Fax: 703-524-9094
Website: www.nami.org
E-mail: info@nami.org

National Safety Council (NSC)
1121 Spring Lake Dr.
Itasca, IL 60143-3201
Toll-Free: 800-621-7615
Phone: 630-285-1121
Fax: 630-285-1434
Website: www.nsc.org
E-mail: customerservice@nsc.org

National Scoliosis Foundation (NSF)
5 Cabot Pl.
Stoughton, MA 02072
Toll-Free: 800-NSF-MYBACK
(800-673-6922)
Fax: 781-341-8333
Website: www.scoliosis.org
E-mail: nsf@scoliosis.org

Palo Alto Medical Foundation (PAMF)
Toll-Free: 888-398-5677
Phone: 650-321-4121
Website: www.pamf.org

Pan American Health Organization (PAHO)
525 23rd St., N.W.
Washington, DC 20037
Phone: 202-974-3000
Fax: 202-974-3663
Website: www.paho.org/hq

Radiological Society of North America (RSNA)
820 Jorie Blvd., Ste. 200
Oak Brook, IL 60523-2251
Toll-Free: 800-381-6660
Phone: 630-571-2670
Website: www.rsna.org/ContactUs.aspx

INDEX

INDEX

Page numbers followed by 'n' indicate a footnote. Page numbers in *italics* indicate a table or illustration.

Index

Index

Index

Index

Index

693

Index

P

pacemakers
electrocardiogram test, 169
healthcare expenditure, 35
light therapy, 395
magnetic resonance imaging
(MRI), 175
remote patient monitoring, 84
virtual colonoscopy, 210
pain management
health technology assessment
(HTA), 27
rehabilitation engineering, 411
virtual reality (VR), 581
Palo Alto Medical Foundation
(PAMF), contact, 674
Pan American Health Organization
(PAHO), contact, 674
pandemic
advanced molecular
detection, 140
augmented reality (AR), 577
COVID-19, 3, 257
telemedicine, 16
3D printing, 603
pathologist
disabilities, 496
tumor surgery, 298
patient management, mobile medical
applications, 99
patient portals
COVID-19, 20
electronic personal health
records, 537
Health Insurance Portability
and Accountability Act
(HIPAA), 625
healthcare expenditure, 34
Patient-Centered Outcomes Research
(PCOR), blockchain technology, 41
patient-derived xenografts (PDX),
described, 311

patient-specific devices, 3D
printing, 603
pedometer
rehabilitation engineering, 414
remote patient monitoring
(RPM), 85
personal health record (PHR)
defined, 663
described, 530
Health Insurance Portability
and Accountability Act
(HIPAA), 625
See also electronic personal health
records
personal protective equipment (PPE)
COVID-19, 19
nanotechnology, 335
point-of-care diagnostic
testing, 235
3D printing, 605
personalized medicine. *See* precision
medicine
PHI. *See* protected health formation
photoacoustic imaging
nanotechnology, 352
optical imaging types, 194
photodynamic therapy (PDT)
nanotechnology, 346
optical imaging, 194
photon
artificial intelligence (AI), 571
defined, 663
light therapy, 397
nanotechnology, 360
nonlinear optical imaging, 226
nuclear medicine, 188
optical imaging, 193
photonic dosimetry,
overview, 611–14
PHR. *See* personal health record
physical prosthetics, rehabilitation
engineering, 410

Index